Counseling in Sports Medicine

Richard Ray, EdD, ATC
Hope College, Holland, Michigan

Diane M. Wiese-Bjornstal, PhD
University of Minnesota–Minneapolis

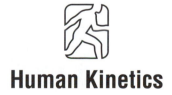

Human Kinetics

Library of Congress Cataloging-in-Publication Data

Counseling in sports medicine / [editors], Richard Ray, Diane M. Wiese-Bjornstal.
        p.   m.
    Includes bibliographical references and index.
    ISBN 0-88011-527-0
    1. Athletes—Counseling.   2. Athletes—Mental health.   I. Ray,
Richard, 1957– . II. Wiese–Bjornstal, Diane M., 1958–
RC451.4.A83C68   1999
616.89'14'088796—dc21

ISBN: 0-88011-527-0

Acquisitions Editor: Loarn Robertson, PhD
Developmental Editor: Christine Drews
Assistant Editor: John Wentworth
Copyeditor: Karen Bojda
Proofreader: Denelle Eknes
Indexer: Sheila Ary
Graphic Designer and Graphic Artist: Judy Henderson
Photo Editor: Boyd LaFoon
Cover Designer: Jack Davis
Illustrator: Mick Greenberg
Printer: Edwards Brothers

Printed in the United States of America   10 9 8 7 6 5 4 3 2 1

Human Kinetics

Web site: http://www.humankinetics.com/

United States: Human Kinetics
P.O. Box 5076
Champaign, IL 61825-5076
1-800-747-4457
e-mail: humank@hkusa.com

Canada: Human Kinetics
475 Devonshire Road Unit 100
Windsor, ON N8Y 2L5
1-800-465-7301 (in Canada only)
e-mail: humank@hkcanada.com

Europe: Human Kinetics, P.O. Box IW14
Leeds LS16 6TR, United Kingdom
(44) 1132 781708
e-mail: humank@hkeurope.com

Australia: Human Kinetics
57A Price Avenue
Lower Mitcham, South Australia 5062
(088) 277 1555
e-mail: humank@hkaustralia.com

New Zealand: Human Kinetics
P.O. Box 105-231, Auckland 1
(09) 523 3462
e-mail: humank@hknewz.com

To my children,
Richard, Sarah, and Matthew.
Each different, each special,
each loved, forever.

Richard Ray

I dedicate my work on this book to my husband, Carl,
and to our children, Christine and Ryan, for being
constant reminders of where life's priorities should be.
I thank them for bringing balance and joy to my life.

Diane M. Wiese-Bjornstal

Contents

Preface

As athletic trainers, physical therapists, and other sports health care professionals, we have long recognized that our patients are more than the sum of their injuries or disabilities. One of the most fundamental qualities that typifies successful sports health care practitioners is the ability to effectively interact with patients. We are confronted daily with patients who need more than our physical medical treatments can provide. Our patients often require guidance, encouragement, support, and reinforcement—in other words, counseling. Indeed, sports medicine professionals are often the most influential people in the lives of injured patients as they attempt to recover from their injuries and return to a physically active lifestyle. The purpose of *Counseling in Sports Medicine* is to help you maximize your ability to interact effectively with your patients by improving your counseling skills. This book will also help you to recognize those psychological conditions of your patients that would be best addressed by someone professionally trained in counseling.

WHY IS THIS TEXT NEEDED?

Counseling skills are, unfortunately, among those competencies that we often develop only after many years of practice. Educational programs in athletic training and physical therapy have provided only limited instruction in counseling and other patient interaction skills. We have therefore been left to our own experience to develop patterns of patient interaction that often leave us ill equipped to counsel our clients in the most effective way possible. This book will help both students and young practitioners in sports medicine professions develop appropriate psychosocial interaction skills in a counseling context without having to experience the difficult problems associated with acquiring these skills through trial and error. *Counseling in Sports Medicine* will also help athletic training and physical therapy educators by providing a comprehensive and practical alternative to the course packs now used for most courses dealing with counseling issues in sports medicine. This book brings together the body of knowledge on counseling in sports medicine and presents it in a manner that allows you to make an immediate connection between the theory of sport and injury psychology and the practical problems involved in applying this theory with real patients. This book is different from the few other books that deal with the psychology of sports injuries because of its pragmatic counseling orientation. Although well grounded in theory, *Counseling in Sports Medicine* is designed to help you develop your counseling and referral skills in a way that will enable you to implement effective patient interaction strategies right away. In addition, the chapters in part III, "Specific Counseling Issues in Athletic Health Care," provide information on the topics about which athletic trainers, physical therapists, sports physicians, and other sports medicine professionals are most concerned.

WHO SHOULD READ THIS BOOK?

This book is written primarily for these three groups of readers:

- Undergraduate and graduate sports medicine students, especially athletic trainers and physical therapists

- Athletic trainers, physical therapists, and other allied health care providers who want to improve their knowledge and skill in counseling the injured, physically active patient
- Physicians who work with athletes and other physically active patients and who want to enhance their ability to frame their medical advice in a context that is likely to be most useful to their patients

HOW IS THIS TEXT ORGANIZED?

The content of this book is organized into three parts designed to provide an overview of counseling in athletic health care, practical concerns and strategies for effective counseling, and coverage of counseling in specific health care topics. Part I provides an introduction to the counseling role that medical and allied health professionals must perform as a part of their day-to-day practice. This material provides a foundation for the actual counseling skills that will be developed in later sections of the text. The chapters in part II provide readers with an introduction to the skills that they need to become effective counselors to their injured patients. The skills outlined in the chapters of this section are generic in nature (unlike the specific counseling skills for particular counseling problems contained in part III) and apply to most counseling situations. Part III of the text helps readers develop specific strategies for counseling patients in the most common situations found in typical sports medicine settings. Anecdotes, practical suggestions, and case studies are used liberally to help integrate the theory into strategies that are likely to improve patient interaction skills.

Special Features

We hope these features will guide you through the book with as much ease as possible.

- *Chapter Objectives.* Each chapter opens with a list of expected learning outcomes. These objectives are broad enough to form the behavioral objectives for an entire course in counseling in sports medicine.

- *Case Studies.* A case study is included at the end of each chapter to help you understand how the concepts discussed in the text can be applied under actual practice conditions. Each case is accompanied by questions that test your ability to synthesize the most important concepts in the chapter.

- *Chapter Summaries.* The most important concepts of each chapter are summarized at the end of most chapters.

- *Glossary.* A running glossary defines key words and phrases in the margins near their use in the text. For convenience in locating them, glossary terms appear **bold** in text.

- *Annotated Bibliography.* An excellent bibliography of important references commonly cited in the sports medicine, sport psychology, and counseling literature appears at the end of the book. For greater ease, the bibliography is organized by chapter. The most important citations are accompanied by a brief annotation to help you decide whether to do any additional reading on any given topic.

- *Index.* An index of the entire text by author and subject facilitates easy reference.

Acknowledgments

Many people helped us bring this book to completion, and we are grateful for all their assistance. We would especially like to thank our colleagues at Hope College and the University of Minnesota who freely gave of their time and expertise in helping us develop the book. The staff of the VanWylen Library at Hope College was an invaluable source of support. We appreciate the thoughtful reviews of Robert Moss, PhD, ATC, and Mark Andersen, PhD. Their comments were very helpful in tightening and refining the text. The professionals at Human Kinetics deserve our praise for accepting our idea and helping us bring it into being. Finally, we offer our public thanks to our families, whose support of our careers has encouraged and strengthened us in our work.

I

Introduction to the Counseling Role

The first part of the book will help you answer the question, "What is my role in counseling the athletes under my care?" The sole chapter in this part of the book, "The Role of the Sports Medicine Professional in Counseling Athletes," is intended to provide an introduction to the counseling role that athletic trainers, sport physical therapists, and team physicians must perform as a part of their day-to-day practice. This material provides a foundation for the actual counseling skills that will be developed in later sections of the text. This part will also help you recognize some of the pitfalls associated with counseling the athlete.

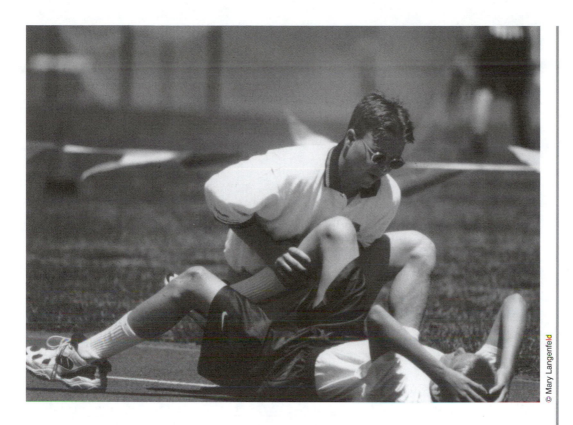

© Mary Langenfeld

The Role of the Sports Medicine Professional in Counseling Athletes

Richard Ray, EdD, ATC, *Hope College, Holland, Michigan*
Tom Terrell, MD, MPhil, *University of Maryland School of Medicine*
David Hough, MD[1], *Michigan State University*

CHAPTER OBJECTIVES

Understand the nature of counseling as practiced by sports medicine professionals

Understand why sports medicine professionals should counsel their athletes

Understand the groups sports medicine professionals should counsel

Understand the limitations sports medicine professionals should place on themselves in their counseling roles

---

[1]Dr. Hough has passed away since the time this chapter was written.

mental health professional—A person who is professionally trained (and frequently licensed) to provide psychological services in a variety of settings. Examples include psychiatrists, psychologists, psychiatric social workers, and mental health nurses.

The importance of sports medicine professional's role in counseling should not be underestimated. In many cases, they are the first ones to attend to an injured athlete, allowing them to provide counseling during the time when pain and confusion are at their worst (Wiese-Bjornstal & Smith, 1993). The role that athletic trainers, physical therapists, and team physicians play as counselors to injured athletes is made more evident when one considers the fact that **mental health professionals** are not a part of the sports medicine team in most athletic health care settings (Wiese-Bjornstal & Smith, 1993). Although most sports medicine professionals have a wealth of experience in this area, they often lack formal educational preparation in counseling skills (Wiese, Weiss, & Yukelson, 1991). This is unfortunate, since it can often lead to difficulty in providing the holistic care that most injured athletes both want and need (Etzel & Ferrante, 1993). The purpose of this chapter is to help sports medicine professionals—primarily certified athletic trainers, physical therapists, and team physicians—to understand what their role should be in counseling their patients.

WHAT IS COUNSELING IN SPORTS MEDICINE?

Before a discussion of the sports medicine professional's role in counseling can be meaningfully attempted, we should first be clear about the question, What is counseling? Many definitions exist. Health care and mental health professionals hold divergent views based on their level of training, the techniques they use to interact with patients, and the limitations placed on them by both ethical standards and the rules of their professional associations. This is an important issue for sports medicine professionals, since the ability to define the nature of counseling will influence the limits we place on ourselves in this role.

The formal practice of counseling is defined by Biggs (1994) as "a helping process in which one person, a helper, facilitates exploration, understanding, and actions about developmental opportunities and problem conditions presented by a helpee or client" (p. 63). Although Biggs's definition is useful for a wide variety of counseling professions and situations, you should realize that there is no universally accepted definition of counseling. The most typical distinctions revolve around differences in who is providing the counseling and the nature of the problems being experienced by the person being counseled. At one end of the spectrum you will find psychiatrists providing psychotherapy to patients with serious mental illnesses. At the other end of the spectrum are those with no medical or psychological training providing advice to people who just want to know what options are available to them on some question or issue. For many in the health professions, the line between counseling and education can become difficult to discern. For the sports medicine professional, the very act of discharging our duties will force us into a counseling role, irrespective of the artificial limits delineated in a formal definition.

What follows are a few of the most widely understood and accepted conceptions of counseling. They represent the broad range of opinion previously described, and elements of each conception are often used in sports health care settings.

psychotherapy—A method of working with patients or clients to assist them in modifying or reducing factors that interfere with effective living (Corsini, 1994).

Psychotherapy

Around 1940 counseling began to be viewed as a form of **psychotherapy** (Corsini, 1994). This view was largely influenced by the well known psychotherapist Carl Rogers. He emphasized a focus on an individual's problems in isolation from the influence of society or the environment in which those problems existed. He viewed counseling as a process in which the therapist, without attempting to direct or influence, attempts to develop a therapeutic relationship with the client in an effort to help work through emotional problems. This definition of counseling is not very useful for most sports medicine professionals for a variety of reasons, not the least of which is that we are neither trained nor licensed as psychotherapists. Nevertheless, *psychotherapy* and *counseling* are often used interchangeably in the literature—to the dismay of some mental health professionals.

Helping

One of the most pervasive—and vague—definitions of counseling is one of **helping** (Ivey & Authier, 1978). Helpers assist people in identifying and defining social–emotional problems, developing goals for ameliorating these problems, and implementing action plans to eventually solve problems. Egan (1986) categorizes helpers according to four levels of involvement:

helping—A goal-oriented act intended to benefit another person.

- First-level helpers (counselors, psychiatrists, psychologists, social workers)
- Second-level helpers (consultants, health care professionals, lawyers, clergy, police, probation officers, teachers)
- Third-level helpers (managers, supervisors, bartenders, hairdressers)
- Fourth-level helpers (relatives, friends, acquaintances)

As second-level helpers, sports medicine professionals are called on to counsel athletes with problems. This definition and subsequent categorization implies that sports medicine professionals should refer athletes with serious social–emotional problems to first-level helpers. This conception of counseling is one with great potential application for athletic trainers, physical therapists, and team physicians.

Education

Various authors view counseling as education or teaching (Ivey & Authier, 1978; Wiese-Bjornstal & Smith, 1993). Sports medicine professionals are certainly called upon with great frequency to educate their patients. Injured athletes require education about their physical problems at several stages during their recovery. Effective athletic trainers and team physicians discuss the nature of the injury with the patient as soon as possible after the injury has occurred. The process of rehabilitation from injury is one of teaching athletes what to do and how to do it.

Another element of counseling as teaching occurs when sports medicine professionals educate athletes, in groups or individually, about health-related concerns that they are likely to face during the course of their athletic careers. Problems relating to nutrition, substance use and abuse, and training techniques are common topics for counseling by sports medicine professionals of their healthy and unhealthy patients. This image of counseling is important because it expands the concept beyond the realm of patients or clients who have problems to those who could potentially develop problems. The idea of counseling as education, then, is one that embraces prevention as a central focus. At the same time, it is important to recognize that not all education is counseling. These are two different concepts that tend to overlap when sports medicine professionals interact and develop therapeutic relationships with athletes.

Rapport and Communication

Another viewpoint is that counseling is what happens when **rapport** is established and clear and effective communication is maintained between the sports medicine professional and the athlete (Wiese & Weiss, 1987). Even the inexperienced sports medicine professional can recognize the value of these two elements in the patient–practitioner relationship. **Communication**, which involves the process of sending,

rapport—A state of relationship between two or more people characterized by trust and confidence.

communication—
The process of sending, receiving, and understanding information.

receiving, and understanding information, is arguably the most elemental aspect of counseling in any setting. Athletic trainers, physical therapists, and team physicians who counsel athletes as part of their daily practice will be more effective in this role if they improve their communication skills. Simply enjoying rapport and communicating effectively with athletes does not mean, of course, that you are counseling them. But when counseling situations arise, these elements are crucial for a successful outcome.

Heil, Bowman, and Bean (1993) define rapport as a feeling of being comfortable or in harmony with another person. This feeling can obviously lay the foundation for effective communication between the sports medicine professional and the athlete. These authors assert that the sports medicine professional builds rapport through a process of active listening, matching sensory language, and implementing a variety of utilization techniques. Some authors restrict this definition of counseling to those individuals who do not have a vested interest in returning the athlete to competition (Brewer, Jeffers, Petipas, & Van Raalte, 1994). This obviously creates a dilemma for those sports medicine professionals who are employed by institutions or professional athletic organizations and whose jobs involve treating and rehabilitating injured athletes for the specific purpose of returning them to competition.

Emotional First Aid

A simplistic but potentially useful conception of counseling is provided by Stewart (1989), who characterizes counseling as "emotional first aid." First aid, in the physical, medical sense, is the immediate, short-term treatment provided to those who have suddenly become ill or injured. It usually involves both the provision of a service by a caregiver and instruction to allow the ill or injured person to help him- or herself. The idea of counseling as emotional first aid is appealing, especially for sports medicine professionals. Most counseling conducted by sports medicine professionals is short-term. Exceptions to this general rule exist, of course, especially in cases where counseling is provided in the context of a lengthy rehabilitation program. Sports medicine professionals are in a position to provide counseling (or at least to recognize problems) at an earlier stage than mental health professionals because they spend more time with the athletes, often interacting with them on a daily basis. In addition, sports medicine professionals can be trained to teach athletes some relatively simple techniques that they can use to help themselves during times of stress or anxiety. The problem with this definition, of course, is that it is rather simplistic. Mental health professionals who spend their entire careers counseling patients for a variety of problems would no doubt argue that effective counseling involves far more than the application of "emotional first aid."

A Unified Definition for the Sports Medicine Professional

With the exception of counseling as psychotherapy, all the definitions just discussed have appeal for the sports medicine professional. What they lack, however, is a sense of completeness, which is required to help professionals who work with athletes understand their counseling role. The conception of counseling that we think is most appropriate for sports medicine professionals—and the one on which the rest of this book is based—is actually borrowed from the career counseling literature. Holland, Magoon, and Spokane (1981) assert that the critical elements involved in counseling include

social support—
The benefits to well-being that people derive through their relationships with others (Corsini, 1994).

- provision of **social support**,
- providing information about choices,
- helping the patient establish goals, and
- encouraging decision making based on identified alternative choices.

In addition to these four counseling functions, sports medicine professionals should also consider the following two elements as important in their counseling role: (1) screening for more serious psychoemotional problems and (2) referral to mental health professionals.

Placed in a setting of athletic injury, this definition helps sports medicine professionals understand what their role should and should not be when counseling both healthy and unhealthy athletes (see figure 1.1). It implies that counseling is what happens when we lend an ear to athletes who want to talk about their problems. It implies that counseling is what happens when a sports medicine professional provides information to athletes regarding the nature of their injuries. It acknowledges the importance of involving the athlete in the establishment of goals—not just rehabilitation goals, but personal development goals as well—rather than imposing goals on the athlete. Finally, it suggests that part of counseling is action- and future-oriented. In some cases counseling may lead to advances in the athlete's rehabilitation program. In others it may involve helping the athlete to accept referral to a mental health professional for more advanced psychological intervention. When we talk about counseling in the remainder of this chapter, these are the critical elements to which we refer.

This definition is admittedly broad and may be viewed as too all-encompassing by some. We feel a broad definition is essential, given the range of professionals who are involved in the physical and mental health care of the athlete. A narrower conception would limit the range of services provided to athletes and would deny athletes choice in whom to turn to when they experience difficulty. Finally, the broad definition we propose reflects the reality that athletes will turn—often as a first

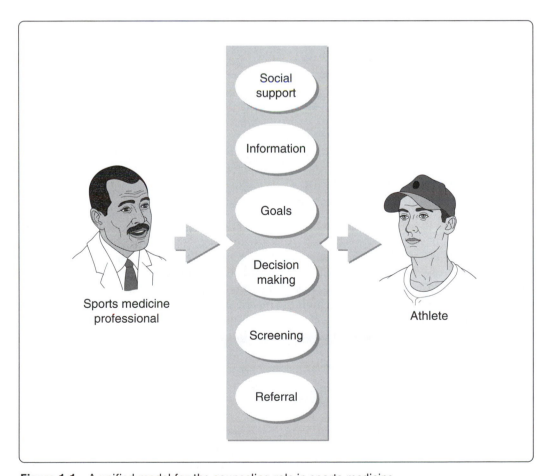

Figure 1.1   A unified model for the counseling role in sports medicine.

choice—to the sports medicine professional with whom they already have a relationship.

WHY SHOULD SPORTS MEDICINE PROFESSIONALS COUNSEL?

Although we have already established that sports medicine professionals are in an excellent position to counsel their patients on a wide variety of subjects, some may wonder why athletic trainers, physical therapists, and team physicians should counsel. Isn't it enough to simply attend to the physical needs of our patients as we were trained to do? Shouldn't everything related to mental health be the province of the mental health professional? There are a number of reasons why sports medicine professionals should be involved in counseling their patients. We have legal and ethical responsibility in this area. Our patients want us to counsel them. We often act as the first line of defense in the recognition of psychological problems. Above all, counseling helps us improve the effectiveness of our practice as measured by patient outcomes. Indeed, the argument can be made that we simply cannot do our jobs without counseling patients. It is integral to nearly every job function. Athletic trainers, physical therapists, and primary-care team physicians are—first and foremost—helpers. With some exceptions, our primary responsibility is to help injured athletes heal themselves.

Legal and Ethical Duty

informed consent—*The process by which a health care provider explains the risks and benefits of a specific treatment and obtains written documentation from the patient that the patient understands and accepts the risks, benefits, and alternative treatment options and agrees to the treatment.*

Sports medicine professionals have both a legal and an ethical duty to counsel their patients within the scope of their training and license to practice. Failure to do so almost always breaches a central duty to provide their patients with the information they require to make informed choices. Indeed, two common areas of negligent behavior on the part of health care professionals are failure to warn and breach of duty. A critical component of warning patients involves obtaining their **informed consent** before initiating treatment. Informed consent includes the following elements (American Physical Therapy Association [APTA], 1995):

- Description of the treatment or medical intervention
- Risks of the treatment or medical intervention
- Expected benefits of the treatment or medical intervention
- Explanation of the risks of forgoing the treatment or medical intervention
- Explanation of alternative treatments

Each of these activities involves a substantial counseling component. They require clear communication between the sports medicine professional and the patient. They require the sports medicine professional to educate patients, answer their questions, and develop treatment plans consistent with their goals—goals they wouldn't even know about unless they listen to patients and help them clarify their objectives for treatment. These are all components of counseling.

Breach of duty is another common legal trap that may snare sports medicine professionals who fail to counsel their patients. To prove a charge of negligence, an aggrieved patient must be able to prove that the health professional failed to perform a legally required duty (Ray, 1994). Duty can be codified in many ways. Employment contracts, employee handbooks, and job descriptions often delineate the employer's expectations for the job activities of the employee. Duty can also be established by the professional standards to which sports medicine professionals are obliged to adhere. Such standards are found in codes of ethics, role-delineation studies, and state statutes. These documents delineate specific counseling functions that the sports medicine professional is expected to perform. Failure to comply with these counseling functions may constitute a breach of duty.

Sports medicine professionals also have an ethical responsibility to counsel their patients. The codes of ethics the American Physical Therapy Association (APTA), National Athletic Trainers Association (NATA), and American Medical Association (AMA) require the practitioner to place the patient's welfare above all other considerations. This would be difficult, if not impossible, unless the sports medicine professional enters into a relationship with the patient that is characterized by rapport, effective interpersonal communication, and empathy—all critical elements of counseling behavior. Athletic trainers may, in fact, be held to a higher standard in this regard since a major focus of their professional practice is supposed to revolve around the prevention of injury and illness. One of the ways that athletic trainers can help prevent injuries is by being alert for the signs of stress-related attentional deficits in their athletes (Henderson & Carroll, 1993). The appropriate action may be low-level counseling by the athletic trainer or referral to a mental health professional. Another, and perhaps the primary, factor in injury and illness prevention undertaken by all sports medicine professionals is the ability to convince patients—or potential patients—to alter their behavior. This involves both individual and group education on an ongoing basis. Sports medicine professionals have an ethical responsibility to prevent injuries and illnesses. They cannot do this without educating athletes. Education is a critical element of counseling. Sports medicine professionals have an ethical responsibility to counsel.

Patients' Expectations for Counseling

One of the reasons that sports medicine professionals should fill a counseling role is simply because the patient wants, and in many cases expects, to be counseled. The work of Brewer, Jeffers, Petipas, and Van Raalte (1994) demonstrated that college students regard some psychological interventions during injury rehabilitation positively. Goal setting, a crucial counseling element in rehabilitation planning and evaluation, is held in particularly high regard. The subjects in this study were grateful for the opportunity to discuss their emotions related to their rehabilitation. Additional support for the notion of patient expectation is provided by the work of Brody and his colleagues (1989). They discovered that patients who were provided with education, stress counseling, and the opportunity to discuss ideas about how to best treat their problems were significantly more satisfied than patients who were not provided with this type of counseling. The provision of technical interventions alone, such as examinations, tests, and therapy, were unrelated to patient satisfaction. It seems logical to conclude that patients, presumably including injured athletes (Miller & Moore, 1993), are not only open to the idea of counseling during their treatment and rehabilitation, but actually prefer it to the provision of services normally associated with athletic injury treatment without such counseling. Patient satisfaction seems to be strongly linked to the presence of effective communication and good interpersonal relationships (Guccione & DeMont, 1987).

First Line of Defense

Athletic trainers, physical therapists, and team physicians should involve themselves in counseling injured athletes because they often represent the first line of defense in the identification of psychological conditions that range from mild to severe (Heil, Bowman, & Bean, 1993; Smith, Scott, & Wiese, 1990). Early intervention in psychological or emotional problems is usually most effective (Stewart, 1989). This requires identification of minor problems before they can become more severe (Murray, 1992). The problems that athletes experience are similar in many ways to those of the general public, including employment problems and relationship discord. In addition, they have the extra pressure of dealing with other stressors related specifically to their athletic involvement. Injured athletes are at significant risk of depression because of their sudden separation from sport (Ermler & Thomas, 1990).

Most patients with depressive symptoms seek the advice of a nonpsychiatric health professional before eventually being referred to a mental health professional (Henderson, Pollard, Jacobi, & Merkel, 1992). Because sports medicine professionals are in such frequent contact with both injured and healthy athletes, they are often called on to provide the initial stages of counseling on a wide variety of health-related topics (Furney & Patton, 1985). Although the issues that the sports medicine professional addresses in counseling should be chosen with care and should be based on his or her level of expertise, Henderson and Carroll (1993) point out that the sports medicine professional is in a good position to influence the athlete to accept referral to a mental health professional. Sports medicine professionals are particularly well suited for this role since they so often are familiar with the athlete and are viewed with respect, authority, and trust (Kane, 1982, 1984). Sports medicine professionals are in a position to emphasize that seeking help is a sign of maturity and self-direction, not weakness. The sports medicine professional can then help the athlete secure an appointment with a knowledgeable mental health professional. Because sports medicine professionals are often the only medical practitioners with whom some athletes have regular and frequent contact, they are in the best position to help the athlete with this important process.

Improved Effectiveness of Practice

One of the most persuasive arguments for establishing a counseling role for sports medicine professionals is that it will improve the effectiveness of their practice. Unfortunately, much medical advice is ignored by patients (Janis, 1983). Many, if not most, patients fail to take their medication, do their home exercises, or follow their prescribed diets—at least some of the time. Although counseling is not the answer to all of sports medicine's noncompliance ills, there are at least two areas in which an increased level of effective counseling holds promise for improved outcomes: prevention and rehabilitation.

Counseling for Prevention

Most of the data on counseling effectiveness in the prevention of injury come from studies that employed primary-care physicians as counselors. These studies have demonstrated that counseling can help patients—and their families—alter their behavior in a manner consistent with injury and accident prevention (Bass, Mehta, Ostrovsky, & Halperin, 1985). Counseling is associated with increased patient knowledge, improved behavior, and—most important—decreased injury rates (Bass, Christoffel, et al., 1993). These data are intriguing in light of the significant role in prevention that is incumbent on sports medicine professionals. It would be interesting to see whether the same results shown by these studies could be obtained using athletic trainers or physical therapists as counselors—especially in high school settings where the opportunity to counsel the young athlete's parents is the greatest.

Counseling for Rehabilitation

There is a wealth of information that demonstrates the effectiveness and importance of counseling in improving rehabilitation outcomes in a variety of settings. Although the specific techniques used to improve rehabilitation adherence are discussed later in this book, a brief discussion for the purpose of justifying the sports medicine professional's role in counseling is appropriate.

Sick and injured people often experience a physical benefit from counseling (Viney, Clarke, Bunn, & Benjamin, 1985). They often require less pain medication after surgery, and they tend to achieve a faster physical recovery. Even those patients who do not receive formal counseling after injury or illness tend to exhibit improved compliance with medical prescriptions if the health care provider can develop and maintain an effective personal relationship (Saunders & Maxwell, 1988). One of the theories that attempts to explain this phenomenon is provided by Ramsden and Taylor (1988), who postulate that counseling helps reduce the high level of anxiety often present in patients suffering from injury or illness. If left unaddressed, this anxiety can prolong rehabilitation and lengthen the recovery process. With specific regard to rehabilitation, the quality of athlete–practitioner interaction seems to be an essential ingredient for successful rehabilitation (Fisher, 1990). In addition, social support, encouragement, goal setting, and effective communication all seem to enhance adherence to the rehabilitation plan (Byerly, Worrell, Gahimer, & Domholdt, 1994; Fisher, Scriber, Matheny, Alderman, & Bitting, 1993). Sports medicine professionals are in an ideal position to enhance the effectiveness of rehabilitation through these simple counseling components (Fisher, Mullins, & Frye, 1993).

WHOM SHOULD SPORTS MEDICINE PROFESSIONALS COUNSEL?

Although the question of whom the sports medicine professional should counsel may seem obvious, the list is actually longer than might be assumed. Injured athletes are not the only ones who can benefit from our counseling skills. Although the normal cautions about not exceeding our level of expertise apply, a case can be made for a counseling role for the sports medicine professional with injured athletes, uninjured athletes, parents, and students in the health professions (see figure 1.2).

Injured Athletes

The injured athlete is the most obvious beneficiary of the sports medicine professional's counseling. Our primary focus is on this population. We spend most of our time with injured athletes. As previously noted, a significant body of research supports a counseling role for the sports medicine professional with this group.

Uninjured Athletes

Sports medicine professionals play an important role in helping healthy athletes avoid injury. Counseling uninjured athletes, alone or in small groups, is one important function in this role. In addition, sports medicine professionals can also provide physically healthy athletes who have minor social–emotional problems with a vehicle for sharing their concerns and feelings. This may be particularly important when athletes must deal with the death of a teammate (Pedersen, 1986; Ray, Hanlon, & Van Heest, 1989).

Parents

Injured student athletes exist in the context of families. As any sports medicine professional who has worked at the high school level will readily attest, parents are a large part of the high school sports culture. Their presence often manifests even more when their child becomes injured. As the first health care professional to attend to their child's injury, the athletic trainer, physical therapist, or team physician is often called on to explain the nature of the injury, give advice about referral, and

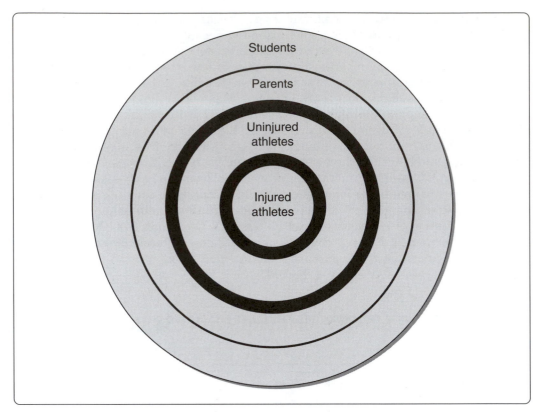

Figure 1.2   Counseling relationships of the sports medicine professional.

serve as a sounding board for parental concerns. Indeed, it is incumbent upon sports medicine professionals to be sure that parents understand enough about the injury that they can take the appropriate follow-up steps.

Students in the Health Professions

Some of us work with students in professional preparation programs as part of our normal job responsibilities or on an occasional basis during clinical rotations. Anyone who has ever worked with students can attest to their frequent need for advice and counsel. The questions, issues, and problems that students ask about are usually related to education or professional preparation. Students, however, like all young people, look to their teachers for advice on a wide range of issues, some of which are only minimally connected to their teachers' role as educators. Issues of professional and social adjustment, along with financial and relationship problems, are commonly addressed to sports medicine professionals who work with students. The counseling we provide is very important to these students. An important and valuable service that we can provide to students, which they cannot get anywhere else, is counseling in the context of the culture of our various professions. Students may wonder, "How do athletic trainers, physical therapists, or physicians feel about or handle this issue that I'm dealing with?" Who better to advise them than those who have experienced similar situations in the same social context that the student is in?

COUNSELING ROLES WE SHOULD AVOID

One of the dangers of preparing and defending the argument that health professionals who work in sports medicine should counsel athletes as a function of their jobs is

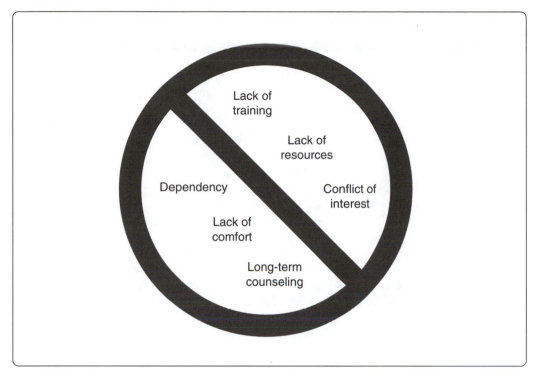

Figure 1.3   Counseling traps the sports medicine professional should avoid.

that some may take the argument too far and attempt to supplant the role of the mental health professional. This is a danger because of the very real limits sports medicine professionals are ethically bound to place on their counseling role. Although sports medicine professionals may be first-line counselors for many problems faced by athletes, they are clearly not qualified to handle some situations. Athletic trainers, physical therapists, and team physicians have often been trained in a culture that treats the ability to "do it all" as a virtue, although this is beginning to change. This "do it all" philosophy has led to a smaller number of referrals from sports medicine professionals to mental health professionals than might be expected (Etzel & Ferrante, 1993). Although a list of the problems sports medicine professionals ought to refer would always be incomplete, those discussed in the following six sections should help guide decision making in this area.

Lack of Training

Sports medicine professionals who lack training for specific problems should refer athletes with those problems to an appropriate mental health professional. Although we all should become competent to deal with normal, routine, minor psychoemotional problems that our patients face, more serious pathological behaviors should quickly raise a red flag. The same rules that apply for referral of physical problems ought to apply for mental health problems. Although some sports medicine professionals may experience personal regret at the loss of control that comes with referral, they should understand that they still have an important follow-up role to play in the athlete's eventual recovery. One of the most important roles you can play after referring the athlete is supplying the mental health professional with objective health history information (Heil, 1993). This is critical because it allows the mental health professional to compare actual health and performance data with those presented by the athlete.

Lack of Comfort

We hope that sports medicine professionals of the future will be provided with more counseling education than those of the past and that they will be better prepared to handle a wider variety of low-level counseling functions than they are today. Even so, all sports medicine professionals will be confronted from time to time with an athlete who has a problem that they are trained to handle but for which they have very little experience and little personal comfort. Such cases should be referred. Just as sports medicine professionals are ethically bound to refer patients with physical problems with which they are uncomfortable, so should they refer mental health problems if they lack the requisite amount of experience or comfort in dealing with the difficulty. This is not to suggest that we should shirk our responsibilities to our patients. Referring a patient who requires counseling on the basis of racial prejudice, for example, is obviously poor professional practice. Similarly, referring patients who present with problems or viewpoints with which we disagree is also an abrogation of our responsibilities. The pregnant student athlete who approaches her athletic trainer for advice because she is considering an abortion is a good example. The athletic trainer has a professional responsibility to provide the patient with all the information she needs to make a choice that is right for her, the patient—even if the athletic trainer is personally opposed to abortion or, conversely, thinks that completing the pregnancy is a poor decision.

Ongoing or Long-Term Counseling

Athletes requiring ongoing or long-term counseling should be referred. Although sports medicine professionals may serve as important resources for follow-up with mental health professionals, most are not trained to engage in a long-term counseling relationship with their patients—whether injured or uninjured (Makarowski & Rickell, 1993). An exception to this general rule may exist for the counseling provided during a long-term rehabilitation program.

Lack of Resources

Athletic trainers, physical therapists, and team physicians are busy people. Quality counseling takes time and requires a significant expenditure of personal energy (Kottler, 1986). It is understandable that from time to time the sports medicine professional will lack both the time and the personal energy required for effective counseling. Since the need for counseling does not disappear just because the sports medicine professional lacks resources, we have an obligation to make sure that an appropriate referral is arranged.

Conflict of Interest

Sports medicine professionals have an ethical obligation to refer athletes requiring counseling when it would conflict with the practitioner's interest were he or she to provide it personally. This is an especially thorny problem for athletic trainers and team physicians, many of whom are employed by educational or professional athletic organizations. Although most sports medicine professionals would say that their first allegiance is to the athlete, many do, in fact, have an obligation to communicate with coaches and other members of the organization. When this communication would force the sports medicine professional to break the confidentiality of the practitioner–patient relationship, the athlete would be better served by being referred to an unconflicted third party.

Dependency

Any counseling that causes the athlete to become overly dependent on the sports medicine professional is potentially harmful to both the athlete and the practitioner. An athlete who becomes dependent on the sports medicine professional for psychological support may lose his or her capacity for independent decision making. **Dependency** can be difficult to identify before it is too late. Two of the best ways to prevent dependency are to ensure that counseling remains short term and that the limits of the counseling relationship are defined and understood in advance.

dependency—Habitual reliance on another person for comfort, guidance, and decision making.

THE COUNSELING ROLES OF VARIOUS SPORTS MEDICINE PROFESSIONALS

The different counseling roles played by the athletic trainer, physical therapist, and team physician can be established in many ways. Legislators, administrators, and institutions all have an opinion on the nature of the work that sports medicine professionals ought to be doing. Codes of ethics and other standard-setting documents of professional organizations also help define the counseling roles of sports medicine professionals. In many cases the counseling roles of these three groups overlap significantly. The responsibility to provide counseling in the form of patient education, for example, is a role that athletic trainers, physical therapists, and team physicians share. Nevertheless, some counseling roles, while similar, are emphasized differently depending on the professional's training, experience, and license.

Counseling Role of the Athletic Trainer

The elements of the athletic trainer's role that involve counseling have been fairly well defined. For example, the NATA's *Competencies in Athletic Training* (1992) mandates proficiency in counseling and related skills regarding the following entities:

- Psychological and emotional factors related to injury and rehabilitation
- Injury and illness risk reduction
- Physiological effects of physical activity
- Principles of nutrition
- Recognition of eating disorders
- Weight control
- Effects of drugs and ergogenic aids
- Personal hygiene
- Personal protection from exposure to infectious disease
- Recognition of signs and symptoms associated with common mental disorders
- Personal and community health issues
- Referral to mental health and social services
- Education and provision of health care information to athletes, coaches, parents, and the general public

The NATA Board of Certification's *Role Delineation Study* (1995) also cites the following counseling activities for practicing athletic trainers:

- Educational programs for both healthy and injured athletes, including general health, alcohol and drug use, and performance-anxiety information

- Effects of acute injury and illness
- Psychological responses to trauma, healing, and exercise
- Motivation in rehabilitation
- Psychological readiness to return to competition
- Communicating appropriate information to the rehabilitating athlete
- Problem solving
- Signs and symptoms of emotional, behavioral, and physical status
- Referral to appropriate health care and mental health professionals
- Interpersonal communication for the purpose of motivating, instructing, and eliciting information

Counseling Role of the Physical Therapist

Many of the counseling roles assumed by athletic trainers are similar to those performed by physical therapists. While athletic trainers are required to perform counseling activities in a wide variety of settings and under many different conditions, physical therapists typically counsel their patients on some aspect of their rehabilitation for injury or illness in the context of acute inpatient care or in clinically based outpatient facilities. While the APTA has not defined the counseling roles and responsibilities of the physical therapist in as detailed a manner as the NATA has for athletic trainers, it has provided some direction. For example, the APTA's *Guide for Professional Conduct* (1991) specifies that physical therapists must be guided in part by the psychological welfare of their patients. The standards for patient care as established by the APTA (1995) require physical therapists to

- educate patients regarding their proposed treatment plans,
- explain the benefits and risks of the plan, and
- obtain informed consent before beginning therapy.

Educational requirements for physical therapists also help define their counseling role. The social and behavioral sciences are recognized as basic to physical therapy education (APTA, 1992). Learning experiences in the areas of education and consultation are required. Physical therapy education programs are evaluated in part based on the following abilities of their graduates:

- Professional practice consistent with a caring manner
- Collaboration with patients, their families, and other individuals who may be responsible for the patient
- Interaction with the patient for the delivery of psychosocial support
- Effective communication with patients and their families
- Effective interpersonal relationships

Counseling Role of the Team Physician

It is interesting that the person on the sports medicine team who arguably has the greatest responsibility for effective and comprehensive counseling—the team physician—has a role not well defined in the sports medicine literature. Physicians are, of course, trained in the basic and applied behavioral sciences. The patient interview is an important part of their medical training. Team physicians must draw on their prior training experience and comfort level with the counseling role, which varies in focus by medical specialty, when determining their niche. The Residency Review Committee in Family Practice has defined basic competencies in issues of human behavior and mental health for family practice physicians. Some requirements include emotional aspects of nonpsychiatric disorders, counseling skills, and the physician/patient relationship. Each medical specialty values and requires some level of training in counseling.

In fact, the *Program Requirements for Residency Education in Family Practice,* established by the Residency Review Committee in Family Practice (1996), stipulate that there must be instruction in the following areas:

a. Diagnosis and management of psychiatric disorders in children and adults

b. Emotional aspects of nonpsychiatric disorders

c. Psychopharmacology

d. Alcoholism and other substance abuse

e. The physician/patient relationship

f. Patient interviewing skills

g. Counseling skills

h. Normal psychosocial growth and development in individuals and families

i. Stages of stress in a family life cycle

j. Sensitivity to gender, race, age, sexual orientation and cultural differences in patients

k. Family violence including child, partner, and elder abuse (physical and sexual), as well as neglect, and its effect on both victims and perpetrators

l. Medical ethics, including patient autonomy, confidentiality, and issues concerning quality of life

m. Factors influencing patient compliance

Heil (1993) points out three major counseling roles of the physician: counselor, educator, and protector. These roles are inextricably woven and interchangeable. The role as counselor includes education of the student-athlete about the nature and severity of the illness or injury, its anatomical location, rehabilitation management, prognosis, and potential long-term complications. The more a patient is educated about his or her injury or illness, the more capable that individual is in future prevention, rehabilitation, and management and the better the eventual outcome will be. For example, an asthmatic patient who does not understand the chronicity of his or her condition may have difficulty adjusting to daily use of medications. If proper administration of inhaled asthma medications is not accomplished, this athlete may experience impaired exercise performance and potentially diminished self-esteem. Describing to the patient the role that social and family relationships play in asthma flare-ups illustrates the utility of applying family systems theory stress management strategies as part of the patient education process. Education empowers the athlete to direct a goal-oriented, autonomous management and rehabilitation style.

Serving as a patient advocate or protector is a traditional part of the team physician's role. Athletes face pressure to return to play. Some pressure originates from their own risk-taking, goal-focused nature, while some comes from peers, coaches, or family encouraging them to return to play (Heil, 1993). Providing treatment or a safe haven for an injured athlete through negotiation with the coach about return to play is protective. Often, rehabilitation does not go as planned, and athletes need encouragement and backing.

Hendrickson and Rowe (1990), while cautioning that the team physician's counseling role should be dictated by his or her qualifications and the nature of the athlete's problems, state that the team physician should be involved in the following counseling activities:

• Crisis intervention

• Stress management

- Psychological skills training
- Referral for serious psychoemotional conditions
- Group and individual psychotherapy
- Pharmacotherapy
- Patient education
- Psychological assessment and diagnosis
- Treatment planning
- Development of a working alliance with the patient

SUPERVISION FOR COUNSELING

Because sports medicine services are so frequently provided by a team of health care professionals, it is important to consider the supervisory roles that one member of the team may play for others when they counsel athletes. Establishing the proper supervisory lines of authority for counseling can be especially difficult. There are many factors that may determine who requires supervision for his or her counseling activities and under what circumstances such supervision should be provided. Do athletic trainers—who technically perform their work under the supervision of physicians—need to be supervised when they counsel athletes? Do they require supervision for every athlete they counsel? In every situation? For every problem? Does the team physician still retain supervisory authority over a psychologist to whom he or she has referred an athlete for counseling services? Does a physical therapist whose license allows treatment without referral require supervision for counseling? What about the physical therapist who practices in a state where prescriptions from physicians are required? The answers to these questions are not always readily apparent.

Rather than provide a strict set of rules for counseling supervision that would be unlikely to function well under all circumstances, it seems more appropriate to propose a few simple guidelines that sports medicine professionals can use to determine whether supervision is required and what form it should take. Sports medicine professionals should be supervised when they counsel athletes if these conditions exist:

- Supervision is required by law, codes of ethics, established professional standards of practice, or employment contracts
- The athletes' best interests would be served by involving other professionals in their counseling care
- The sports medicine professional providing the counseling has questions or is unsure of how to proceed

Formal supervision for counseling is probably not required under these conditions:

- The counseling provided is "low level" advice or nontherapeutic in nature
- Counseling occurs on a one-time or infrequent basis
- The counseling provided is part of a routine patient education program
- Athletes refuse to waive their rights to confidentiality

What form should counseling supervision take after it has been established that it is required? The answer to this question can vary, depending on the situation. Although exceptions can exist, the team approach to provision of sports medicine services that has worked so well in many environments is probably appropriate for many (but not all) counseling situations as well. The composition of the counseling team may differ slightly from the traditional sports medicine team. For example, the typical university-based sports medicine team might comprise an athletic trainer, primary-care team physician, and specialist physicians who are called on for specific problems. When an anorexic athlete is identified at that university, a counseling team made up of the athletic trainer, the primary care team physician, a nutritionist, and a consulting psychiatrist or other mental health professional may be employed. These people should all work together in the care plan for this athlete. In order for this to occur, of course, the athlete would have to agree to allow the mental health professional or team physician to communicate with other members of the team. Communication regarding the athlete's counseling should be limited to a summary of the mental health professional's interview with the athlete along with the goals for treatment (Wiese-Bjornstal & Smith, 1993). Such communication is important because it allows for more effective coordination of care. The weakness of this approach, however, is that the athlete may have difficulty developing an effective therapeutic alliance with the physician or mental health professional if he or she thinks they will be discussing his or her case with others. Providing a completely confidential working relationship with an outside mental health professional may be empowering for the athlete dealing with particularly sensitive issues such as substance abuse. In the team approach to coordination and supervision of counseling, it is critical that only the information that is likely to lead to resolution of the problem is shared with others, that the athlete is informed about what will be shared, and that he or she provides permission for the sharing of information (Thompson & Sherman, 1993). The counseling team must carefully guard against sharing confidential information with coaches and certain members of the sports medicine team.

CASE STUDY

Jane Whitcomb was the only freshman on her college volleyball team. She came to the east coast school from a small farm in Nebraska. Although she liked college well enough, there were a few problems. Her roommate was unfriendly and was rarely home, having made friends with students in a dorm across campus. The courses in college were much more difficult than in high school. Jane had to stay up much later than she was used to in order to keep up with the work. This was made even more difficult by the fact that Jane was so tired after rushing to the dining hall before it closed after her three-hour volleyball practices. Perhaps she would have felt differently about everything if she were playing more, but she rarely made it into the games.

Jane's situation went from bad to worse one day when she injured her back diving for a ball in practice. She tried to continue, but the pain was too great, and her coach told her to go to the training room. When Jane shuffled into the training room a few minutes later, she was met by one of the school's certified athletic trainers, Sarah Wick. Sarah evaluated Jane's back, spent about 15 minutes explaining the injury to Jane, and applied ice to the injury. She told Jane that she would like to see her again the next morning. Sarah also gave Jane instructions for how to care for the injury in her dorm room that night. Finally, Sarah gave Jane her business card and told her to call her if she had any questions or concerns.

Sarah received a phone call at home that night from Jane. She was crying and struggled through her tears to tell Sarah how badly her back hurt. She asked Sarah if she would come over to the dorm and look at her back again. Sarah didn't have anything else to do that evening, so she agreed. After she arrived she examined Jane's back again, applied ice, helped her with some mild low-back stretching, and gave her ibuprofen for the pain. While Jane was icing her back, Sarah asked her how things were going for her since coming to college. Although Jane was a little reluctant at first, she eventually told Sarah how unhappy she was and how different everything was from how she expected it would be. Sarah spent three more hours in Jane's room talking to her about her problems.

QUESTIONS FOR ANALYSIS

1. Analyze the various counseling roles Sarah has assumed with Jane. Which are appropriate? Why are they appropriate? Which are inappropriate? Why are they inappropriate? What would you have done differently?

2. What benefits might Jane receive as a result of Sarah's counseling?

3. What potential pitfalls should Sarah avoid in her counseling? What kinds of problems could she face? How should she handle those problems?

4. From the information you have, would you refer Jane to a mental health professional for more advanced counseling? Why or why not? If so, to whom would you refer her? How would you convince Jane to accept the referral?

SUMMARY

The counseling role is an important part of most sports medicine professionals' jobs. Although they often lack formal training in counseling, their effectiveness in this area is often a determining factor in the success of their practice. Counseling has been alternatively defined as psychotherapy, helping, education, rapport building, communication, and emotional first aid. The most useful definition of counseling as practiced by sports medicine professionals involves the provision of social support, information about choices, helping the athlete establish goals, and encouraging decision making. The counseling role of sports medicine professionals is defined both explicitly and implicitly by various codes of ethics, professional associations, standards of practice, and state credentialing laws. Sports medicine professionals should counsel their athletes for a variety of reasons. They may have a legal and ethical responsibility to do so. Their patients generally appreciate their counsel. Sports medicine professionals act as a first line of defense in the identification of psychological conditions in athletes. Counseling can improve the effectiveness of the sports medicine professional's practice, both in terms of preventing injury and in improving treatment outcomes. Counseling can be effective for a variety of people, including injured and uninjured athletes, their parents, and students in professional preparation programs in sports medicine. Sports medicine professionals should exercise caution in their counseling roles by referring athletes who have problems for which the practitioner lacks training, comfort, or resources. Athletes who require long-term counseling should be referred to a mental health professional. When counseling would create a conflict of interest or result in dependency, referral is also appropriate. Although the counseling roles played by athletic trainers, physical therapists, and team physicians overlap significantly, each profession has defined its role in different terms. Supervision for counseling is important in some situations, and the sports medicine professional should carefully consider the athlete's needs when entering into a counseling relationship.

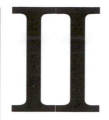

Practical Aspects of Counseling for the Sports Medicine Professional

The chapters in this part of the text provide readers with an introduction to the skills they will need to become effective counselors to their injured patients. The skills outlined in the chapters of this part are generic in nature (as opposed to the specific counseling skills for particular problems contained in part III) and apply to most counseling situations. After reading these chapters you should better understand the psychological processes involved in recovery from injury and the various techniques that can be employed to help the athlete during such difficult times. You will better comprehend the ethical pitfalls associated with counseling athletes, and your referral and documentation skills will be enhanced. Finally, you will be able to discern between the techniques that are effective for one-on-one counseling and those more useful for group settings.

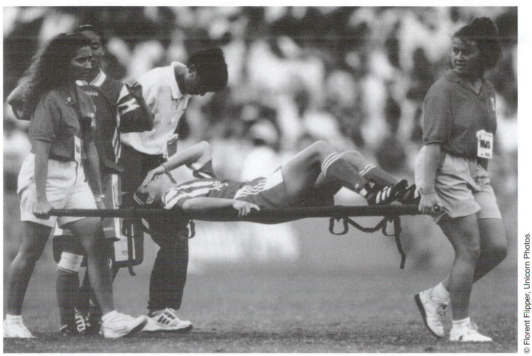

Psychosocial Dimensions of Sport Injury

Diane M. Wiese-Bjornstal, PhD, *University of Minnesota*
Shelly M. Shaffer, PhD, *Pinnacle Health Systems*

Chapter Objectives

Identify influential psychosocial factors that precede sport injury

Discuss ways in which the sociocultural context of sport affects occurrence of and response to sport injury

Explain the stress response mechanisms by which psychosocial factors contribute to occurrence of sport injury

Cite examples of personal and situational factors influencing the responses of athletes to injury

Describe some of the cognitive, emotional, and behavioral responses common among injured athletes

Sports medicine professionals are very comfortable dealing with the physical dimensions of sport injury. The focus of their education and training is on preventing injury and treating the physical consequences once injury occurs. They are less comfortable and familiar with the psychosocial dimensions of sport injury. This is not altogether surprising, since they devote little of their education and training to these dimensions. To address this gap in the education of sports medicine professionals, this chapter outlines psychosocial factors that affect athletes both before and after injury. This knowledge will enhance both injury prevention efforts and your ability to manage the cognitive, emotional, and behavioral consequences of injury.

PSYCHOSOCIAL RISK FACTORS BEFORE SPORT INJURY

One of the most important functions of sports medicine professionals is injury prevention. Thus the identification of factors that predispose athletes to injury is essential in order to develop effective interventions before the actual occurrence of sport injury. Preventing all sport injuries is impossible, but reducing their frequency is a desirable goal. Coaches and athletes embrace preventive strategies recommended by sports medicine professionals. Although sports medicine professionals typically are comfortable recommending physical prevention strategies, it is also to their advantage to recommend psychosocial prevention strategies. To recommend such prevention strategies, sports medicine professionals should first understand the precursors to injury.

Precursors to Sport Injury

Many factors in combination create a situation in which sport injury is more likely. These factors group into four major areas:

- Physical
- Environmental
- Sociocultural
- Psychological

Physical factors are the physical characteristics of individual athletes and include such things as their physical condition, age, experience, existing muscular imbalances, overtraining, and physical fatigue. Environmental factors include the physical and social environment surrounding participation. Environmental situations that might precipitate injury include uneven surfaces, slippery conditions, and unsafe equipment. Environmental factors might also include such influences as the quality of officiating (e.g., do the officials allow more contact than they should?) and the quality and style of coaching (e.g., does the coach teach unsafe techniques?).

Most sports medicine professionals are familiar with physical and environmental risk elements and are comfortable recommending preventive strategies for managing these risks. Most are not as familiar, however, with the sociocultural and psychological factors affecting the occurrence of sport injuries. Therefore we turn our attention to a discussion of these psychosocial precursors.

Sociocultural Factors

sport ethic—A system of principles and beliefs, held predominantly by athletes, that advocates personal sacrifice, risk taking, and playing with pain to promote conformity and adherence to sport norms (Hughes & Coakley, 1991).

The major sociocultural factor influencing injury risk for athletes includes the broadly described **sport ethic** (Hughes & Coakley, 1991) endemic in North American sport participation at all levels. This ethic includes a number of attitudes that contribute to an unhealthy climate for many athletes. These attitudes include acting tough in the face of pain and injury (e.g., "no pain, no gain") and an unwillingness to seek out medical treatment for fear of being labeled as weak. Thus inherent in the sport ethic is the typical expectation to play with pain and injuries. Although these factors are not the cause of injury per se, these attitudes may create a climate that discourages athletes from reporting injuries early or from seeking treatment for injuries.

Frey (1991) discussed elements of the "culture of risk" in sport, describing the socialization process through which athletes learn that accepting physical risks is their only legitimate or viable choice if they want to compete. This cultural belief system reflects the following themes: role pressures and monetary inducements to play with pain and injuries, general cultural values linking pain tolerance to the demonstration of masculine character, management and institutional rationalizations of pain and injuries as "part of the game" and "for the good of the team," the so-called learning experiences of playing hurt and returning from serious injury, and the need to push oneself and accept or ignore the risks of pain and injuries (Frey, 1991).

On the basis of interviews with former male athletes, Messner (1992) also identified external pressures and threats to masculine identity as primary reasons to risk injury. Values of the sports world are such that coaches, teammates, fans, and the media negatively judge the athlete who refuses to play hurt. This external pressure is especially prevalent in the media when they frequently celebrate an athlete's willingness to endure extreme amounts of pain and injury in order to compete. Those who demonstrate the least amount of reaction to pain and injury are glorified (Hughes & Coakley, 1991; Messner, 1992).

An emphasis on masculine identity, such as that which predominates in sport, results in males becoming alienated from their feelings, thus making them more prone to view their bodies instrumentally, as weapons to harm and be harmed (Young, White, & McTeer, 1994), especially in the competitive and insecure world of sport careers (Messner, 1992). Certain sports such as boxing, football, and wrestling are essentially rule-bound combat, likely to produce high rates of injury. Played almost exclusively by males, these sports perform an important role in shaping a masculine identity (Messner, 1990). For athletes to question the decision to "give up" their bodies would be to question the entire system of rules through which they had successfully formed relationships and their sense of identity. Because such questioning is considered too threatening, athletes instead are more likely to rationalize their own injuries as "part of the game" and to claim that the pain contributed to "character development," thereby gaining them the respect of others (Messner, 1992). Serious injury is viewed as a masculinizing experience (Young et al., 1994). These internalized ideas about masculinity work in conjunction with external factors (such as pressure from coaches) to influence athletes to "choose" to play hurt (Nixon, 1993).

Curry's case study (1992, as summarized by Coakley, 1996) of a wrestler's competitive career clearly illustrates this socialization process as an athlete learns to deal with pain and injury. The athlete's early observations of other wrestlers taught him to define pain and injury as routine parts of the sport. Progressing to higher levels of competition demonstrated that endurance of injury was commonplace. To be successful a wrestler had to adopt the following beliefs, attitudes, and actions: "(1) to "shake off" minor injuries, (2) to see special treatment for minor injuries as a form of coddling, (3) to express desire and motivation by playing while injured or in pain, (4) to avoid using injury or pain as excuses for not practicing or competing, (5) to use physicians and trainers as experts whose role was to keep him competing when not healthy, (6) to see pain-killing anti-inflammatory drugs as necessary performance-enhancing aids, (7) to commit himself to the idea that all athletes must pay a price as they strive for excellence, and (8) to define any athlete (including himself) unwilling to pay the price or to strive for excellence as morally deficient" (Coakley, 1996, p. 358). Finally, through a combination of injuries to his spine, knees, and ears, this wrestler became a role model for younger wrestlers (Coakley, 1996; Curry, 1992).

As increasing numbers of girls and women enter the competitive arena, they are no longer immune from the expected norm of playing with pain. Every bit as determined and tough as their male counterparts, these female participants are equally reluctant to take time out for injuries to recover fully. Females are also somewhat more likely to abuse their bodies in other ways, such as through the development of disordered eating habits (see chapter 12). Accommodation of a certain level of pain—from the marathoner "hitting the wall" to the acute pain associated with contact sports—is often a necessary condition of sport (Thornton, 1990). The system of rewards and punishments attached to playing with pain as well as the unstable nature of athletic careers, however, make it difficult to take oneself out of competition when injured or to avoid competition until an injury is fully healed. Even more disturbing is that some sports medicine professionals who treat competitors unknowingly promote playing with pain. This is particularly worrisome in the case of young athletes.

For example, as attending physicians at a wrestling tournament, Strauss and Lanese (1982) noted that 9- to 14-year-old wrestlers "overreported" their injuries because they sought medical attention for muscle strains and contusions—injuries that would have been ignored by older wrestlers. "The children seemed to have less tolerance for discomfort" and reported their pain "more readily" in comparison to the older competitors (p. 2018). This view of young athletes as "overreporting" their injuries—therefore implicitly not being tough enough to compete with injury—and failing to model the behavior of the older, more experienced wrestlers is one of the very reasons that adolescents are at risk for incurring permanent physical damage. Their natural desire is to emulate the more physically and psychologically mature high school and college athletes. If these youngsters perceive that it is not acceptable within the culture of wrestling to report injuries, they could be learning a costly lesson.

Young athletes train and compete without the benefit of mature musculoskeletal or physiological systems and without much historical background against which to compare their sport experiences (Lord & Kozar, 1989). Overuse injuries seen in this age group may reflect the growth characteristics of the immature skeleton or may be of the type seen in adult athletes undergoing rigorous training schedules. This second type of overuse injury is uncommon among children in neighborhood or free-play activities, and its incidence rises in proportion to the expected achievement or performance level. These types of overuse injuries are particularly common if the young athlete is excessively intent on **modeling** the workout intensity of older, more physically mature athletes.

modeling—The process of imitation; learning by observing others.

It is paramount that coaches and athletic trainers involved in youth and adolescent sport programs pay close attention to the training habits of young athletes, especially in light of the fact that younger athletes do not always make the wisest long-term health decisions. Adolescents' sense of immortality (Thornton, 1990), coupled with pertinent developmental issues, significantly relates to their frequent unwillingness to comply with medical advice (Cromer & Tarnowski, 1989). For example, level of cognitive ability represents one of the most important developmental differences between adolescents and adults (Ginsberg & Opper, 1979). The age at which formal thinking abilities develop differs from child to child; thus a normal adolescent may lack the ability to foresee the potentially negative implications of his or her behavior (Friedman & Litt, 1986). Young athletes functioning at a lower reasoning level therefore would have greater difficulty complying with preventive health or medical treatment recommendations than their teammates who have well-developed abstraction abilities (Cromer & Tarnowski, 1989). Compounding the risk for injury in this scenario is the prevailing sport ethic of playing with pain.

Pain in children, however, should always cause concern, given the potentially irreversible damage that may occur if they ignore their bodies' own warning device (Kozar & Lord, 1988). All adults who value the overall well-being of children above their athlete status must recognize children's inexperience and limited cognitive ability to make judgments about pain and injury severity. Sports medicine professionals must intervene on behalf of the well-being of child athletes, even if their recommendations are not popular among coaches and parents. It is incumbent upon sports medicine professionals, and all adults who work with athletes, to fully consider the long-range health and best interests of the athlete when making the decision whether to allow the athlete to compete with injury. Chapter 3 presents strategies for intervening in the face of such opposition.

Psychological Factors

Andersen and Williams (1988) outlined several injury-predisposing psychological factors, based primarily on the stress-response model of athletic injury. These authors initially relied on research examining the relationship between stress and health, which provided evidence for links between stress and negative health consequences (Rice, 1992). More recently, they have outlined the sport-specific research supporting various components of their model (Williams & Andersen, 1998). A detailed discussion of the research supporting this model is presented in chapter 14; this section will serve as an overview to that review.

Figure 2.1 presents a simplified illustration of the major predictions of this model (Andersen & Williams, 1988). **Personality, history of stressors,** and **coping resources** interact to increase or decrease the likelihood of a stress response—including both cognitive and physiological or attentional changes—which in turn affect the occurrence of sport injury when the athlete participates in a potentially injurious sport situation. Athletes' stress histories directly affect their stress response; however, personality factors and coping resources can affect the stress response either directly or through a moderating influence on stress histories (Williams & Andersen, 1998).

Personality

Personality differences influence whether or not individuals are likely to perceive situations as stressful, as well as their susceptibility to the effects of stressors. Factors such as self-concept, introversion or extroversion, psychological hardiness, sen-

personality—The blend of dispositional characteristics that make a person unique.

history of stressors—An individual's personal stress factors, including major life events, chronic daily problems, and previous experience with injuries.

coping resources—A wide variety of behaviors and social networks that help individuals deal with life, including personal attitudes, beliefs, and attributes, as well as social support networks.

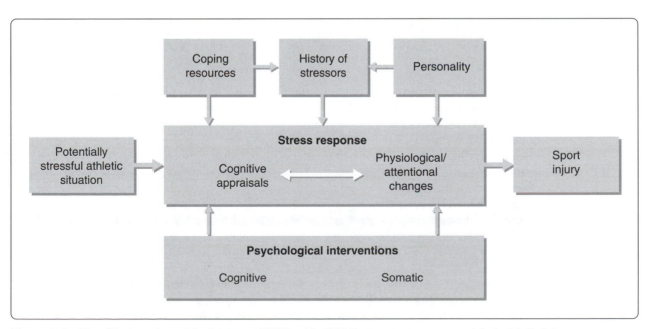

Figure 2.1 Simplified version of Andersen and Williams's (1988) stress-response model of athletic injury.

Adapted with permission from Andersen & Williams (1988). A model of stress and athletic injury: Prediction and prevention. *Journal of Sport and Exercise Psychology, 10,* 294-306.

sation seeking, competitive trait anxiety, and locus of control are personality factors thought to be likely candidates that affect the risk of sport injury.

Although belief in the role of personality in the occurrence of sport injury is intuitive, the research has provided somewhat mixed results. The general health literature has documented a variety of personality variables related to health outcomes (Andersen & Williams, 1993; Rice, 1992). Research specific to sport, however, has typically failed to consider how personality might interact with other components of the model to influence the stress response (Williams & Andersen, 1998). Further research in the unique context of sport needs to clarify the role of personality in injury. It seems likely, however, that personality factors may interact with sociocultural factors to result in increased injury risk. To illustrate this interaction, as an example, one might think of a perfectionistic young athlete who constantly tries to live up to both personal and parental expectations for success, thus pushing herself to the point of injury and beyond.

History of Stressors

life stress—Major life events and changes that can result in feelings of stress.

A second major psychological factor predicted by the Andersen and Williams (1988) model as affecting the stress response is the athlete's history of stressors. These include major life events, chronic daily problems, and previous experience with injuries (Williams & Roepke, 1993). Major life events—also known as **life stress**—consist of major changes in a person's life, such as death of a family member, divorce of parents, or extended illness. In addition to these more negative factors, however, major life events can also include positive changes such as marriage, birth of a child, or starting a new job. It is important to remember that even positive life changes can be stressful and that a major life change that is negative for one person may be viewed as positive for another (e.g., the breakup of a relationship). The general research findings have been that high levels of life stress are associated with more frequent injuries (Williams & Roepke, 1993) and that the risk of injury increases in proportion to the level of life stress (Williams & Andersen, 1998).

The other major category of stress levels includes chronic daily problems, also known as daily hassles. These are more minor stressors that can accumulate to be as problematic as the more major life events. Daily hassles for athletes, for example, might include disagreements with coaches, school difficulties, transportation problems, or financial worries. Although these examples are negative, also considered in combination with daily hassles are daily uplifts, which reflect more-positive minor events such as interactions with family members, socializing with friends, and doing well in school. Research on this element of stress history is more limited; however, the available evidence suggests that daily hassles should be included as a factor related to injury vulnerability (Williams & Andersen, 1998).

Understanding the role of each athlete's stress history is essential because research has shown that higher levels of stress are often associated with greater frequency of sport injury. In other words, athletes who have experienced a greater number of major life events—particularly negative ones—or who have high levels of daily hassles are at particular risk for injury. Chapter 14 presents a more extended discussion of this research. The relationship between stress history and injury occurrence seems particularly strong when compounded with low coping resources, as described in the next section.

Coping Resources

Coping resources, the third group of factors affecting the stress response both directly and through the links with stress history and personality, consist of a wide variety of behaviors and social networks that help individuals deal with life. Access to and use of these resources seem helpful in dealing with the stresses of life. There is evidence that athletes' coping resources affect injury outcome both directly and indirectly (Andersen & Williams, 1993). For example, use of coping resources may act directly on the perception of an event as stressful or not or may act indirectly as a factor that buffers the effects of stressful life events through various coping mechanisms. One study of high school athletes, for example, found that those low in both social coping mechanisms (e.g., **social support**) and personal coping skills (e.g., ability to concentrate, keep a positive attitude, and control arousal levels) were at greatest risk for sport injuries (Smith, Smoll, & Ptacek, 1990). In general, evidence from sport populations indicates that social support as a coping resource can directly affect injury outcome and moderate the relationship between life stress and sport injury (Williams & Andersen, 1998).

Stress Response

Two primary mechanisms—attentional disruption and increased muscle tension—operate in an elevated stress response, which places certain individuals at greater risk for sport injury (Andersen & Williams, 1988). Research has demonstrated that stress disrupts athletes' attention by reducing peripheral attention or increasing central vision distractibility (Williams & Andersen, 1998). This is particularly problematic in open-environment sports. Most team sports—in which athletes must have access to the full field of view and focus their vision on this view to forestall unwanted collisions with other participants, equipment, or apparatus—fall into this category. A second related attentional factor is more cognitive. Increased **state anxiety**—a situation-specific form of anxiety—causes internal distraction by irrelevant thoughts. Under high-stress conditions athletes thus pay too much attention to what is going on in their own heads and not enough attention to what is happening on the field of play. Again, if they are not attending to critical environmental cues, they may be at greater risk of injury because of failure to recognize and avoid potentially injurious situations.

The second operative mechanism in a high-stress condition is a more physiologically based response of increased muscle tension. This increased muscle tension interferes with normal coordination and increases chance of injury. Thus athletes who are tense are often less fluid in their play. Muscular co-contractions associated with inefficient motor performance can lead to greater fatigue and the sense of muscles fighting each other rather than working together smoothly. Again, it is important for sports medicine professionals to recognize the mechanisms by which psychological and social factors might increase the likelihood of injury, so that they can engage in preventive efforts.

Interactions Between Precursors

Figure 2.2 presents a summary of how the four categories of factors just described (physical, environmental, sociocultural, and psychological) might influence injury occurrence. Although these injury precursors are not necessarily the immediate cause of injury, they may interact to increase the likelihood of an injury occurring, given the specific situation.

The following case example illustrates how this model might work:

*Jasmine had a weak left knee from a sprain last year during her Junior Olympic volleyball season. During the off-season the athletic trainer had recommended exercises to strengthen both knees, since she seemed to have ongoing problems with them, but she really hadn't done much exercise. Her parents and her coach were really pressuring her to have a good season this year so that she could get a college scholarship. She wanted to please them and valued her reputation as a tough player, but she told them that her knee was still giving her trouble. They told her that she "just **had** to play" in the tournament this weekend because the college scouts were watching. She decided that she should just get used to playing with the pain. After all, everyone did*

social support—
"An exchange of resources between at least two individuals perceived by the provider or the recipient to be intended to enhance the well-being of the recipient" (Shumaker & Brownell, 1984, p. 13).

state anxiety—*A fluctuating emotional state of subjective feelings of apprehension and tension associated with activation of the autonomic nervous system* (Weinberg & Gould, 1995).

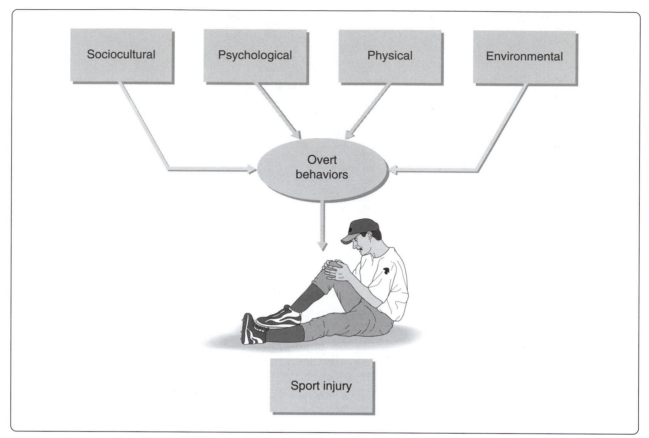

Figure 2.2 Precursors to sport injury.

it. Jasmine's teammates said they really needed her; after all, she was the starting setter.

The day of the tournament arrived. The scouts were in the gym, and the pressure was mounting. The court space was a little cramped, and the spectators were lined up along the sidelines. Jasmine knew that she had to play her best, but she felt very nervous, and her stomach was jittery. When a deflected block off her teammate headed way out of bounds toward Jasmine's defensive zone, she instinctively launched herself to make the play. Under all the pressure, she had forgotten about the chairs and spectators on the sideline. Her legs became tangled with those of the chair, and she felt a sharp, stabbing pain in her knee.

Although the proximate cause of Jasmine's injury was actually her dive to get the ball and her collision with the chair, several factors set the scene for the impending disaster. Physically, she had some existing problems with her knee. Environmentally, the physical space was crowded and dangerous. Socioculturally, she felt pressure from her parents, coaches, and teammates to play even though her knee was hurting. Psychologically, she was the type who wanted to please others and who was proud of her identity as an athlete. She was nervous and perhaps distracted during play, which may have led her to dive for a ball she otherwise would have known to be untouchable. These factors in combination may have indirectly led to her reinjury of the knee.

Injury Prevention

There are several implications derived from a review of sport injury precursors. First, sport injuries occur as a direct result of physical or environmental factors or both. As supported by the literature, however, a subset of injury causality is indirectly attributable to underlying psychological factors. For example, when asked to identify what they thought was the major cause of their most recent injury, intercollegiate track-and-field and cross-country athletes included such perceived causes as "too many things going on" and "not paying attention," reinforcing the idea of attentional distraction as leading to injury occurrence (Brown, 1995).

Sociocultural factors can also affect the potential for injury. A shift in the way society thinks about and glorifies playing with pain and injury is needed. This is particularly important for young, physically and cognitively immature athletes who do not yet have the frame of reference from which to make sound, long-term decisions about their health. It is imperative that all those involved with sport truly place the best interest of the athlete above the need to win and neither encourage nor reinforce young athletes' playing with injury. Athletes should be evaluated by medical professionals who do not have a vested interest in returning the athlete to sport if the risk of further injury or long-term impairment is too great. Chapter 3 extends the discussion of what we have termed *philosophical intervention* and further describes ways in which sports medicine professionals might intervene on behalf of their athletes who do not wish to adopt the expected norm of playing with harmful pain and injury.

From a psychological standpoint on injury prevention, alertness to signs of stress-related attentional problems helps identify athletes who could benefit from the use of stress management strategies (see chapter 14) or from psychological intervention by the appropriate practitioner (see chapter 8). Signs of stress-related attentional problems include the following (Heil, 1993):

- Inability to perform routine tasks

- Changes in patterns of behavior

- Somatic complaints (e.g., upset stomach, dry or "cotton" mouth, rapid heartbeat)

- Irritability and mood swings

- Diminished motivation

Sports medicine professionals who notice these signs in their athletes should seek appropriate help early, before the problem becomes compounded by an injury as described in the next section.

PSYCHOLOGICAL RESPONSES TO SPORT INJURY

Once injury occurs, it becomes yet another potential stressor for the athlete to manage. Remember that most preinjury stressors do not disappear; the occurrence of injury often compounds them. Athletes, however, respond to and deal with injury in many different ways.

Wiese-Bjornstal and colleagues (Wiese-Bjornstal & Smith, 1993; Wiese-Bjornstal, Smith, & LaMott, 1995; Wiese-Bjornstal, Smith, Shaffer, & Morrey, 1998) have developed a model of response to sport injury, which extends the preinjury model of Andersen and Williams (1988) into the postinjury phase. The most recent version of this developing model is presented in figure 2.3. It depicts the factors that influence athletes' responses to injuries as well as the actual responses themselves (cognitive, emotional, and behavioral). Although the model has not been tested in its entirety, there is research to support each individual component of the model.

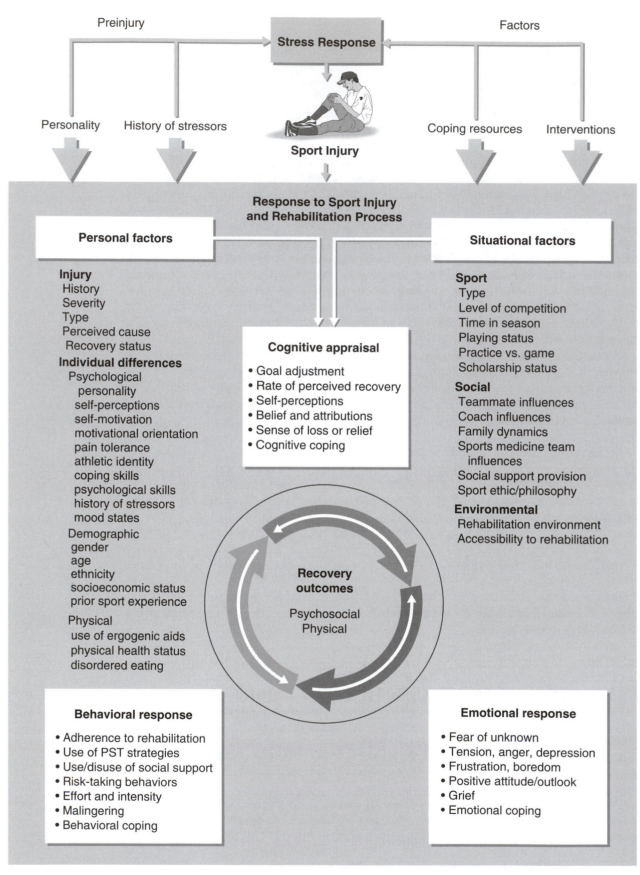

Figure 2.3 Model of psychological response to sport injury.

Reprinted with permission from Wiese-Bjornstal, Smith, Shaffer, and Morrey (1998). An integrated model of response to sport injury: Psychological and sociological dynamics. *Journal of Applied Sport Psychology,* 10(1), 46-69.

Factors Moderating Psychological Responses

A number of physical and psychological factors affect psychological response to sport injury. Although empirical support for many of the specific factors is lacking, anecdotal and tacit knowledge supports their mention. In an interactional approach these moderators fall under the broad categories of personal and situational factors, as outlined in figure 2.3. These moderators certainly do not operate in isolation but interact to influence the dynamic responses of athletes to injury throughout the injury and rehabilitation process.

From a temporal standpoint there are two major groups of moderators: those that exist before the injury and those that arise subsequent to injury and during the recovery process. The first category, preinjury moderators, includes major factors identified by Andersen and Williams (1988) in their model of stress and athletic injury (see top portion of figure 2.3). These include primarily factors that involve individual differences—such as demographic, psychological, and physical factors—but also tap into other categories such as injury factors (especially injury history), sport factors, and social factors as identified in figure 2.3.

The second category, postinjury moderators, includes those that arise subsequent to injury, many of which likely will change dynamically throughout the injury recovery process. Situational factors involving the social and physical environments change throughout the recovery process, but many of the personal psychological and physical factors can change during this time as well.

Some examples of how these factors moderate the responses of athletes to injury and rehabilitation, through the interaction of personal and situational factors, are described next. For a further discussion of research supporting the role of these moderators, see Wiese-Bjornstal et al. (1995). Keep in mind that understanding moderators is important because of their direct influence on the thoughts, feelings, and behaviors of injured athletes, which are the focus later in this chapter.

Personal Factors

The first category of personal factors includes prior experiences of injury as well as characteristics of the current injury. The severity of injury, for example, relates to elements of cognitive appraisal (e.g., perceived rate of recovery) and emotional response (e.g., mood state). To illustrate this dynamic, research has observed negative relationships between perceived recovery status and mood disturbance for severely injured athletes (A.M. Smith, Scott, O'Fallon, & Young, 1990; A.M. Smith et al., 1993). Another study noted that an overestimation of injury severity related to reports of more pain, higher state anxiety, and greater feelings of anger, apathy, loneliness, and inadequacy (Crossman & Jamieson, 1985).

The perceived cause of injury (i.e., who or what caused the injury) may influence emotional responses. For example, players may react more negatively—in particular, with greater anger—if they feel injury occurred as a result of illegal or unacceptable behavior on the part of an opponent rather than being an accidental occurrence. This is consistent with attribution theory (Weiner, 1985), which suggests that perceived causes of events and behaviors are related to affective (emotional) responses.

The second category of personal factors includes individual differences. Individual-difference factors are grouped under three subheadings: psychological, demographic, and physical. Among the psychological individual-difference factors, for example, is personality. The role of personality was discussed earlier as a precursor to injury. We now consider personality as a possible moderator of postinjury responses. For example, a study by Grove (1993) noted a relationship between personality and postinjury mood states. He examined three personality variables—**pessimistic explanatory style**, **dispositional optimism**, and **hardiness**—chosen because recent literature has connected these personality variables with health behaviors and

pessimistic explanatory style—*Tendency to explain negative events as personally caused, stable over time, and global in nature and to explain positive events as externally caused, unstable over time, and specific in nature.*

dispositional optimism—A general expectancy for good rather than bad outcomes to occur, which is thought to determine the extent to which an individual is willing to initiate health-oriented behaviors and persist with them in the face of difficulties.

hardiness—The combination of commitment, challenge, and control.

athletic identity—An individual's identity that is entirely contingent on her or his role as an athlete to the exclusion of other important roles (Brewer, 1993).

adherence—Conforming to a standard of behavior in order to meet some goal.

pain tolerance—The ability to manage and endure the sensory, emotional, and physical experience of pain.

cognitive appraisal—Mental estimation of one's own abilities.

self-efficacy—A situation-specific form of self-confidence.

consequences. Among 21 sport patients with anterior cruciate ligament (ACL) injuries, depression and anger were greatest in the first month of rehabilitation for athletes with a pessimistic explanatory style. Athletes high in dispositional optimism had less depression and less confusion, whereas those high in total hardiness reported less overall mood disturbance than those low in hardiness.

Another psychological individual-difference factor is **athletic identity** (Brewer, 1993). This construct represents the degree to which an individual's identity is predominantly contingent upon her or his role as an athlete. Athletes high in athletic identity see injuries as a threat to their very core identity and self-worth. In a sample of injured athletes, Brewer (1993) found that athletic identity related positively to depressed mood in the context of injury. In other words, athletes who more strongly identified with their athletic role suffered more depression when injured than athletes who did not identify as strongly with their athletic role. To discourage this unidimensional focus on the athletic role only—and the consequent effects on emotional health in the face of injury—both athletes and others (e.g., sports medicine professionals, coaches, parents) must recognize and encourage the multidimensional character of athletes' lives.

Motivational differences also relate to athletes' responses. For example, athletes who were more self-motivated better adhered to rehabilitation programs (a behavioral response) in one investigation (Fisher, Domm, & Wuest, 1988). Other research has shown that athletes demonstrating greater treatment **adherence** place more emphasis on mastery or task-involved goals in sport (Duda, Smart, & Tappe, 1989). Those athletes who best adhered were more interested in mastering challenging tasks than in competitive or ego-related goals of proving superiority to another.

Pain tolerance is an example of a moderating factor affected by both psychological and physical individual differences. Athletes' different capacities to deal with pain relate to their **cognitive appraisal** of the situation, **self-efficacy**, and coping skills. One study has shown that athletes who better adhered to rehabilitation programs—a behavioral response to injury—have reported themselves to tolerate pain better than do those less adherent (Fisher et. al., 1988). Chapter 15 discusses dimensions of rehabilitation adherence in greater detail.

Demographic-difference factors have not been the focus of extensive research. Nonetheless, given some evidence of sex differences, for example, in preinjury relationships (Williams & Andersen, 1998) and of sex differences in type and frequency of injury in comparable sports, it is important to at least consider their possible moderating role. Age and prior sport experience have been found to be related to such things as cognitive assessment of injury severity (Crossman & Jamieson, 1985).

Situational Factors

Situational factors have also been found to affect postinjury cognitive, emotional, and behavioral responses of athletes. Three categories of situational factors are identified in Figure 2.3: sport, social, and environmental.

Among the sport-related factors, for example, is the level at which the athlete competes. Physiotherapists rated intensity of athletic involvement as one of the top two factors affecting degree of psychological response to injury (Pearson & Jones, 1992). A study of National Football League (NFL) players noted very high stress levels among these elite injured athletes (Lewis & LaMott, 1992). One recent study of athletes who underwent ACL reconstruction noted that the competitive-level athletes experienced greater mood disturbance at the time of return to sport than did recreational-level athletes (Morrey, 1997).

Among the situational social factors, relationships with coaches and teammates are influential in determining how an athlete responds to injury. Rehabilitating athletes need support from significant others, including teammates and coaches; this support can improve adherence. Support from the coaching staff and continued involvement with team activities were very important to injured athletes in one study (LaMott et al., 1989). The support of family members is also critical in enhancing the recovery of injured athletes, particularly during a long and arduous rehabilitation. Chapter 7 discusses the role of social support in greater detail.

In addition to support from personnel related to the sport, interactions with members of the sports medicine team can influence the cognitive, emotional, and behavioral responses of athletes. Athletes report believing that sports medicine professionals have considerable potential to influence their moods during rehabilitation (Pearson & Jones, 1992). A study of NFL football players, however, found that coaches and athletic trainers were considered less supportive than other support providers examined (Lewis & LaMott, 1992). This suggests that although support from sports medicine professionals is important, there is room for improvement in the actual provision of support by this group.

The category of environmental factors considers both the physical and social environments, particularly those of the sports medicine setting. The research of Fisher and colleagues (described in chapter 15), in particular, has identified the environment and accessibility of the training room as important influences, particularly on the behavioral responses of adherence.

Overall, these personal and situational moderators influence the dynamically changing cognitive, emotional, and behavioral responses of athletes to injury. It is these thoughts, feelings, and actions that are next described.

Psychological Response to Sport Injury

Preinjury and moderating factors affect the postinjury responses of injured athletes. Figure 2.3 provided a global view of the ways in which these elements interact to influence the cognitive, emotional, and behavioral responses of athlete to injury. The lower circular portion of the model depicts the dynamic process next discussed. This postinjury **stress process** (Wiese & Weiss, 1987) is more simply illustrated in figure 2.4. The actual incident, or stressor, in this case is the sport injury (What?), which triggers associated thoughts (Think?), feelings (Feel?), and actions (Do?).

Evidence, for example, of the stressful nature of injury and the associated rehabilitation has been examined by Gould, Udry, Bridges, and Beck (1997a) among elite-level skiers. They found eight major categories of stress sources associated with season-ending injuries: psychological, social, physical, medical/rehabilitative, financial, career, missed nonsport opportunities, and other. Furthermore, those skiers who did not have a successful return to sport following injury were more likely to identify social concerns (e.g., lack of attention or empathy, negative relationships) and physical concerns (e.g., poor performance, inactivity) than were those who made a successful return to sport. Many new challenges are presented in the context of injury than were present beforehand; the athlete must learn to manage them in order to rehabilitate successfully.

stress process— *A perceived imbalance between physical or psychological demands and response capability, particularly in situations when failure to meet the demands is perceived to have important consequences.*

Cognitive Appraisal

The cognitive component encompasses the thoughts of injured athletes, both immediately postinjury and dynamically throughout the rehabilitation and recovery cycle. Many things are "appraised" by athletes postinjury. For example, athletes think about the perceived cause of injury, their perceived recovery status, the availability of social support, and their perceived ability to cope with injury. Athletes can also appraise that they have lost something due to the injury (e.g., loss of starting position, loss of status afforded athletes, financial loss, scholarship loss, etc.). The key element of appraisal consists of an assessment of the demands of the injury situation and one's perceived resources to meet these demands (i.e., ability to cope). These thoughts affect both subsequent emotions and behaviors. One study, for example,

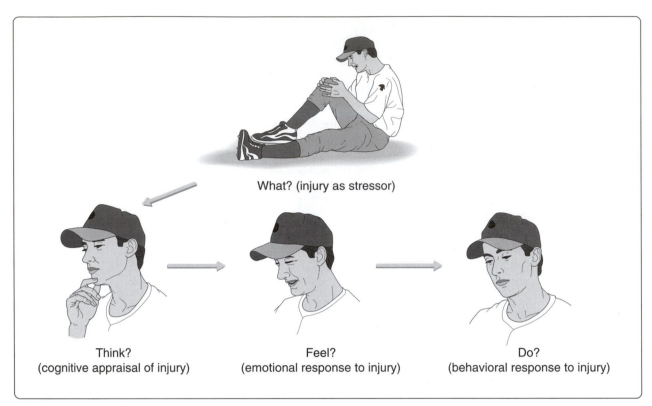

Figure 2.4 Stress response to sport injury.

Reprinted with permission from Wiese & Weiss (1987). Psychological rehabilitation and physical injury: Implications for the sportsmedicine team. *Sport Psychologist, 1,* 318-330.

found that lower levels of perceived ability to cope with injury were associated with higher levels of mood disturbance and lower levels of attendance at rehabilitation (Daly, Brewer, Van Raalte, Petitpas, & Sklar, 1995). Thus the connections between cognitive appraisals, emotions, and responses were demonstrated. The sports medicine professional's responsibility is to help athletes be as realistic and proactive about their appraisals as possible.

self-perceptions—*The view one has of oneself.*

Another dimension of postinjury thoughts is that of **self-perceptions**. Essentially, self-perceptions encompass the views an individual has of him- or herself. An individual's perceptions of self, capabilities, and worth can all be affected by sport injury. Sport psychology researchers have examined specific dimensions of postinjury self-perceptions, including self-esteem, self-confidence, and self-efficacy (for a review, see Wiese-Bjornstal et al., 1998). For example, a reduction in self-esteem has been noted in some groups of injured athletes when they are unable to participate (e.g., Chan & Grossman, 1988). Sport injury may have greater influence on more-specific aspects of self-perceptions, such as physical self-efficacy (athletes' situation-specific confidence for a particular physical task). Since specific physical skills are hampered by a sport injury, it is logical that athletes' perceptions of their specific physical abilities suffer at this time. This further validates such commonly used assessments as functional evaluations, because in addition to providing the sports medicine professional with information about athletes' physical recovery status, they also psychologically reinforce to athletes themselves their abilities to perform specific physical activity tasks. Athletes can also document their progress through frequent evaluations—employing a form of goal setting—as they return to full capacity.

Recent work by Udry, Gould, Bridges, and Beck (1997) has elaborated on the cognitive, emotional, and behavioral responses of elite skiers to season-ending injuries. Athletes' cognitions regarding the nature and extent of the injury and the associated negative consequences were common. Emotionally, athletes in this investigation described feelings such as being emotionally agitated (e.g., angry, panicky, worried) and emotionally depleted (e.g., disappointed, depressed). Emotional responses such as these are described in the next section.

Emotional Response

Athletes' emotional responses to injury often stem directly from their thoughts. Athletes' postinjury feelings change dynamically throughout the injury and recovery process. The most common means of assessing athletes' postinjury feelings is to evaluate their **mood state**. Some of the most commonly noted postinjury mood states include anxiety or tension, depression, and frustration (see reviews by Smith, 1996, and Wiese-Bjornstal et al., 1998). Other emotions commonly observed include boredom (particularly during long rehabilitative periods), anger, and fatigue. Many athletes, however, also respond to injury with more positive emotions, such as optimism, vigor, and relief (e.g., Udry et al., 1997).

mood state— Transitory presence of specific emotional states.

Some research literature has illustrated the importance of examining the patterns in which these changing moods occur during the recovery cycle. For example, studies of more severely injured athletes have shown mood-state improvements paralleling rates of perceived physical recovery (McDonald & Hardy, 1990; Smith et al., 1990). Longitudinal studies of athletes who underwent ACL reconstruction have demonstrated a curvilinear pattern of changing positive and negative mood states over time (LaMott, 1994; Morrey, 1997). In particular, these two studies observed that athletes who underwent ACL reconstruction show high negative and low positive mood states about the time of surgical intervention, progress to a more positive and less negative mood state during the next few weeks postsurgery, and then return to a more negative and less positive mood state at about three to six months postsurgery (particularly as they are about to return to sport). These studies illustrate the dynamic nature of mood-state fluctuation throughout the injury process.

With respect to some of the more extreme emotional responses, a minority, rather than a majority, of injured athletes have been shown to experience serious or clinical levels of depression, ranging on the order of approximately 10 to 19 percent (Brewer, Petitpas, Van Raalte, Sklar, & Ditmar, 1995). Even this number, however, is certainly a cause for concern. Chapter 5 presents a further discussion of the warning signs associated with seriously disturbed athletes in the context of recognizing suicidal tendencies.

Sports medicine professionals should avoid the assumption that all injured athletes will react "negatively"; many appear to handle the injury situation quite well (e.g., Udry et al., 1997). On the other hand, some injured athletes express relief at being able to escape what to them is an unbearable situation. This is of concern, since it is unfortunate that some athletes view injury as their only escape from sport demands. Ideally, athletes would feel able to express and act on their desire to disengage from sport without having to sustain an injury to do so. Unfortunately, this is not always the case, as athletes may fear being viewed as "quitters" if they decide to leave sport. Sports medicine professionals would be wise to avoid the assumption that all athletes want to return to their sport as soon as possible. Some may not have this as their goal; in fact, some may not want to return at all.

Behavioral Response

Behavioral responses, such as use of coping mechanisms and adherence to rehabilitation, stem from athletes' thoughts and feelings about the injury. Like injury rehabilitation as a dynamic process, the types of coping mechanisms employed may change over the course of a lengthy rehabilitation (Udry, 1997). Recent investigations with elite skiers, for example, have noted that athletes employ a wide variety of coping mechanisms (Gould et al., 1997a). Thus it is important to provide a variety of coping skills and resources (such as personal psychological skills, described in chapter 3, and social support networks, described in chapter 7) to adapt to these changing needs. Athletes tend to prefer active coping strategies rather than passive ones (Smith, Scott, O'Fallon, & Young, 1990; Gould et al., 1997a). This is not surprising, given the action-oriented nature of sport and the types of individuals it attracts.

One specific type of behavior essential for successful rehabilitation is adherence behavior. Several factors have been suggested as influencing adherence behavior, including personal factors (e.g., anxiety, confidence), social factors (e.g., training room climate, social support), and physical factors (e.g., pain, recovery progress) (Fisher, Mullins, & Frye, 1993; Fisher, Scriber, Matheny, Alderman, & Bitting, 1993). Heil (1993) has suggested that poor adherers may be more somatically anxious, have psychological adjustment problems, be less confident about treatment, lack a sense of social support, be less self-motivated, and be less goal oriented. Factors predicting successful adherence, according to Heil (1993), include the athlete's perception of the need for a particular intervention, expectation of a positive outcome, belief that the benefits of rehabilitation outweigh the costs, and a sense of active involvement in treatment. Chapter 15 provides a much more detailed analysis of the factors related to rehabilitation adherence.

malingering—
Adaptive response to adverse circumstances that requires an external incentive for being injured.

A final consideration in behavioral response involves **malingering** behavior. Malingering behavior is an adjustment to negative circumstances that requires an external incentive for being injured (Rotella, Ogilvie, & Perrin, 1993). In other words, malingering athletes are those who intentionally deceive sports medicine professionals and coaches about their injury—by consciously faking symptoms of discomfort or physical distress—in order to avoid practice or competition. Most athletes who have a repeated habit of malingering do so primarily as a result of fears, a need for attention, or both (Rotella et al., 1993). Sports medicine professionals certainly need to believe athletes' claims of injury but must also recognize that there are many reasons for malingering behavior related to the moderating factors, cognitions, and emotions described earlier. These reasons include rationalizing the loss of starting status, playing-time reduction, or poor performance; personal realizations of limited ability; attracting needed attention not elsewhere received; using injury as an escape from sport pressures; and avoiding rigors of practice to save oneself for game day (Rotella et al., 1993). An alertness on the part of the sports medicine professional to malingering behavior can allow a chance to identify and remedy the underlying cause of the behavior.

In sum, athletes' postinjury thoughts, feelings, and actions are influenced by a number of moderating factors. These cognitions, emotions, and behaviors continue to fluctuate in a dynamic process throughout the injury and rehabilitative process. By understanding athletes' responses to injury, sports medicine professionals are better prepared to handle them as they occur and seek appropriate help as needed (see chapter 8).

Sports Medicine Professionals' Perceptions

Several studies have examined the perspective of sports medicine professionals such as physical therapists (Gordon, Milios, & Grove, 1991), athletic trainers (Crossman & Jamieson, 1985; Fisher, Mullins, & Frye, 1993; Kahanov & Fairchild, 1994; Wiese, Weiss, & Yukelson, 1991), and physicians (Brewer, Linder, & Phelps, 1995; Brewer, Van Raalte, & Linder, 1991) about athletes' psychological responses to injury. Two studies have compared the perceptions of athletes, coaches, and medical professionals (Brown, 1995; Crossman, Jamieson, & Hume, 1990). Those studies that best illustrate the advantages and disadvantages of relying on the perceptions of sports medicine practitioners about athletes' responses are next highlighted.

Kahanov and Fairchild (1994) studied 50 injured athletes and six athletic trainers to determine the similarities of perception in comprehension of injury and rehabilitation, objective aspects of rehabilitation, athlete's frame of reference, communication, short- and long-term goals, and rehabilitation strategy. Fifty-two percent of the athletes did not understand the process of rehabilitation from injury. Significant discrepancies existed between the athletes' and athletic trainers' perceptions for all but one area examined. The authors concluded that athletic trainers need to develop better communication skills (see chapter 4). Other studies have also found that the communication skills of athletic trainers influence athletes' responses to injury and effective rehabilitation (Fisher, Mullins, & Frye, 1993; Fisher, Scriber, et al., 1993).

Brewer et al. (1991) surveyed sports medicine providers to assess their perception of the frequency with which mood disturbance was associated with athletic injury. Physicians reported that postinjury behavioral and psychological problems occurred with some frequency. They were moderately positive about involving sport psychologists in the recovery process. Brewer, Linder, and Phelps (1995) used the physician's rating of the patient's injury severity and current injury status as situational correlates of the athlete's emotional adjustment to athletic injury. Somewhat surprisingly, and more indicative of chronic-injury and chronic-pain patients, physician-rated injury severity was unrelated to athletes' depression. Physician-rated current injury status had a significant but modest negative relationship with depression. Brewer, Petitpas, et al. (1995), however, found no correlation between the physical therapist's and athletic trainer's rating of the patient's behavior during rehabilitation sessions and the patient's self-reported ratings of psychological distress. This finding speaks to the importance of communication between sports medicine professionals and patients about levels of psychological distress and the associated intervention, if any.

Crossman et al. (1990) compared 35 athletes, their coaches, and their medical professionals to assess the disruption, seriousness, and short-term effects of sport injuries. Relative to the opinion of the medical professionals, athletes significantly underestimated the disruptive effects of injury, although athletes participating at lower levels overestimated the disruptive effects of injury.

This interpretation of under- or overestimation, however, begs the question of whose assessment is most accurate. Although medical professionals' assessment of athletes' postinjury responses is helpful, erroneous assumptions of another person's subjective experience can occur (Dugan, 1987). On the other hand, the unwillingness of many athletes to admit to weakness (Carmen, Zerman, & Blaine, 1968) suggests that in some cases the medical practitioner's assessment may be more accurate. The lack of a relationship between physical therapists' and athletic trainers' psychological distress ratings and those of their patients (Brewer, Petitpas, et al., 1995); the lack of a relationship between the physician's rating of injury severity and the athlete's postinjury depression (Brewer, Linder, & Phelps, 1995); the discrepancies between athletes', physicians', and coaches' ratings of the causes, seriousness, and disruptiveness of injury (Brown, 1995; Crossman et al., 1990); and the discrepancies in perceptions held by injured athletes and athletic trainers during the initial injury evaluation (Kahanov & Fairchild, 1994) support the need for caution in completely accepting the perceptions of either athletes or sports medicine professionals. Steps should be taken to enhance the insight of and clarity of communication between the injured athlete and all members of the sports medicine team to provide a complete picture of the athlete's emotional states.

Pierre is a 14-year-old Canadian figure skater, the son of English-speaking parents. He presented with an "entrance complaint" of back pain, aggravated by landing jumps. He has been skating since he was four years old and in the past three years has lived in three American cities. He has a younger sister whom he never

CASE STUDY

sees. Although his parents are married, they don't get along, and according to Pierre, they frequently argue about money and the cost of skating. He sees little of them because he is away training in different cities. This is expected if he intends to be an elite skater; he must pay the price for glory by living away from his family and pushing through pain, pressure, and fatigue.

Pierre's mother had been a skater but had not realized her ambitions, primarily for financial reasons. She had an obsession that her son would represent Canada as a figure skater in the Olympics. Pierre had initially loved skating and according to his coaches was talented. He is on the ice for seven hours a day (5:00 to 9:30 A.M. and 4:30 to 7:00 P.M.), and since the cost for ice time and coaching fees is enormous, he isn't allowed time off to rest. He attends class with a tutor on weekends to make up what he misses during the first two hours of school. He has few friends, his school grades are slipping, and he has started to dislike skating. Competitors, previously well behind him, are now landing jumps that he has not mastered. As he falls behind the competition, the pressure from his coach and his parents has increased. He questions his skating abilities and feels frustrated, anxious, and discouraged. Pierre shows little interest in putting much effort into his rehabilitation protocol but continues to skate eight hours a day even though he is in much pain.

QUESTIONS FOR ANALYSIS

1. What are some of the antecedent psychosocial factors evident in the case study?

2. Are there any moderating factors evident in the case that might be affecting how Pierre copes with his injury?

3. Can you identify any cognitive, emotional, and behavioral responses to sport injury in Pierre's case?

4. Do any elements of the sport ethic appear to have influenced Pierre's thoughts, emotions, and behaviors?

Case study from A.M. Smith, personal communication, September 2, 1992.

SUMMARY

Understanding psychosocial factors can enhance the work of sports medicine professionals. Psychosocial factors clearly influence incidence of injury, responses to injury, and injury rehabilitation processes. Athletes' responses to injury occur in a constantly changing, dynamic process. Although most athletes certainly prefer to avoid injury, when it does occur, it is helpful to remember that there can be positive psychosocial and physical gains, which might include returning to sport physically and mentally stronger than before the injury and having a renewed sense of appreciation and motivation for participation. It is helpful for the sports medicine professional to encourage athletes to think about these positives while recovering from injury. Certainly, negative psychosocial consequences are associated with injury as well, such as reduced self-perceptions and increased negative mood states. It is therefore essential that professionals in sports medicine be prepared to initiate teaching strategies aimed at helping prevent sport injuries, assisting with coping resources, countering the sport ethic, and providing a supportive environment.

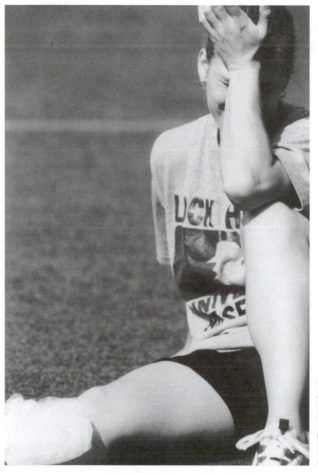

© 1997 Terry Wild Studio

Psychosocial Intervention Strategies in Sports Medicine

Shelly M. Shaffer, PhD, *Pinnacle Health Systems*
Diane M. Wiese-Bjornstal, PhD, *University of Minnesota*

CHAPTER OBJECTIVES

Explain the importance of psychosocial intervention strategies in pre- and postinjury sports medicine programs

Identify mental-skills approaches suitable for use in sports medicine settings

Develop and implement appropriate psychosocial intervention strategies to enhance injury prevention and rehabilitation programs

Sports medicine professionals know well the challenges of dealing with the spectrum of athletes' health conditions. From preventive strengthening programs for those free of injury, to protective taping for those whose participation is limited, to postsurgery rehabilitation for the completely incapacitated, even the most advanced techniques can have only limited success if the athlete is unmotivated to perform. In ongoing efforts to keep athletes practicing and competing, psychosocial interventions may be the most valuable tool since 1 1/2–inch tape. The use of mental skills can enhance traditional techniques (e.g., ultrasound, electrical stimulation) employed in the prevention, care, treatment, and rehabilitation of injury.

Many sports medicine professionals have embraced psychological techniques as an important modality for enhancing performance; others view them with the same skepticism directed at *Breathe-Rights*. It seems viable, however, to suggest that the same models employed to explain the **psychophysiological** and **psychomotor** processes (e.g., skill acquisition, visualization) used in athletic performance can be applied to the healing processes associated with rehabilitation (Green, 1994). The same mental energies and techniques used for competitive preparation can be channeled into injury prevention and treatment.

This chapter will introduce several psychosocial approaches that sports medicine professionals potentially can employ with healthy athletes to keep them injury-free and with injured athletes to facilitate the healing process. Many of these approaches will be discussed in greater detail in later chapters of this book; this chapter is intended to provide a survey of the psychological strategies and interventions most manageable for sports medicine professionals. It is important to acknowledge that as yet research on the effectiveness of these interventions with injured athletes is limited; thus these interventions should be viewed as suggested strategies at this point. Several strategies have potential application as both pre- and postinjury interventions; consequently, they are discussed in both sections of this chapter. The following information will provide a starting point from which sports medicine teams can develop preventive as well as therapeutic programs incorporating psychosocial strategies. Sports medicine teams that include a sport psychology consultant would benefit greatly from this consultant's expertise in developing and implementing these strategies. Not all sports medicine settings will have such expertise available; thus we have focused our attention on those strategies most easily learned and implemented by the sports medicine professional.

psychophysiology—The study of the interrelationship between the body's physical and psychological functioning.

psychomotor—Relating to muscle movement initiated by conscious mental activity.

PREINJURY INTERVENTION STRATEGIES

social support systems—Network of significant others to whom the athlete turns for insight and guidance in troubling times.

stress—Perceived imbalance between the demands of a situation and one's abilities to meet those demands.

Sports medicine professionals can be considered "sport psychologists" of sorts, in that they are often the first to hear of events affecting athletes' lives. During an ankle taping or ultrasound treatment, athletes trust and share very personal information: career aspirations, family problems, roommate arguments. Consequently, this provides the perfect opportunity to teach athletes to handle stressful events, to reach goals, and to identify and overcome barriers to success by using skill development, knowledge acquisition, and **social support systems** (Danish, Petitpas, & Hale, 1993). Spending extra time and effort to psychologically strengthen the athlete can have a powerful effect in minimizing injury occurrence as well as reducing negative responses should an injury occur.

As discussed in chapters 2 and 14, Andersen and Williams (1988) developed a model from which to examine the interplay between various psychosocial precursors to athletic injury and the stress response. The basic premise of their model is that the aggregation of **stress** stretches athletes' coping resources, consequently increasing their risk of injuries through physiological and cognitive changes in functioning. The coping resource and intervention components of their model suggest several specific approaches aimed at reducing the incidence of injury (Yukelson & Murphy, 1993). In particular, stress management strategies have been proposed as having potential to reduce injury rates. For example, Davis (1991) explored the role of stress intervention on injury rates for university swimmers and football players. He reported a 52 percent reduction in injuries among swimmers and a 33 percent reduction in serious injuries among football players during the year in which the psychological intervention was conducted compared with the previous year's injury statistics. Kerr and Goss (1996) examined the effects of a stress management program on injuries and stress levels of male and female gymnasts. Athletes in the stress management program reported significantly less negative athletic stress than did the control group, but there were no differences in time injured (likely due to small sample sizes).

Given at least some preliminary evidence that mental-skill strategies can help athletes cope with stress and possibly reduce injury rates, the next section briefly discusses specific mental-skill strategies that can be incorporated into injury prevention programs.

Coping

Intensely training athletes struggling to find and maintain balanced lives often experience high amounts of stress, creating a susceptibility to reduced immune system functioning and increased risk of injury or illness (Yukelson & Murphy, 1993). Coping behaviors and social support systems can minimize the effects of stressors (such as adjusting to higher levels of competition, coaching change) (Danish et al., 1993), thereby reducing the likelihood of injury occurrence (Yukelson & Murphy, 1993). Athletes need to practice dealing with stress in the same manner in which they practice for their sport (Suinn, 1987).

Coping has been defined as cognitive and behavioral efforts to master, reduce, or tolerate demands (Folkman & Lazarus, 1980). From a preventive standpoint, coping methods might include such things as avoiding stressors through making life adjustments, lowering demand levels, and developing **coping resources**. Coping resources represent "a wide variety of behaviors and social networks that help the individual deal with the problems, joys, disappointments, and stresses of life" (Andersen & Williams, 1988, p. 302). This broad category includes such elements as general coping behaviors, social support systems, and stress management and mental skills (Andersen & Williams, 1988).

Developing preventive coping resources (i.e., avoiding stress before it become a problem) might include enhancing one's psychological or social assets or both (Rice, 1992). Psychological assets, for example, might encompass enhanced levels of confidence and increased sense of control over one's life. Other cognitive assets such as developing time management skills and improving academic competence can also be preventive coping methods (Rice, 1992). Social assets include the ability to form and maintain friendships, to have and be able to access social support networks, and to have a wide range of friends and acquaintances both within and outside of the sport network. Once athletes perceive themselves to be "stressed out," other strategies might be employed to combat the triggering stressors. Suggested methods for coping with existing stress include attacking stressors through problem solving or assertiveness training, tolerating stressors through cognitive restructuring, or lowering arousal through the use of relaxation strategies (Rice, 1992).

Sports medicine professionals can actively intervene when athletes' coping mechanisms seem inadequate. They can identify coping strategies (e.g., talking with teammates, friends, or family; keeping a journal) and assist athletes in applying these strategies to their present situation. Educating athletes to increase their personal competencies in dealing with life events can be seen as a forward-looking health care delivery system. Such intervention fosters self-reliance, life-planning abilities, and

coping—All cognitive and behavioral efforts to master, reduce, or tolerate demands (Folkman & Lazarus, 1980).

coping resources—"A wide variety of behaviors and social networks that help the individual deal with the problems, joys, disappointments, and stresses of life" (Andersen & Williams, 1988).

the confidence to approach significant others when feeling stressed and overwhelmed (Yukelson & Murphy, 1993).

Athletes should be encouraged by sports medicine professionals to expand their range of coping skills. This shifts the emphasis of interaction from treatment of injury to an educational approach designed to help prevent injury (Yukelson & Murphy, 1993). Psychological interventions aimed at teaching athletes how to manage themselves more effectively and to feel as if they are in control are key aspects to injury prevention (Yukelson & Murphy, 1993).

Relaxation

relaxation—The process of controlling muscle tension to produce a calm, restful state.

cue—A word, image, or behavior that triggers a desired response.

While **relaxation** techniques (e.g., autogenic relaxation, progressive muscle relaxation) vary in their appropriateness for athletic settings, all approaches share the common outcome of teaching athletes how to control their muscles by releasing muscular tension, thus producing a deeply relaxed state. Repeating a **cue** word associated with feeling relaxed (e.g., "calm," "focus," "relax") while practicing the relaxation technique can hasten the athlete's response and enhance the overall effect of the technique. Controlling their own bodies through relaxation can send a powerful, confidence-building message to both novices and seasoned athletes who are struggling with their performance. The ability to consciously relax also enhances the muscles' capability to recuperate after a physical training session. With regular practice, athletes can relax on command, thereby maximizing recovery from fatiguing workouts while minimizing the potentially injurious effects of competitive stress and anxiety. Table 3.1 provides an example of a relaxation technique that might be used by athletes.

Imagery

imagery—The process of using sensory stimulus to create or recreate an experience in the mind (also known as visualization, mental practice, and mental rehearsal).

Also known as visualization, **imagery** involves mentally rehearsing desired performance outcomes, such as executing sport skills and learning new plays. Ideally, relaxation training precedes imagery because controlling excess tension in the body allows the mind to fully focus on the intended images. In a sports medicine setting, imagery may be used to facilitate strengthening and conditioning programs (e.g., imagine muscle hypertrophy), enhance training motivation (e.g., picture achieving goal time), and provide athletes with a method for coping with the stresses of sport participation (e.g., visualize giving 100 percent effort despite being second string).

Using imagery as a form of preventive medicine can lessen the influence of stressors and thus reduce the potential for injury. Imagery techniques that enhance relaxation and provide perspective on specific stressful situations can be developed and implemented throughout the season as needed (Green, 1994). Imagery is also an effective postinjury strategy that is discussed later in the chapter.

Positive Self-Talk and Stopping Negative Thoughts

Athletes who react to stress with negative thoughts are often unable to properly determine the necessary physical and mental adjustments; instead, these athletes become preoccupied with the negative musings, thus disrupting performance. Sports medicine professionals can help athletes identify meaningful cues that will quiet the interfering, useless thoughts. Cues can be verbal (e.g., "Stop!" or "Shhh"), visual (e.g., imagine a flashing stop sign or see the word *no*), or behavioral (e.g., clap hands or shake head). Once athletes effectively stop the negative thoughts, they can replace them with positive statements. At times, athletes will struggle to find something positive about the situation; sports medicine professionals can be particularly valuable in these instances by gently reminding athletes of the day's accomplishments (e.g., "You played hard all practice," or "You didn't give up!").

Table 3.1 Sample Relaxation Method

1. Find a quiet, comfortably warm room where distractions are minimal.

2. Attention must be focused on something, such as your breathing.

3. It is essential to have a passive attitude and to let thoughts and images move through your mind in a passive manner. Gently bring your attention back to the object of focus when your mind wanders.

4. A comfortable position is essential, but you should not be so comfortable that you fall asleep.

5. Instructions:

   a. Sit in a comfortable position and close your eyes.

   b. Contract your muscles as hard as possible, even harder, for a count of 10.

   c. Muscles are contracted one group at a time for a count of 10, starting with the toes. Start by pulling your toes up toward your nose (tightening calves), tighten quadriceps (thighs), tighten abdominals, grip hands, tighten biceps and triceps ("make a muscle"), and last pull your shoulders up toward your ears.

   d. Feel the relaxation that follows—the warm feet, the warm hands.

   e. Allow the muscles to remain deeply relaxed.

   f. Now settle in to the deep-breathing phase. The breaths are slow, deep. As you breathe out, say the word *calm* to yourself.

   g. Allow all the air to escape so that you feel like a deflated balloon. Continue this practice for about 10 minutes. Keep your mind on the movement of air in and out of your lungs, gently bringing your attention back if your mind wanders.

6. Practice this technique at least once daily. Gradually use it as a form of emotional and arousal control for sport or stressful life situations. Learn how to use it to help you maintain an optimal flow zone for sport.

Adapted from Wiese-Bjornstal & Smith (1993). Counseling strategies for enhanced recovery of injured athletes within a team approach. In D. Pargman (Ed.), *Psychological bases of sport injuries* (pp. 149-182). Morgantown, WV: Fitness Information Technology.

POSTINJURY INTERVENTION STRATEGIES

Many athletes accept the premise that injuries are an inherent aspect of sport participation. The rigorous, physical, competitive nature of organized sports creates a situation ripe for injury occurrence (Pargman, 1993), despite the most diligent of physical and mental-skills training programs. To ensure the success of any postinjury intervention, sports medicine professionals must attend to the person and not just the injury (Petitpas & Danish, 1995).

Helping athletes plan strategies to cope with their unstructured time after injury is often critical to the success of the psychological intervention. Some athletes need continued active involvement with the team through activities such as scouting, charting, or practice coaching (Wiese & Weiss, 1987). Other athletes need to get their exercise "fix" through alternative sports or cross-training (Petitpas & Danish, 1995). Being an active participant and having responsibility and expectations for success minimize passivity and encourage positive involvement in rehabilitation (Yukelson & Murphy, 1993).

Ievleva and Orlick (1991) in their research with athletes recovering from knee or ankle injuries noted that those athletes who experienced the most rapid recoveries were more likely to use psychological strategies such as goal setting, positive self-talk, and healing imagery. Their research was based on the belief that the mind plays a substantial role—within the integrated mind–body system—in overcoming disease and pain. Strategies for enhancing the recovery of injured athletes include the following practical recommendations applicable to the work of sports medicine professionals: Maintain regular contacts with injured athletes, point out the positive side of taking a time-out from intensive sport training, reinforce to athletes their capacity to control and influence their own rehabilitation, assist athletes in setting rehabilitation goals, and encourage athletes to transfer the mental skills they have previously used to excel at sport to excel at recovery (Ievleva & Orlick, 1993).

Social Support

Often sports medicine professionals are the first responders when injury occurs. What they say and, perhaps more important, how they say it are crucial to the athlete's thoughts surrounding the incident (Wiese-Bjornstal & Smith, 1993). Since lack of knowledge is often the first major barrier to successful recovery, it is imperative to provide athletes with accurate information about the injury, the injury process, and the ensuing rehabilitation. Furthermore, sports medicine professionals must discover what the injury means to individual athletes so that they feel understood and accepted. If athletes feel that they are understood, there is a much greater chance that they will share their fears and insecurities (Petitpas & Danish, 1995).

social support—
"An exchange of resources between at least two individuals perceived by the provider or the recipient to be intended to enhance the well-being of the recipient" (Shumaker & Brownell, 1984, p. 13).

Since **social support** is a multidimensional construct (Udry, 1996) there are not only many possible providers of support but also many forms. These include such forms as emotional, informational, and tangible support. All three forms of support can be provided by sports medicine professionals. Emotional support, for example, could best be provided by other members of the athlete's social network, such as teammates, friends, and family (e.g., Udry, Gould, Bridges, & Tuffey, 1997). This does not mean that the sports medicine professional should not be sensitive to the athlete's emotional states and provide encouragement and support when possible. Sports medicine professionals would be wise to set boundaries for providing this form of support, however, to minimize the risk of overdependence on medical personnel. Informational support falls well within the purview of sports medicine professionals; in fact, patient education is among their primary responsibilities. Providing information about the nature of the injury and rehabilitation program, worded in a way that athletes can understand, is a very basic yet often overlooked form of support. Tangible support can also be provided by sports medicine personnel, in such forms as providing necessary medical supplies (e.g., crutches, ice packs, braces) or scheduling convenient rehabilitation sessions. Providing support to injured athletes can have positive effects on athletes' morale and behavior. For example, preliminary research has demonstrated that social support is positively related to rehabilitation adherence (Duda, Smart, & Tappe, 1989; Fisher, Domm, & Wuest, 1988).

Health care professionals are in an excellent position to identify athletes who are having difficulty adjusting to an injury. In many cases, doubts lead to behaviors that adversely affect the healing process. Athletes may push too hard or attempt short-cuts in their rehabilitation programs if they do not make continuous progress. Helping injured athletes regain a sense of control often becomes the primary counseling goal (Petitpas & Danish, 1995).

Ideally, rapport between athletes and sports medicine professionals will have been forged prior to injury occurrence. If not, the supportive relationship should be initiated by the sports medicine professional who administers medical care and should be maintained throughout rehabilitation. Because of close daily contact with injured athletes, sports medicine professionals are able to provide positive feedback while monitoring athletes' emotional well-being.

Another effective use of social support is the pairing or grouping of athletes who are at different stages of recovery from similar injuries (Udry, 1996; Weiss & Troxel, 1986). Those further along in their rehabilitation can share their experiences and give a sense of what athletes with newer injuries can expect as they progress through treatment. If social support and sports medicine systems are skillful at helping injured athletes feel understood, the physical and emotional rehabilitation process will be greatly enhanced (Petitpas & Danish, 1995).

Relaxation

From a therapeutic standpoint, relaxation can be used for flexibility improvement and pain reduction. First, to increase muscle length during active or passive range-of-motion exercises, athletes should engage in a relaxation technique, focusing particular attention on muscles targeted for stretching. Seeing—and feeling—definite gains in flexibility produces a sense of accomplishment and also facilitates recovery. Second, muscular tension stemming from anxiety or the pain–spasm–pain cycle of the specific injury can increase sensations of pain. Relaxation can reduce the pain response by minimizing muscular as well as mental stress.

Imagery

With the mind's eye, athletes often picture themselves performing the feats of their respective sports. In the event of an injury, sports medicine professionals can encourage injured athletes to tap into this skill and apply it to the various facets of the recovery process (e.g., while receiving treatment, to attain rehabilitation goals). Using imagery can return a sense of control to injured athletes: When they cannot physically perform an activity, envisioning a successful performance is the next best thing.

Used as an adjunct to therapy, imagery allows athletes to achieve specific mind-sets for maintaining a positive outlook, controlling stress, using positive and descriptive self-talk, and sustaining belief in the rehabilitation process. Incorporating imagery into rehabilitation sessions improves confidence and instills a sense of control over the injured body part. Many of the mental exercises can be performed during therapies such as whirlpool, bike riding, ultrasound, and electrical muscle stimulation (Granito, Hogan, & Varnum, 1995) to better cope with internal and external pain, to expedite the recovery process, and to keep physical skills from deteriorating (Richardson & Latuda, 1995). An example of an imagery exercise is presented in table 3.2.

Table 3.2   Sample Imagery Exercise

Close your eyes. Breathe in and out slowly and deeply. Relax your whole body by whatever method works best for you. Then let your ideas of your injury symptoms become like bubbles in your consciousness. Now imagine that these bubbles are being blown out of your mind, out of your body, out of your consciousness by a breeze that draws them away from you, far into the distance, until you no longer see them or feel them. Watch them disappear over the horizon.

Now imagine that you are in a place that you love. It may be the beach, in the mountains, on the desert, or wherever else you feel fully alive, comfortable, and healthy. Imagine the area around you is filled with bright, warm light. Allow the light to flow into your body, making you brighter and filling you with the energy of health. Enjoy basking in this light before gradually returning to the present.

Adapted from Samuels & Samuels (1975). *Seeing with the mind's eye.* New York: Random House; Berkeley: Bookworks.

When introducing an imagery program into the treatment regimen, sports medicine professionals can employ three complementary types of imagery to facilitate recovery: injury, skill, and rehabilitation imagery (Richardson & Latuda, 1995).

Injury Imagery

With the use of anatomical models, X rays, and photographs, athletes can visualize the bones and soft tissue involved in the injury. Understanding the body's inner workings and the structural damage caused by the trauma can help athletes gain control over the injury (Richardson & Latuda, 1995). Additionally, explaining the body's reactions to injury (e.g., causes of discoloration, edema, limited range of motion) provides valuable information and saves athletes from engaging in negative thought patterns based on the unknown (e.g., Why is there so much swelling?). Athletes are very in tune with their bodies; preparing and encouraging them to "read" and understand their physical selves can strengthen their psychological selves.

Skill Imagery

This strategy involves injured athletes' mentally rehearsing sport-related activities during practices and competitions (Green, 1994). Athletes should attend team meetings, practices, and games when possible, paying particular attention to plays and strategies specific to their positions (Richardson & Latuda, 1995). Practicing mentally allows athletes to remain in an actual sports situation and to rehearse desired results without making mistakes. Underlying these benefits are other potential advantages, such as instilling confidence in the athlete, enhancing feelings of control, and fostering more relaxed performances (Warner & McNeill, 1988).

Rehabilitation Imagery

Sports medicine professionals can facilitate achievement of rehabilitative tasks and outcomes by helping athletes visualize the desired effect of exercises (Green, 1994). Viewing skeletal models and photos imparts understanding of the involved anatomy and empowers athletes to use visualization to enhance the efficacy of prescribed exercises (e.g., envisioning the musculature of the shoulder joint can enhance the efficacy of Codman's exercises). During the actual rehabilitation program, the purposes of imagery are to (1) facilitate the healing process, (2) promote the development of a positive and relaxed outlook toward recovery, (3) create the mind-set required for optimal performance, and (4) bring closure to the injury experience (Green, 1994).

Athletes' mental images as well as their mental attitudes greatly influence physical functioning (Warner & McNeill, 1988). Improper use of visualization (e.g., dwelling on images of the injurious event) can hamper the recovery process: Athletes do not seem to recognize and appreciate their power to enhance—or impede—their recovery through the use of imagery. This strategy is most effective when athletes believe it will assist the healing process; consequently, they will look to sports medicine professionals for reinforcement that visualization is a valuable use of time.

systematic desensitization—The process of combining relaxation and imagery to overcome progressively stressful or fearful events.

Systematic Desensitization

Combining injured athletes' training in relaxation and imagery, they can be instructed in **systematic desensitization** (Wolpe, 1973) to effectively cope with any anxiety-provoking feelings associated with the injury. First, the relaxation method is taught and must be mastered before proceeding. Once relaxed, athletes develop a hierarchy detailing sport-related fears (e.g., Will the pain go away? Will I ever race again?). Each fear is progressively imagined while maintaining a deeply relaxed state. When fear or anxiety is experienced during visualization, athletes focus on relaxing until the fear subsides. The process of visualizing fearful situations is repeated until the list of fears has been covered and no anxiety is felt. At this point, athletes are better prepared psychologically for the eventual return to competition.

Cognitive Restructuring

For athletes who have difficulty keeping their minds off negative thoughts, assistance with reframing these negative thoughts into a more positive mind-set may be helpful. Ievleva and Orlick (1991) found that faster-healing athletes were more likely to use self-talk that was positive and self-encouraging, as compared with the slower healing athletes whose thought patterns reflected whining and self-pitying. According to Ievleva and Orlick (1993, p. 231), "thinking and acting in positive ways contribute to personal well-being and enhanced health." Table 3.3 provides a sample activity for restructuring negative postinjury thoughts into positive ones.

Goal Setting

Setting **goals** is a natural—and controllable—part of an athlete's daily routine. In the event of injury, the skill of establishing goals for athletic performance may be easily transferred to rehabilitation. Goal setting allows athletes to actively engage in their treatment, thus restoring a sense of control in the injury situation.

goal—*A desired objective toward which effort is directed.*

Preseason baseline data of physical and sport-specific parameters can serve as guides for establishing long-term goals. Such data can provide the target criteria to which athletes can compare their progress during rehabilitation. Teaching goal setting is a means of empowerment that encourages athletes to take responsibility for their healthy return to sport (Danish et al., 1993).

To implement an effective goal-setting program, athletes and sports medicine professionals should consider the following principles to ensure optimal effectiveness:

Table 3.3 Cognitive Restructuring Activity

Self-defeating thoughts	Change to self-enhancing thoughts
Example. There's no sense in going to rehabilitation; I'll never get back to my old self.	Example. I've seen good players recover from a similar injury; I can get back to my old self if I work hard at it.
1. The coach has given up on me; since I can't play she thinks I'm useless.	1.
2. I don't want to fail at rehabilitation.	2.
3. This surgery is really going to be painful, and all I'll have to show for it is a big scar.	3.
4. I'll take it easy in rehabilitation today and go hard at the next session.	4.
5. Who cares whether I recover from my injury or not anyhow?	5.
6. This hurts; I don't know if it's worth it.	6.
7. _____	7.

Adapted from Bunker, Williams, & Zinsser (1993). Cognitive techniques for improving performance and building confidence. In J.M. Williams (Ed.), *Applied sport psychology* (pp. 225-242). Mountain View, CA: Mayfield.

1. Goals should be specific and measurable. Individuals demonstrate more commitment to specific, concrete goals that clearly state what they need to do to achieve the desired result (Yukelson & Murphy, 1993). In addition, goals must be measurable so as to provide feedback regarding progress. "I will do 3 × 25 straight-leg raises, three times a week" exemplifies a straightforward, easily measured goal.

2. Goals should be challenging. If goals are too easy, athletes will become bored; if too difficult, athletes may feel frustrated. Sports medicine professionals can guide the setting of reasonable yet challenging goals.

3. Goals should be realistic. Athletes are accustomed to pushing their bodies during sport participation and often apply the same vigor to their rehabilitation. Unfortunately, some athletes do not appreciate the extent of their injuries and the time necessary for a full recovery; consequently, they may set impractical goals and risk reinjury. If goals are unrealistic, the athletes will likely feel frustrated when their bodies do not respond as anticipated and they fail to achieve the established goal.

4. Goals should be reinforced and rewarded. As injured athletes advance through the goal-setting program, they should regularly receive information on proximity to goal attainment. The quantifiable factors of attendance, weight-lifting sets and repetitions, exercise frequency, and time illustrate how easily goals can be measured and monitored. Athletes should be encouraged to reward themselves for achieving an established goal, particularly one that was especially challenging. Going to a movie or buying a new CD are fun ways to celebrate a rehabilitation success.

Table 3.4 presents a sample goal-setting activity to evaluate your goal-setting abilities based on the principles just described.

While these psychological strategies have the power to greatly facilitate physical recovery from injury, bear in mind that not all techniques work for all athletes. As previously mentioned, athletes have to believe in the importance of the method to

---

Table 3.4   Sample Goal-Setting Exercise

Select a specific sport injury in your mind, and write five goals that you think would be appropriate for an athlete with that injury. Remember to answer the following questions in each goal: "Who?", "will do what?", "by when?". Then rate the five goals according to each of the goal-setting principles by placing a check mark in the appropriate column if the goal conforms to that principle.

	Specific	Measurable	Challenging	Realistic
Example. I will be able do three knee extensions with 5-lb (2.3-kg) resistance using my injured leg by this Friday.	✓	✓	✓	✓
1.	___	___	___	___
2.	___	___	___	___
3.	___	___	___	___
4.	___	___	___	___
5.	___	___	___	___

Adapted from Martens (1987). *Coaches guide to sport psychology.* Champaign, IL: Human Kinetics.

accrue any mental, and consequently physical, health benefits. Undoubtedly, some athletes will scoff at the suggestion of using any of the aforementioned techniques. These athletes may also resist the traditional preventive and rehabilitative approaches (e.g., whirlpool, cross-training, rest) employed in sports medicine settings. It is with these athletes that sports medicine professionals may need to intervene philosophically.

PHILOSOPHICAL INTERVENTION STRATEGIES

As described in chapter 2, athletes train and perform within a social system that emphasizes physical and mental sacrifice, toughness, endurance, and fortitude. Although these are certainly laudable characteristics in some ways, the negative effect of these characteristics is that many athletes are unwilling to cease participation regardless of the pain they experience. The **socialization** experiences of many competitors' careers illustrate aspects of what has been termed the **sport ethic** (Hughes & Coakley, 1991). As athletes are socialized into sport, this normative ethic provides the framework within which athletes learn to define sacrifice, risk, pain, and injury as the prices that must be paid to be competitive athletes. One need only look at chronicles of life in elite sport, such as in the National Football League (Huizenga, 1994), gymnastics, and figure skating (Ryan, 1995), to realize the extraordinary risks being taken with athletes' health and even lives in the name of sport.

> *socialization—The process of learning and adapting to one's social environment or to a particular group's behaviors and beliefs.*

Sports medicine professionals are often in a position to deal directly with coaches as well as injured athletes. Unfortunately, the following scenario described by a former elite female gymnast is all too common:

> *[Coach] would get mad if I got an injury. He would be so pissed off. He'd be like, "oh no, not again," and then he'd want me in the gym working out and everything. . . . [He] thought that [an injury] was a lack of concentration. So, he was mad at me because if I was concentrating better, I wouldn't have [gotten injured]. (Krane, Greenleaf, & Snow, 1997, p. 59)*

> *sport ethic—A system of principles and beliefs, held predominantly by athletes, that advocates personal sacrifice, risk taking, and playing with pain to promote conformity and adherence to sport norms (Hughes & Coakley, 1991).*

Although this young elite gymnast sustained repeated injuries and was told by medical personnel that she should quit participating (or at the very least spend more time in rehabilitation), this advice was ignored by the gymnast, her parents, and her coaches.

Recognition of the "playing with pain" phenomenon provides sports medicine professionals with insight into the motivations of the frustrating, noncompliant athlete. Injured athletes' reactions of denial and dismissal of pain and injury can be understood and appreciated for their true origin: the fear of appearing weak and vulnerable in front of teammates and coaches who expect absolute physical and mental toughness. Unfortunately, these unhealthy responses prevent athletes from using available coping and social support networks at a time when such resources are most needed. A **philosophical intervention** initiated by the sports medicine professional might be of assistance in encouraging athletes to report injuries early, when there is still a chance to prevent further damage.

> *philosophical intervention—An intervention directed toward countering the influences of the prevailing sociocultural climate of sport (which encourages playing with pain and injury).*

Acceptance of the sport ethic by young athletes is particularly distressing. Desiring to emulate the more physically and psychologically mature athletes in the high school, college, and professional ranks, youngsters perceive that it is not acceptable within the sport culture to report injuries. Unfortunately, many young participants therefore do not report seemingly small injuries for fear that they will be replaced or accused of being "babies." This attitude could teach them a costly lesson. Shaffer's (1996) findings with high school wrestlers noted that pressure to perform with injury transcends competitive level and ability. The desire to succeed for themselves and for significant others motivated the young wrestlers she interviewed to endure great amounts of physical discomfort. Sadly, the adults responsible for protecting the athlete—parents and coaches—often played the role of motivator when obstacles such as injury threatened competitive success. Unless taught early to exercise power to protect themselves from influences that promote team welfare before personal welfare, young athletes will be subject to considerable pressures to risk their bodies and health for athletic success. If injured athletes believe that they can rely only on a support network that abides by the credo "no pain, no gain," playing with pain and injuries despite advice to the contrary will unfortunately continue.

Thus, to intervene philosophically, the sports medicine professional may need to stand up for the physical and mental health of athletes as top priority, which supersedes the desire to compete and perform. This stance needs to be taken even when others (such as parents, coaches, and administrators) may not reinforce it. Although challenging the widespread and persuasive power of the sport ethic may be difficult, sports medicine professionals must remain proponents for athletes' health and well-being—even in cases when athletes are not advocates for themselves.

Sports medicine professionals can easily identify competitors who resist medical intervention or those who use sports medicine only as a means of performance enhancement. By allowing ailing athletes to "save face" with teammates and coaches, sports medicine professionals can deliver necessary medical treatment, and athletes can avoid being negatively labeled (e.g., "faker" or "lazy"). For example, depending on the sport requirements (e.g., heavy pounding, high contact, high repetitions), it may be acceptable to mandate that all athletes ice down after practice for preventive reasons. This allows athletes who are injured to receive cold therapy as well as additional modalities without being the only team members in the training room.

Encouraging young athletes to be sufficiently sensitive to the difference between discomfort that is a routine part of training for sport and pain that serves as a warning of possible damage to the body is another strategy that sports medicine professionals can employ. However, young athletes' inexperience with assessing pain severity, their impatience to resume normal participation, and their sense of immortality greatly contribute to their unwillingness to comply with medical advice, thereby testing the patience of even the most mild-mannered sports medicine professional! Additionally, parents, coaches, and teammates can, knowingly or not, exert pressure or induce feelings of guilt to keep the injured athlete competing, further compromising the likelihood of a successful recovery. Sports medicine professionals must educate parents, coaches, and young athletes about accurate recognition of injury and appropriate selection of responses and behaviors directed toward long-term, rather than short-term, athletic participation (Wiese-Bjornstal, Smith, & LaMott, 1995).

Following are some situations in which it might be up to the sports medicine professional to intervene philosophically:

- When athletes are reluctant or fail to report obvious injuries for fear of losing their spot
- When coaches want injured athletes to play because winning is all-important
- When parents pressure their youngsters to play when injured, whether for scholarships, status, or acclaim
- When organizations treat athletes as expendable commodities to maintain profits

At these times like these, it is helpful for sports medicine professionals to remind themselves of their overriding responsibility for the physical and mental health of athletes. The most direct strategy is to talk with the involved athlete, coach, or parent about the possible health-related consequences of continuing to compete with injury. It is particularly important for the sports medicine professional to outline the risks of permanent damage. Encouraging coaches to maintain regular contact with injured athletes may help keep coaches apprised of athletes' injury status and sensitive to athletes' fears and concerns about returning to sport too soon after injury.

Parents, particularly those of child athletes, should be challenged to question their own motives for encouraging their children to participate when injured. Often parents live vicariously through the sport successes of their youngsters rather than allowing their children to make their own choices in life. Sports medicine professionals would be wise to speak with the athlete alone, beyond earshot of the pushy parent, to ensure that it is the athlete's—not the parent's—wish to return to sport.

Of course many athletes (and parents and coaches) are so conditioned by the sport culture and by their feelings of invincibility that these arguments will fall on deaf ears. Recognizing that these strategies alone may not be enough to sway the decision toward caution rather than risk, sports medicine professionals thus might ultimately reach the point where they have to refuse to go along with a decision to "patch up" an injured athlete one more time so that he or she can play. For every performer who is lucky enough to succeed with injury (e.g., Kerry Strug at the 1996 Summer Olympic Games in Atlanta), there are many lost to injury along the way (e.g., Julissa Gomez, as described in Ryan, 1995). The price is far too high.

CASE STUDY
Part I

Christie is a 21-year-old Division I cross-country and long-distance runner. During the outdoor track season, she complained of low-back pain and some muscle tightness in her legs and back. As a distance runner, Christie is accustomed to training through pain, so she doesn't believe she has an injury. She feels that the team has simply put in a lot of miles lately and her body is just sore. She expressed frustration and annoyance, however, at the interference this pain has placed on her ability to prepare for and compete in the conference meet.

Questions for Analysis

1. What is the first thing the sports medicine professional should do?

2. Discuss Christie's situation from a psychological standpoint.

3. What preinjury strategies could the sports medicine professional use to help Christie maintain her training regimen until she races?

Part II

Christie's back pain worsened to the point where it radiated down the length of her right leg. She experienced increased muscle tightness and spasms as well as occasional numbness in her right leg. She no longer could tolerate sitting for long periods of time, which interfered with her studies. Pain management techniques were not effective in decreasing the pain, forcing Christie to stop running. The team orthopedic surgeon stated that her symptoms were consistent with an L5-S1 disk herniation and, because she was not responding to noninvasive procedures, recommended retirement from running. A second opinion suggested surgery but made no promises that she'd be able to run again. Christie felt depressed and confused, especially with conflicting opinions from her doctors. She became easily irritated and obstinate, especially with the sports medicine professionals with whom she was working.

Questions for Analysis

1. Discuss Christie's psychological response to her back injury.

2. What postinjury strategies could the sports medicine professional use to help Christie manage her pain and regain lost functions?

3. What factors might help or hinder Christie's acceptance of the sports medicine professional's suggestions?

SUMMARY

In the social climate of sport today, with more pressure and stress being placed on athletes, sports medicine professionals may have to assume guidance and counseling responsibilities if other services are unavailable. Recognizing the potential benefits of using the athletes' minds to prevent and manage injury provides additional prevention and rehabilitation options. This chapter introduced several techniques that use an integrated mind–body perspective and serves as a springboard for more in-depth examinations of these strategies to be presented in later chapters. For example, chapter 7 provides more detailed explanations about social support, and chapter 14 describes some specific interventions for athletes who have problems dealing with stress and anxiety.

Each sports medicine professional must individually decide the value of psychological skills for injury prevention and treatment. Although these methods may be used as infrequently as a CPR pocket mask or as often as a pair of scissors, they should be included in every sports medicine professional's "training kit."

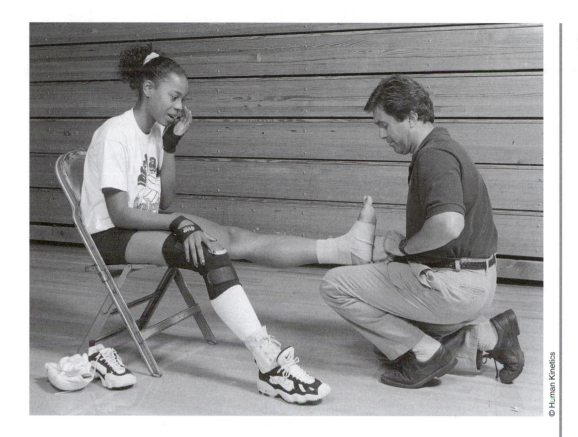

© Human Kinetics

Effective Interaction Skills for Sports Medicine Professionals

Diane M. Wiese-Bjornstal, PhD, *University of Minnesota*
Diane M. Gardetto, MA, *University of Minnesota*
Shelly M. Shaffer, PhD, *Pinnacle Health Systems*

CHAPTER OBJECTIVES

Describe the role of rapport, empathy, and trust in working with injured athletes

List elements essential to educating athletes about their injury and rehabilitation

Explain the importance of effective communication skills to the work of sports medicine professionals

Illustrate types of nonverbal communication common in sports medicine settings

Outline characteristics of active listening

Identify strategies for enhancing communication between sports medicine professionals and injured athletes

From recording the results of an injury evaluation to explaining the nature of the rehabilitation protocol, virtually all of a sports medicine professional's work involves some form of interaction with others. The development of effective interaction skills, however, is rarely a central component of sports medicine educational programs (Schultz, Wellard, & Swerissen, 1988). Sports medicine professionals with the greatest of expertise and technical skill may indeed find their efforts wasted if they cannot adequately communicate with the injured athlete and other members of the sports medicine team (Wagstaff, 1982). The purpose of this chapter is to help sports medicine professionals better understand the foundations of effective interaction and the skills of communication as they relate to working with athletes.

FOUNDATIONS OF EFFECTIVE INTERACTION

Within their professional roles, sports medicine professionals engage in education and counseling activities (Wiese-Bjornstal & Smith, 1993). These interpersonal and group interactions must abide with the ethical standards of their professions and must be limited to their areas of expertise. These interactions involve relationships that should be caring, honest, respectful, and accepting (Kottler & Brown, 1996) because they often involve dealing with the very sensitive thoughts, feelings, and behaviors of injured athletes. Sports medicine professionals interact with others in ways such as establishing rapport with athletes and coaches, providing information concerning physical condition and progress, sharing information with other sports medicine professionals, and giving instructions to a patient.

Even before the actual interactions occur, sports medicine professionals must clear their minds of other distractions and adopt a helping attitude (Kottler & Kottler, 1993). This alone is often a challenge amid the hectic schedules of today's society, but it is worth the effort because it enhances the quality of the interaction. Indeed, the success of these interactions depends to a large extent on the following (Purtilo & Haddad, 1996):

- Attitude and mind-set of the sports medicine professional
- Tone and volume of voice used
- Readiness of the speaker and receiver to listen effectively
- Way in which material is presented

The foundation of effective interactions hinges on the abilities of sports medicine professionals to develop rapport, empathy, and trust in their relationships with athletes.

Rapport

rapport—A relationship of mutual trust and emotional affinity.

The importance of developing **rapport** between the sports medicine professional and the injured athlete is readily apparent (Wiese & Weiss, 1987). If athletes do not feel comfortable with their sports medicine professionals, maximum benefit cannot be obtained from their interactions.

Some sports medicine professionals, particularly athletic trainers, are in a position to develop rapport with athletes before injury occurs. Familiarizing themselves with all athletes in their purview—not just the star athletes—will be of benefit later on. By developing rapport, sports medicine professionals can also learn about individual differences among their athletes, such as personality dispositions, emotional stability, and behavioral tendencies, that might later be of help in interpreting and managing their responses to injury, should it occur.

Building rapport with athletes forms the foundations from which further interactions stem, such as those that occur after injury. The rapport-building phase postinjury involves the following considerations for the sports medicine professional (Petitpas & Danish, 1995):

- Understanding injury from the athlete's perspective
- Using a tentative approach immediately after injury
- Enlisting athletes as collaborators in planning the next steps
- Implementing the treatment strategy

Thus sports medicine professionals should take the time both before and after injury to get to know their athletes and what makes them tick. Asking them about their days, their sports, their lives; sharing lighthearted joking with them; and sharing a bit of yourself with them can—besides making work much more enjoyable—reap benefits in providing effective treatment.

Empathy

One central component of rapport development is the **empathy** displayed by the sports medicine professional, as empathic behavior conveys a message of support and acceptance to the injured athlete. Empathy involves a capacity to view the world through the eyes of others, accurately sense their feelings, and skillfully listen to hear not only the obvious message but the subtle shadings of which the patient may not even be aware (Cormier & Hackney, 1993). The basis of empathy is genuine caring for the other person (Martens, 1987). Empathy is vital to the effectiveness of communication skills because the development of trust occurs within an empathic context (Martin, 1983; Okun, 1992).

empathy—"Communicated understanding of the other person's intended message" (Martin, 1983, p. 3).

Ensuring that the other person feels understood is the key to developing empathy. The sports medicine professional must comprehend the athlete's intended message, which sometimes may not be the overt, but rather the implicit, meaning of the message. One strategy is for the sports medicine professional to put into words what he or she thinks the athlete actually meant by the communication. In this way athletes can either reinforce that the sports medicine professional "got it" or restate their concerns so that the sports medicine professional can again try to understand the underlying message.

For example, when Kirby mentions that he doesn't care whether he recovers from his knee surgery or not, the implicit message might actually be that Kirby perceives that the coach doesn't care whether he returns to the team or not. The sports medicine professional might say to Kirby, "How do you think your coach and teammates would feel if you did not recover from your injury and return to the team?" If Kirby replies, "Oh, they won't care," this reinforces the sports medicine professional's perception of the real meaning of Kirby's original communication. If Kirby says, however, "They will be very disappointed if I don't return," then perhaps Kirby himself either has no desire to return to the team or lacks confidence in his own ability to successfully rehabilitate. Further probing by the sports medicine professional could lead to the underlying reason why Kirby made his statement.

Whether empathy can be learned easily seems subject to debate (Davis, 1990). The chances of improving one's ability to be empathic, however, are enhanced through experience. Davis (1990) suggested that physical therapists and other helpers have plenty of opportunity to practice in situations in which empathic interaction can occur. In other words, helping professionals must practice empathy skills just as they would practice taping techniques. Experience is often the best teacher, and attempting to imagine oneself in the athlete's place during each and every interaction can only improve the ability to be empathic.

One of the first steps toward becoming more empathic is to become aware of and analyze your own communication behaviors. Table 4.1 provides some examples of behaviors that either display empathy or discourage empathic interaction. Reviewing these examples may encourage sports medicine professionals to thoughtfully choose the ways in which they interact with others.

The following case study provides an example of how a sport injury scenario was originally handled in a nonempathic manner and proposes a revised ending to the scenario in which greater empathy is displayed toward the athlete.

Case Study: Empathy

Tonya was a college freshman playing in her high school alumni basketball game over Christmas break. She was working to earn a spot on the college varsity squad but was still playing junior varsity. With a wide-open, fast-break layup in front of her, Tonya ran full tilt toward the basket. As she made a strong, final plant to drive upward for the shot, a foot suddenly appeared underneath her leg from behind. With a sickening twist of her ankle, she went down hard. All was silent as the ankle swelled. No one around knew anything about how to evaluate or care for the injury, so Tonya watched the remainder of the game from the sideline before deciding she needed to visit the doctor. Tonya was frustrated and upset that she had needlessly suffered an injury as the result of an incompetent and unnecessary defensive play.

Scenario Displaying Lack of Empathy

"Just a sprain," the doctor said, although the ankle swelled to twice its normal size, "just stay off it for a month." He gave her some anti-inflammatory medication. Tonya mentioned that she was on the basketball team, but no treatment or rehabilitation regimen was prescribed. When Tonya returned to college, she quietly showed her ankle to the athletic trainer. The athletic trainer somewhat jokingly declared that Tonya had "elephantiasis" of the ankle and that it was the worst ankle sprain she had ever seen. Finally, some minimal treatment was given, but Tonya wasn't attended to as carefully as the stars of the team. The coach rarely asked about her; after all, Tonya wasn't a starter. The coach didn't care whether Tonya attended practice or not. Tonya began to get the feeling that she wasn't much worth their time.

Questions for Analysis

1. How could the physician have displayed more empathy for Tonya's role as an athlete?

Table 4.1 Displaying Empathic Behavior

Behaviors Conveying Empathy	Behaviors Inhibiting Empathy
Seating yourself beside the athlete	Seating yourself behind your desk while the athlete sits across from you
Maintaining an open posture, such as leaning forward with arms held loosely	Closing your posture, such as folding arms across your chest and leaning back
Looking the athlete in the eye and giving the athlete your full attention	Looking around or at other paperwork when speaking with the athlete
Stopping what you are doing to give the athlete your full attention	Continuing to work while you speak with the athlete
Allowing athletes the freedom to express their concerns and emotions	Asking athletes to "suck it up" and be tough

2. How might the athletic trainer's evaluation and depiction of Tonya's injury have been changed to be more empathic?

3. Can you describe some specific behaviors that the coach might have exhibited to display greater empathy?

Scenario Displaying Empathy

"Just a sprain," the doctor said, although the ankle swelled to twice its normal size, "but you'll need to stay off it for a month." He gave her some anti-inflammatory medication. Tonya mentioned that she was on the basketball team. Recognizing that Tonya was an active woman, the doctor gave her crutches to move around on for the first few days. He suggested some active range-of-motion ankle exercises that she could do until she was able to bear weight on the ankle. When Tonya returned to college, she quietly showed her ankle to the athletic trainer. The athletic trainer evaluated Tonya's ankle and noticed that it was still swollen. He asked Tonya to come into the training room daily for cold whirlpool and exercise sessions. Tonya could come in before practice, when the varsity players also were being treated. The coach checked in with Tonya and the athletic trainer daily and arranged for Tonya to participate in those practice drills in which she was able. The coach also asked her if she would be interested in keeping stats for the games until her ankle was better.

Trust

Trust is another essential component of rapport development. Maintaining a climate of mutual trust and concern is vital to the work of sports medicine professionals, particularly as they enter into the cognitive and emotional domains associated with sport injuries. Abiding by the ethical standards of a profession provides a strong foundation on which trust may be based. For sports medicine professionals, this means clearly delineating for athletes the boundaries of your expertise; clarifying the confidentiality of interactions and specifying which types of information will be shared with coaches, parents, media, or others; and keeping athletes' needs and best interests above all else.

Because interpersonal interaction is a two-way street, sports medicine professionals in turn should clearly identify for athletes what is expected of them. Honest reporting of their injuries, levels of pain, and completion of rehabilitation activities must be provided by athletes to maintain the sports medicine professional's trust. Table 4.2 provides a summary of reminders for developing trust between sports medicine professionals and athletes.

Table 4.2 Developing Trust Between Sports Medicine Professionals and Athletes
Keep information shared by the athlete confidential if you don't have his or her permission to share it.
Clearly indicate to athletes the boundaries of your expertise.
Demonstrate that you have the athlete's best interests, rather than your own self-gain, in mind.
Abide by the ethical principles of your profession.
Express concern for the athlete beyond his or her role in sport.
Explain that you, in turn, expect the athlete to be trustworthy and honest in reporting on the injury and rehabilitation activities.

By the same token, sports medicine professionals should work to be perceived by colleagues, coaches, administrators, and others as persons of integrity. By approaching each task and each day with the best of intentions, sports medicine professionals can ensure the trust not only of their athletes, but of their colleagues. Providing accurate information about injuries and rehabilitation, as addressed in the next section, is one component of being a trustworthy professional.

PROVIDING INFORMATION

During the educational phase of interactions with injured athletes, it is important to ensure that injured athletes have as much accurate information as possible about the injury and recovery processes (Petitpas & Danish, 1995). This helps athletes become collaborators in their treatment and reduces exaggerated worry or fear of the unknown (Petitpas & Danish, 1995).

All sports medicine professional should delineate—both for their own sake and for the sake of their athletes—the boundaries of their informational interactions with athletes and the limits of their expertise in providing information. Physicians, physical therapists, and athletic trainers should work as a cohesive, effective team in providing all the informational "pieces of the puzzle" to injured athletes, and they need to ensure that they do not give contradictory messages. They should consider both *what* information should be given and the *manner* in which it is conveyed.

What Information to Provide

Injured athletes want information on a variety of issues related to their injuries (Petitpas & Danish, 1995). These issues include a description of the nature of the injury and medical reasons for initiating the particular treatment. Clarifying the goals of the treatment and identifying possible coping strategies for accommodating the treatment are also helpful to the injured athlete. To a reasonable extent (depending on the age and cognitive developmental level of the athlete), details of the medical procedures that will be performed and possible sensations or side effects should be described. It is also important to discuss the anticipated recovery process and share with the athlete that recovery rarely progresses on a smooth, upward continuum, but rather will likely include setbacks and plateaus along the way. Reassurance that these blips are normal parts of the recovery process helps the athlete mentally prepare for their occurrence. Table 4.3 provides some general suggestions for the contents of injury-education discussions. The specific components will vary on a case-by-case basis.

How to Provide Information

The methods of communicating the preceding information are another skill to be mastered by sports medicine professionals (Wiese & Weiss, 1987). When providing information to athletes, it is important to attend to the following points (Purtilo & Haddad, 1996). First, as mentioned earlier, the sports medicine professional's mind must be focused on the upcoming interaction, not on other distractions in her or his life. Second, sports medicine professionals must consider the vocabulary that they use and decide whether it is appropriate to the developmental level of the athlete. In general, it makes sense to limit highly technical jargon and unnecessary information. Third, the organization of content must be considered. Sports medicine professionals must decide in what order to present pertinent information. Important information should be presented first and repeated more than once. They also need to decide what should be given at a later date to avoid confusion and information over-

Table 4.3   Contents of Injury-Education Discussions
Anatomical illustration of injury
Descriptions of diagnostic or surgical procedures
Options for repairing the injury
Options for rehabilitation methods
Purposes and potential side effects of medications
Distinguishing pain associated with healing from pain signaling further injury
Timeline for progressing from passive to active rehabilitation and return to sport
Instructions for using recommended braces, crutches, or orthotic devices
Ongoing care and maintenance of the injured area
Soliciting and answering the athlete's questions

Adapted from J. Heil (1993, p. 141). *Psychology of sport injury.* Champaign, IL: Human Kinetics.

load. Fourth, sports medicine professionals need to be clear and concise in conveying relevant information and in answering questions. Table 4.4 provides a summary of some general guidelines for providing medical information.

Beyond the initial informational meeting, sports medicine professionals should consider using an approach to communication that focuses on the positive (Wiese & Weiss, 1987). Reinforcing those rehabilitation elements that have been performed correctly and providing praise and rewards to encourage the desired recovery behaviors are examples of this focus on the positive (Wiese & Weiss, 1987).

The following case study provides an example of how injury information is often lacking. An alternative scenario is suggested in which information is provided.

Case Study: Providing Information

Returning for her third season as a starting college varsity volleyball player, Maria was a few pounds overweight. All went well in preseason, however, and the regular season began. In a home match, crouching down low on defensive coverage, Maria felt a popping sensation in her right knee. Nothing seemed amiss, however, and she

Table 4.4   General Guidelines for Providing Medical Information
Give the most important instructions first.
Stress how important the instructions are.
Use short words and short sentences.
Repeat important points.
Make advice as specific, detailed, and concrete as possible.
Ask the patient to repeat key points.
Provide simply worded, printed materials to reinforce oral directions.
Ask questions as well as give information.

Adapted from Wagstaff (1982). A small doses of commonsense—communication, persuasion and physiotherapy. *Physiotherapy, 68,* 327-329.

continued to play. A few plays later, she twisted her knee and went down in pain. It was no one's fault—just one of those things—but Maria was frustrated by the injury because it didn't seem as if anything in particular caused it.

Scenario in Which Information Is Not Provided

After the match the doctor at the student clinic immobilized Maria's knee and pre-scribed a couple of weeks of rest, without telling Maria what was wrong. She wanted to stay involved with the team in spite of the injury and continued to go to practices and help out, doing whatever drills she could, even though the coach didn't help her much. Since there was no athletic trainer for the team, no one knew anything about rehabilitation activities, so none were prescribed and Maria designed her own. Jump-ing workouts in the swimming pool and leg lifts in the dorm room using pop cans in hiking boots strapped across her ankle were the best she could do. When she was ready to resume play, there was no athletic trainer to tape her knee, nor was the coach willing to learn how. Maria learned how to tape her own knee by reading about it in a book and returned to finish the season.

Questions for Analysis

1. What additional information should the physician at the student clinic have provided to Maria?

2. What kinds of things should the coach have learned to assist Maria with re-covery?

3. Was it advisable for Maria to tape her own knee? Why or why not?

Scenario in Which Information Is Provided

After the match, the doctor at the student clinic immobilized Maria's knee. He told Maria that she had sprained the medial collateral ligament and that she should ice her knee for 20 minutes, three times a day for the next week. The doctor said that Maria would probably require a couple of weeks' rest before she would be allowed to return to volleyball. He suggested some strengthening exercises that she could do with-out sustaining further damage to the knee. She wanted to stay involved with the team in spite of the injury and continued to go to practices and help out, doing whatever drills she could, as well as keep the score book at matches. Since no athletic trainer was assigned to the team, the coach took it upon herself to gather information about Maria's injury so that she could recommend some rehabilitation activities. On the advice of the sports medicine professionals whom she phoned, the coach showed Maria some gradual mobility and strengthening workouts for the swimming pool, to use after the doctor gave the okay for Maria to resume some activity. When she was ready to resume play, Maria found that the coach had learned the proper taping technique to use for her knee. With the help of the coach, Maria returned to finish the season.

EFFECTIVE COMMUNICATION SKILLS

Now that we have described the foundational elements on which effective interac-tions are based, in this section we outline specific communication skills to be used. To be effective, sports medicine professionals must use interpersonal communication skills that involve hearing verbal messages (i.e., the cognitive and affective content), perceiving nonverbal messages (i.e., the affective and behavioral content), and re-sponding verbally and nonverbally to both kinds of messages (Okun, 1992). Two re-cent surveys of sports medicine professionals have documented the important role played by effective communication skills. In a survey of athletic trainers, Wiese, Weiss, and Yukelson (1991) noted that the athletic trainers themselves rated communication skills among the most important psychological skills for enhancing injury recovery. Ford and Gordon (1993) investigated ways for Australian sport physiotherapists to improve social support provision and found strong evidence for the need to develop effective communication skills. Among their key findings, they noted that sport physiotherapists provided a necessary communication bridge between physicians and injured athletes. Physiotherapists' top-rated recommendations for providing better social support emphasized improving communication between members of the sport rehabilitation team. Clearly the development of improved communication skills is central to the provision of social support (see chapter 7 for a more extensive discussion of social support).

The question remains, however, as to how sports medicine professionals know whether they are communicating effectively. A key consideration is whether the recipient of the message, in most cases the injured athlete, received and understood the message content. Kahanov and Fairchild (1994) examined the discrepancies in the perceptions of athletic trainers and injured athletes about the communication process. Their study examined the nature of communication between the athletic trainer and injured athlete during an initial injury evaluation. Survey results of 50 injured athletes and six athletic trainers indicated significant discrepancies between athletic trainer and athlete regarding the athlete's understanding of the injury and rehabilitation protocol. Specifically, the athletic trainers thought that athletes understood the nature of their injuries and recommended rehabilitation activities much better than the athletes actually did. Given this evidence that vital information was miscommunicated, the authors made several recommendations for enhancing communication during this initial injury phase. For example, they suggested that athletic trainers need to go beyond merely asking whether athletes understand to specifically asking athletes to rephrase and summarize what they have heard from the trainer. In this way, the athletic trainer can check whether the athlete correctly received and understood the message. The athletic trainer also must consider the athlete's frame of reference (e.g., background, experience with a similar injury, mental perspective, and emotional state) to maximize understanding. This involves using active listening techniques and attending to both the verbal and nonverbal messages of athletes (Kahanov & Fairchild, 1994), as earlier mentioned. For example, athletes who are very anxious (see chapter 14) might hear even less of the communicated message than they normally would; thus checks for understanding and repetition by the sports medicine professional are critical.

Since communication plays such a central role in the work of sports medicine professionals, we next turn our attention to the basics of communication.

Communication Basics

In every facet of life, verbal and **nonverbal communication** express thoughts, feelings, and ideas. Two-way communication between sports medicine professionals and athletes as well as among members of the sports medicine team is paramount to job success and satisfaction. People commonly express the importance of communication; however, learning and practicing how to effectively send and receive messages are often neglected. Essential to effective communication are understanding several basic principles and applying them appropriately to given situations.

To ensure that a message is correctly received, it is necessary to understand how communication works. The process involves sending, receiving, and interpreting a message from one individual to another. Martens (1987) described a six-step communication process that occurs when sending a message, as depicted in figure 4.1. These six elements are as follows:

nonverbal communication— *Communication involving facial gestures, eye contact, and body language.*

1. The decision to share information starts the communication process. The information may reflect values, emotions, or decisions.

encoding—
Thoughts one wants communicated, translated into a message.

2. The thoughts intended for communication are translated into a message. This process is called **encoding**.

3. The message is sent to the receiver.

4. The sent message is transferred through a channel. The spoken words produce sound waves that are detected by the receiver. Channels might include the telephone or an audiotape.

decoding—
Receiving a message and interpreting it.

5. The message is received and interpreted, a process called **decoding**.

6. The receiver thinks about the message and experiences some type of internal response. This response could evoke a number of emotional reactions in the receiver (e.g., happy, angry, uninterested).

A conversation between a physical therapist, Keisha, and a distance runner, Carlos, illustrating these elements might go something like this:

1. Keisha, in her own mind, thinks, "I need to talk with Carlos about skipping his rehabilitation sessions." (Decide)

2. Keisha, in her own mind, thinks, "How can I phrase it so he doesn't get angry with me? Which specific behaviors should I focus on? How can I encourage him to be more motivated?" (Encode)

3. Keisha calls Carlos over to the side and says to him, "Carlos, I'm concerned about the rehab sessions you've been missing. Your recovery progress is a bit behind the schedule I've anticipated for you because of these missed workouts. I just wondered if there is anything we can change about the rehab sessions that would help you in completing the workouts?" (Send)

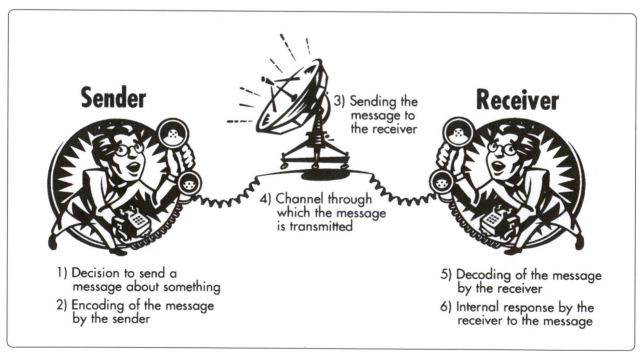

Figure 4.1 Key elements of the communication process.

Adapted with permission from Martens (1987). *Coaches guide to sport psychology.* Champaign, IL: Human Kinetics.

4. Keisha chose to talk with Carlos (a verbal channel) and displayed a sincere expression of concern on her face when delivering the information (a nonverbal channel). (Channel)

5. Carlos thinks to himself, "I have missed quite a few workout sessions, but I just didn't feel like I was making any progress. But Keisha thinks that I'll be able to return to my running sooner if I finish my rehab sessions. Maybe Keisha could let me do more water workouts, since I like those." (Decode)

6. Carlos responds in his mind, "It would be great if I could start running again soon. I'll really try harder in my rehab sessions." (Response)

The subjectivity of this process must be appreciated if a thorough understanding of communication is to be achieved. An individual will receive (i.e., decode) or construct (i.e., encode) a message based on his or her past experiences, emotional mood states, and individuality (Yukelson, 1993). **Noise** occurring in any step of the communication process often garbles the intended message, causing inaccurate reception and misunderstanding. Common sources of noise include

noise—"When the message you intended to communicate is not what [is] heard" (Martens, 1987, p. 49).

- the sender's past experiences (e.g., beliefs, attitudes, and personality),
- the sender's inability to properly encode the message,
- the sender's biases,
- the receiver's psychological state, and
- external sources, such as a bad telephone connection, background noise, or distracting mannerisms of the sender or receiver (Martens, 1987).

Successful communication is difficult but can be accomplished when noise is controlled or eliminated. Recognizing that the receiver of a message has had unique experiences and will approach the sent message with a potentially different frame of reference from the sender will ultimately improve the quality of the interaction.

Verbal Communication

When a message is sent from one person to another, it occurs through verbal and nonverbal communication and can be distinguished in terms of content and emotion. Verbal communication sends messages by way of spoken or written words, whereas nonverbal communication involves facial gestures, eye contact, and body language (Yukelson, 1993). Sports medicine professionals are required in their work to communicate verbally with athletes to accomplish the following (Purtilo & Haddad, 1996):

- Establish rapport
- Obtain information regarding the athlete's condition and progress
- Relay pertinent information to other members of the sports medicine team
- Give instructions to the athlete

In addition, sports medicine professionals are expected to provide social support, offer reinforcement and rewards, relay technical information, educate athletes and coaches, and act in a consulting or counseling role.

In communicating verbally, the sports medicine professional would be wise to consider Purtilo and Haddad's (1996) following recommendations. First, the sports medicine professional should consider the mental status of the recipient of the communication. Factors such as fatigue, anxiety, or fear on the part of the athlete should cause the sports medicine professional to reduce the amount and limit the type of verbiage conveyed. Second, sports medicine professionals should carefully choose the vocabulary best suited to the recipient. Although precise, accurate descriptions should be provided, obviously most patients are not schooled in the technical language of sports medicine; thus highly technical, professional jargon should be avoided. Third, clarity in establishing the purpose of the communication helps establish and focus the discussion on relevant elements. Giving forethought to the upcoming communication can encourage greater clarity and organization in the actual interaction. Fourth, the appropriate use of humor can help patients cope with stress. For example, sports medicine professionals may poke a bit of fun at themselves, thus indicating that humor exists in most situations.

More structured forms of verbal communication occur in interview settings, such as those described in chapter 5. These interview settings typically rely on a planned dialogue to achieve a professional purpose (Purtilo & Haddad, 1996). Sports medicine professionals also engage in extensive written communication, such as giving written instructions to patients, completing informed consent documents for surgery, or documenting the results of an injury evaluation. The process of providing effective written documentation is discussed in chapter 9.

Nonverbal Communication

While written and spoken messages are readily apparent, nonverbal messages are more difficult to detect and accurately interpret. Of messages' total conveyed influence, however, the majority is derived from nonverbal information (Mehrabian, 1971); thus the importance of nonverbal communication should not be underestimated. In fact, when describing the information conveyed by way of "silent messages" (i.e., nonverbal messages), Mehrabian (1971, p. iii) suggested that "in the realm of feelings, our facial expressions, postures, movements, and gestures are so important that when our words contradict the silent messages contained within them, others mistrust what we say—they rely almost completely on what we do."

Nonverbal communication includes three distinct parts: kinesics, proxemics, and paralanguage (Martens, 1987). **Kinesics**, or body language, refers to how people communicate through physical appearance, posture, gestures, touching behaviors, and changes in facial and eye movements. **Proxemics** examines how people communicate through the space they occupy. This can be measured by either body position and distance between individuals or by arrangement of objects in a room. **Paralanguage** refers to voice characteristics such as pitch, resonance, articulation, tempo, volume, and rhythm.

By attending carefully to these three dimensions of nonverbal communication, sports medicine professionals can enhance their understanding of the messages communicated by injured athletes, as well as analyze their own nonverbal messages. Table 4.5 provides specific examples of some common messages conveyed through these three nonverbal means. It also outlines some considerations of these areas as they apply to the work of sports medicine professionals.

kinesics—
Communicating through body language.

proxemics—How people communicate through the space they occupy.

paralanguage—
Voice characteristics associated with communication.

INDIVIDUAL AND CULTURAL DIFFERENCES

It is important to recognize and adjust to individual differences such as social class, sex, ethnicity, and religion when communicating with a diverse population. Sports medicine professionals need to realize that values, beliefs, attitudes, and verbal and nonverbal communication processes may differ from culture to culture (Yukelson, 1993). It is imperative that sports medicine professionals pay close attention to an athlete's response and listen for questions and clarification while also interpreting the various nuances in kinesics, proxemics, and paralanguage. For sports medicine professionals to be successful in working with athletes, understanding and appreciation of individual and cultural differences are imperative. When uncertainty about

Table 4.5 Nonverbal Communication

KINESICS

Nonverbal communication	Message conveyed
Attention to personal appearance, such as manner of dress, grooming, fitness level	Professionalism
Punctuality	Respect (however, some cultures view a certain amount of tardiness as respectful)
Upright, purposeful posture and gait	Enthusiasm and confidence
Gestures such as rubbing hands together	Anticipation and enthusiasm
Gestures such as extending arms out in front, palms up	Sincerity and openness
Firm, positive handshake	Confidence
Holding the other person's hands in yours just in front of your chest	Calming and reassurance
Slight touch on the speaker's arm	Listener would like to interrupt
Both people looking directly into each other's eyes, known as *line of regard,* for a long time	Conflict and anger
Facial expressions such as smiles and "smiling eyes"	Happiness, relaxation
Facial expressions such as a glazed or unfocused look in the eyes	Boredom, distraction, fatigue
Facial expressions such as a furrowed brow	Puzzlement, deep thought, concentration
Smells, such as overpowering cologne or perfume	May be intolerable to patients

PROXEMICS

Communication through use of space	Important considerations
Moving into the *intimate zone* (0-18 in., or 0-45 cm, apart), which is necessary for physical examinations and therapeutic interventions	Be sensitive to the fact that the athlete may feel threatened or embarrassed because this space is usually reserved for lovers and very close friends.
Moving into the *personal zone* (1.5-4 ft, or 0.5-1.2 m, apart), as during a one-on-one meeting with an athlete	Realize that this zone typically is reserved for friends and acquaintances, thus there may be some discomfort with having to share at so personal a level. Allow athletes to back off slightly if they seem more comfortable.
Interactions in the *social zone* (4-12 ft, or 1.2-3.7 m, apart), in which most professional interactions with sports medicine colleagues, coaches, and athletes occur	This seems to be a safe distance from which to conduct most professional business with people from different cultures.
Interactions in the *public zone* (more than 20 ft, or 6 m, apart), as when conducting group education sessions or teaching classes	This distance conveys a more impersonal presence, which may or may not be desired, depending on the purpose of the communication.

(continued)

Table 4.5 (continued)	

PARALANGUAGE

Vocal components of speech	Message conveyed
Pitch of voice lowers	Fatigue, calmness, depression
Pitch of voice rises	Joy, fear, anger
Thin resonance	Insecurity, weakness, indecisiveness
Rich resonance	Firmness, self-assurance, strength
Articulation slightly slurred, drawl	Atmosphere of comfort or intimacy
Articulation crisp and clear	Decisiveness, confidence
Fast tempo	Excitement, persuasion (but may also suggest insecurity or make the listener nervous)
Slower tempo	Sincere, thoughtful
Loud voice	Confidence and enthusiasm (but may also suggest aggressiveness or arrogance)
Softer voice	Trustworthiness, caring, understanding (but may also suggest a lack of confidence)

Adapted from Martens (1987, pp. 57-61). *Coaches guide to sport psychology.* Champaign, IL: Human Kinetics.

how to interact arises, sports medicine professionals can take their cues from the athletes themselves and solicit their preferences for interaction content and style. For example, the acceptability of touching as a form of expressing support varies greatly across diverse ethnic groups. On the other hand, Mehrabian (1971) suggests that due to the narrower scope of nonverbal behavior, there is greater cross-cultural consensus about what actions mean than about the corresponding words used for those same feelings.

In any case, it is important for sports medicine professionals to be aware of and sensitive to diversity when deciding how to handle a particular helping situation. Understanding the fundamentals of communication will greatly enhance your ability to empathically interact with injured athletes from diverse backgrounds. With this basic understanding of the types and content of communication, the next section provides a framework for considering interaction skills specific to the work of sports medicine professionals.

INTERACTION SKILLS

Interpersonal interaction requires the use of both attending skills and responding and action skills (Kottler & Brown, 1996). Attending skills include the ability to elicit information and to listen intently to responses. In turn, responding and action skills focus on developing an action plan for managing the issues being communicated.

Attending Skills

Attending skills encompass both physical and psychological attending. Physical attending involves the arrangement of the physical surroundings as well as nonverbal communicators such as body posture and position, head nods, facial expressions, eye contact, and gestures (Kottler & Brown, 1996). Psychological attending requires the foundational skills of empathy, respect, and acceptance and incorporates reflecting feelings and content back to the communicator to demonstrate concentration and understanding. With the elements of attending in mind, we next describe the specific attending skills of exploration and listening.

Exploration Skills

Several exploration skills have relevance to the work of sports medicine professionals. Exploration skills are helpful in eliciting athletes' concerns, facilitating insight, and examining thoughts and feelings (Kottler & Brown, 1996). These skills include the following (Kottler & Brown, 1996; Kottler & Kottler, 1993):

- *Questioning.* Closed-ended questions have the advantages of eliciting specific information and of being time expedient.
- *Probing.* Open-ended questions have the advantages of eliciting a broader range of possible responses and of encouraging self-examination.
- *Empathy.* Acknowledging both the feelings and the meanings implied in an athlete's statement ascertains whether the sports medicine professional understood the athlete's message.
- *Immediacy.* Immediacy brings the focus back to the present.
- *Self-disclosure.* You may choose to share personal anecdotes or examples to build trust and rapport.
- *Confrontation.* Cautiously identify discrepancies between the athlete's words and behaviors.
- *Summarizing.* Tie together themes that were discussed, and put things into perspective.

Listening Skills

If athletes are to be active participants in their rehabilitation, they must believe that the conveyed messages are worth hearing. People commonly filter some information out of a message, listening only to what they believe is important. This may lead to receiving inaccurate or incomplete information, thereby causing a breakdown in the working relationship. In some instances, if the sent message is perceived as threatening, preachy, or ordering, the receiver may block out the information entirely, resulting in frustrating misunderstandings (Yukelson, 1993). To ensure that athletes interpret information concerning the nature and rehabilitation of their injuries as useful, sports medicine professionals should provide accurate information (Petitpas & Danish, 1995) in language that athletes can understand. Misunderstanding information or experiencing apprehension because of the content of the sports medicine professional's message can sabotage a successful rehabilitation (Wagstaff, 1982), causing frustration for the athlete as well as the training staff.

The sports medicine professional must model **active listening** if the injured athlete is to be a good listener also. Active listening demonstrates that the receiver is concerned about the content, intent, and feeling expressed in the message (Rosenfeld & Wilder, 1990) and requires full participation by all parties involved. If sports medicine professionals expect athletes to hear and understand messages, they must reciprocate active listening behavior and attempt to fully comprehend the athletes' messages. Paraphrasing and asking questions to guarantee accurate understanding of the message provides insights and builds essential rapport. Active listening also involves the use of nonverbal communication to express comprehension and empathy (e.g., making eye contact, leaning forward, and nodding). When the message is not understood, nonverbal cues (e.g., puzzled look, head tilt, body shift) can alert the sender to be more specific, or the situation may require the listener to ask for clarification.

active listening—Listening that demonstrates that the receiver is concerned about the content, intent, and feeling expressed in the message.

Some of the listening skills that promote verbal interaction include the following (Kottler & Brown, 1996; Kottler & Kottler, 1993):

- *Active listening.* Attending to all the messages, both verbal and nonverbal.
- *Parroting.* Repeating the athlete's words to indicate interest or evaluate the accuracy of what was heard.
- *Paraphrasing.* Restating the communication to clarify or to focus attention.
- *Reflection of feeling.* Focusing on the emotional content of messages.

The following case study provides an example of how good attending skills can improve the outcome of interactions. In the original scenario the attending skills are not particularly strong, but they are strengthened in the alternative scenario.

Case Study: Attending Skills

It was Erin's senior year of college, and she was getting close to graduation. As co-captain of the softball team, it was her chance to finish her college career on a high note. After a frustrating season with many cancellations due to weather, her team was finally playing in the state tournament as one of the favorites to win. In a crucial game, a defensive play developed for which she had prepared all year. It was Erin's job to cover third base in a bunt situation. Charging in from her left field position, she was there in time and in good position, straddling the bag and ready to make the tag. The throw was on the money, and Erin's team had the runner dead in her tracks. Little did Erin suspect, however, that the runner would intentionally launch herself into a headfirst tackle and take her out of the play. Erin went down with a knee injury and was out for the remainder of the state tournament. Her injury was evaluated by an athletic trainer and a physician.

Scenario in Which Poor Attending Skills Are Used

Although she was clearly concerned and wanted to know, neither of the medical professionals told her whether she would risk more serious injury by continuing to play. "Just ice your knee three times per day, and keep this immobilizer on when you are walking around" is all the doctor told her. She traveled with the team the next week to the regional tournament. The athletic trainer had her run some figure-eight drills and then asked her whether or not she wanted to play in the game. "I don't know, what do you think?" Erin asked tentatively. The athletic trainer just shrugged his shoulders and said, "It's up to you." Although Erin desperately wanted to play, her knee still caused her quite a bit of pain, so she knew that she was not at full capacity. She also didn't know what was wrong with her knee and whether she would damage it further by playing. Erin decided that the team would be better served by playing her backup, Stephanie, who was at full strength but was just a freshman. Her coach listened quietly as Erin said, "I think that Stephanie should start the game in my place, since it is important for us to win this game." The coach therefore started Stephanie in her spot. Erin got the distinct feeling that rather than interpreting her actions the way she intended them—as a sacrifice of personal desire to do what she thought was best for the team—the coach, athletic trainer, and her teammates saw her as a wimp who couldn't play with pain. No one said much to Erin on the bench, even though she was cheering her loudest for the team. She sat out one game—which her team lost—but then asked to be put in the lineup for the next game because she wanted so desperately to play in what was probably the final game of her career.

Questions for Analysis

1. What concerns did Erin have that the athletic trainer did not address in his response following the functional evaluation?

2. What message was Erin trying to convey that the coach didn't hear?

Scenario in Which Good Attending Skills Are Used

"Erin, you have sprained your lateral collateral ligament [Erin was a physical education major and had taken an anatomy class, so she knew where this was], but I don't think that there is damage to the rest of the knee," said the physician. The athletic trainer told her, "You should ice your knee three times per day, and keep this immobilizer on when you are walking around. I'll check in on you once a day to see how the knee is doing." Erin traveled with the team the next week to the regional tournament. The athletic trainer had her run some straight run and jog drills, completed other functional evaluations, then told Erin that in his opinion she was okay to play in the game—if she felt up to it—without risking further damage to her knee. He suggested that Erin had the option of wearing a knee brace if she felt more confident with one on. Although Erin desperately wanted to play, her knee still caused her quite a bit of pain, so she knew that she was not at full capacity. She wasn't quite sure what to do. Erin finally decided that perhaps the team would be better served by playing her backup, Stephanie, who was at full strength but was just a freshman. Her coach listened quietly as Erin said, "I think that Stephanie should start the game in my place, since it is important for us to win this game." The coach replied, "I can certainly respect your decision. Is it that you don't feel that your knee is ready to go?" Erin responded, "Well, that's part of it, but I also think that it would be cocky of me to think that my play, even when I am injured, is better than Stephanie's. I just want to do what is best for the team." "Well, Erin," said the coach, "I think that the team would best be served by having you, the co-captain, in the game, if you feel up to playing." The athletic trainer provided an encouraging nod as Erin said, "In that case, I'd like to play. But perhaps I'll wear that knee brace just to be sure."

Being a good attender requires adhering to the following principles. When an athlete opens up and shares personal thoughts and feelings, avoid making value judgments. Even if the athlete discusses the same issues every day, demonstrate patience and empathy. Athletes trust their sports medicine professionals and tend to confide issues pertaining to their personal lives as well as to their injuries. Remember, the shared information is confidential, and violating an athlete's privacy could interfere with successful rehabilitation (*Trainers* staff, 1993) and your future relationship with that athlete.

Responding and Action Skills

Once the nature of the concern or problem is established via effective attending skills, responding and action skills are needed to help athletes chart their courses of action for dealing with these issues. The goal at this stage of interaction is to help athletes create more options for successful outcomes, both physical and psychological.

Action skills most appropriate for sports medicine professionals include the following (Kottler & Brown, 1996; Kottler & Kottler, 1993):

- *Reframing.* Helping the athlete think about things in a different light.
- *Goal setting.* Establishing a direction and providing a basis for measuring progress.
- *Problem solving.* Defining the problem, specifying the goals, developing constructive alternatives, evaluating the viability of alternatives and narrowing choices to the most viable, and putting the plan into action.
- *Reinforcement.* Supporting and encouraging desirable behaviors.
- *Directives.* Giving instructions for change.

Interaction Timeline

The foundational elements and basic interaction skills just described guide specific interactions within the sports medicine context. Table 4.6 illustrates some specific recommendations for the times and contents of certain interactions between the sports medicine professional and athlete. The sports medicine professional must be conscious not only of the content of communication at these times, but also of the manner in which information is communicated.

Another strategy that might be helpful in enhancing the quality of interactions between sports medicine professionals and athletes is to ask the athletes to record their thoughts, feelings, and behaviors on an injury timeline, such as that pictured in figure 4.2. This schematic can serve as a basis for discussions that provide a better understanding of the athlete's frame of reference. It also provides a way for athletes to document for themselves changes—and hopefully improvement—in their mental and physical status.

Table 4.6 Interaction Outline for Sports Medicine Professionals

Key incident or time frame	Athlete's possible thoughts and feelings	Interaction with athlete
Preinjury (preventive)	Concerns in other areas of life Lack of support network outside of sport Overwhelmed with school and sport demands	Communicate concern and interest in individual, both as an athlete and as a person. Encourage communication of life stress or other concerns so that appropriate help can be sought before it becomes problematic.
Immediately after injury	Realization of loss Fear Unawareness of injury Embarrassment	Use a calm, controlled communication style. Take charge of the situation, giving directions to teammates and others.
Initial injury evaluation	Concern over extent of injury Uneasiness with sports medicine practitioner Fear of pain Worry about goal achievement being disrupted	Ask athletes to rephrase and summarize what they have heard. Use active listening techniques. Consider the athlete's frame of reference. Give examples of athletes who have recovered successfully from this type of injury.
Presurgery	Uncertainty about ability to cope Need for information about what is going to happen Desire to discuss success rates and possible negative consequences	Provide informative communication regarding injury and surgical procedures. Allow for plenty of questions. Alleviate fears as reasonable.

(continued)

Table 4.6 *(continued)*

Key incident or time frame	Athlete's possible thoughts and feelings	Interaction with athlete
		Reassure athletes that they are receiving skilled care.
Postsurgery	Concern for success of surgical intervention	Provide information on success of surgical intervention.
	Worries about managing day-to-day tasks, such as transportation	Clarify what to expect in terms of pain, mobility, approximate rehabilitation timeline.
During rehabilitation	Boredom with routine	Provide plenty of encouragement.
	Feeling that progress is limited	Evaluate goal attainment and revise goals as needed.
	Thinking him- or herself ready to return to sport even though not allowed	Provide variety in rehabilitative exercises and settings.
During rehabilitative plateaus	Frustration with lack of progress	Refocus on goal achievement to date.
	Discouragement	Reassure athlete that plateaus in rehabilitation are normal.
	Desire to give up	

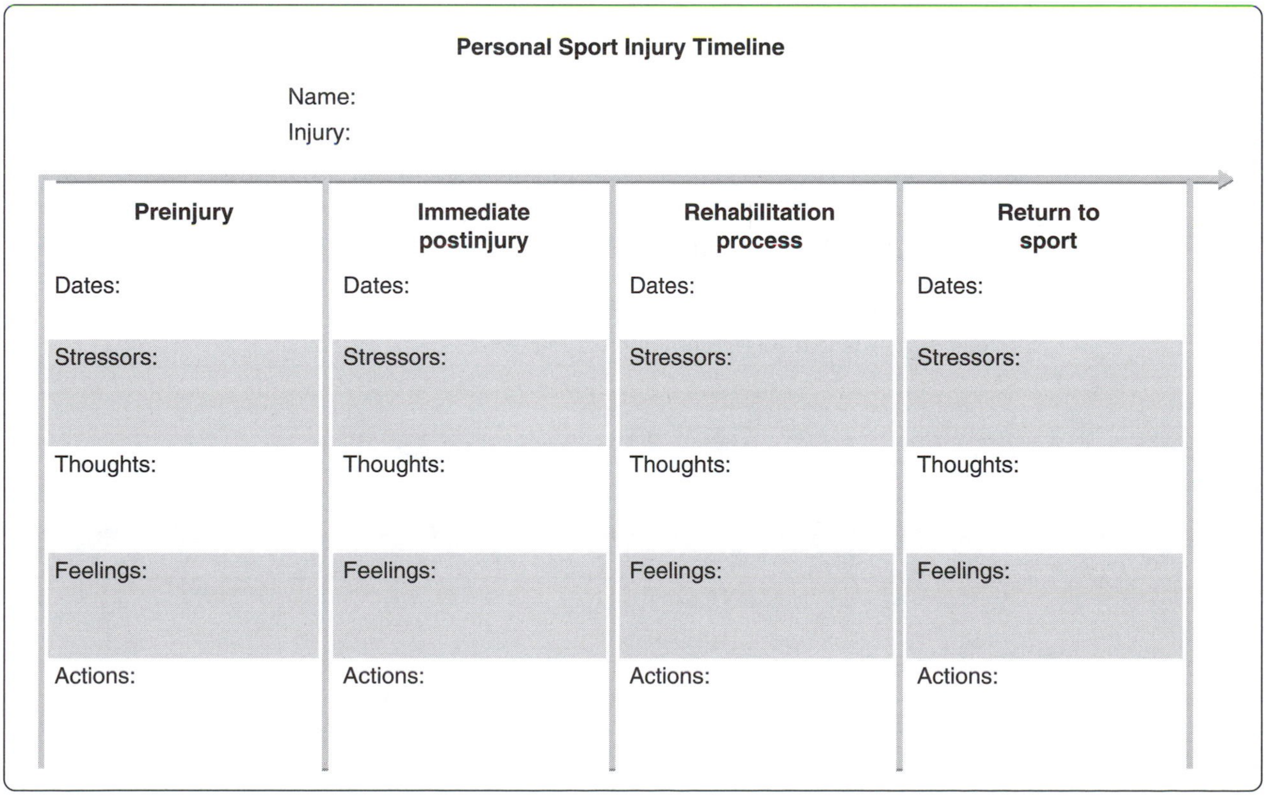

Personal Sport Injury Timeline

Name:

Injury:

Preinjury	Immediate postinjury	Rehabilitation process	Return to sport
Dates:	Dates:	Dates:	Dates:
Stressors:	Stressors:	Stressors:	Stressors:
Thoughts:	Thoughts:	Thoughts:	Thoughts:
Feelings:	Feelings:	Feelings:	Feelings:
Actions:	Actions:	Actions:	Actions:

Figure 4.2 Personal sport injury timeline.

CASE STUDY

It's Thursday afternoon, and Alex, a college freshman soccer player, comes into the training room for treatment of his injured ankle. He experienced a second-degree inversion sprain in last night's game and has expressed that he is "fine" and would like to practice with the team this afternoon. He has a game on Saturday against a very physical team and is determined to play despite his physical status. Mary, the athletic trainer for Alex's team, explains to him that this injury will require rest and rehabilitation for at least one to two weeks. "When I evaluated your injury last night, the bony and soft tissue palpation indicated localized swelling and joint effusion about the medial and lateral malleoli. The positive anterior drawer test suggested that you sprained your anterior talofibular and calcaneofibular ligaments. Returning to practice too soon could cause more structural damage." Alex, frustrated and confused, looks at Mary but doesn't say anything. After explaining the medical reasons for needing rest, Mary describes what his treatment protocol will be for the week. Alex begins to do the exercises prescribed, but Mary notices that he is doing them incorrectly. She asks if everything is okay. Alex states that he is not sure why he is doing these exercises because they don't seem to be helping and asks when he can return to practice.

QUESTIONS FOR ANALYSIS

1. What nonverbal messages are being sent?

2. What information do you think Alex has obtained from this interaction?

3. Based on your understanding of communication, what do you think Mary should have done differently in this situation?

4. What steps can be taken to ensure Alex's return and compliance to the treatment protocol?

5. How can Mary respond empathically to Alex's final statements?

SUMMARY

Strong interaction skills are central to the work of sports medicine professionals. Rapport, empathy, and trust provide the foundation upon which effective sports medicine interactions can be based. A knowledge of both verbal and nonverbal communication helps achieve effective communication. Proficiency in the actual skills of interaction further enhances the ability of the sports medicine professional to facilitate both physical and psychological recoveries.

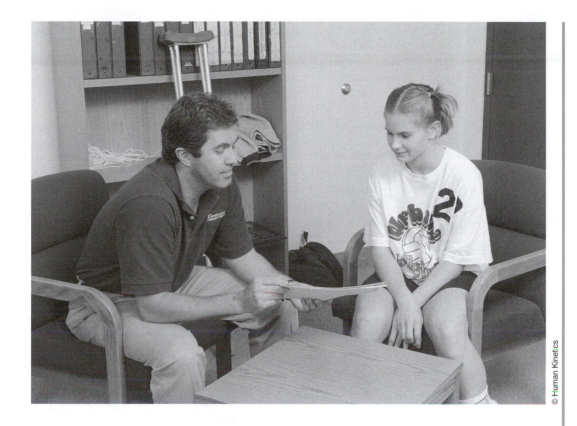

© Human Kinetics

Assessing Athletes Through Individual Interview

Aynsley M. Smith, RN, PhD, *Mayo Clinic Sports Medicine Center*

CHAPTER OBJECTIVES

Describe the purposes of assessment interviews of injured athletes

Specify the personal and professional characteristics essential for sports medicine professionals who wish to become effective in sports medicine counseling

List psychosocial circumstances that might impede a successful therapeutic relationship between the injured athlete and the sports medicine professional

Identify aspects of the sports medicine counseling environment likely to facilitate an effective interview with an injured athlete

Describe how the Emotional Responses of Athletes to Injury Questionnaire: Sports Medicine Professional Form (ERAIQ-SMP) serves as a guide for an assessment interview with an injured athlete *assessment interview*—The assessment interview is usually a one-on-one session between an injured athlete and a sports medicine professional or other counselor. Its purpose is to learn the psychosocial aspects of injury, in contrast to the history and physical examination that the injured athlete receives from the physician or athletic trainer.

The objective of this chapter is to provide guidelines for counseling **assessment interviews**. The impressions formed based on these interviews provide blueprints for verbal interactions between sports medicine professionals and injured athletes. Inherent in these interactions is the necessity to recognize when to refer athletes for professional counseling. Guidelines for making referrals to mental health professionals are presented in chapter 8. It is imperative that sports medicine professionals recognize and accept their limitations in the counseling domain and seek referrals when necessary.

Specifically, this chapter describes factors pertinent to effective assessment interviews. These include characteristics of the counselor, counseling styles used, assessment tools, barriers to effective interviews, and the ideal counseling atmosphere. A detailed discussion of an assessment tool is presented using case examples to illustrate athletes' possible responses. Suicidal ideation is discussed, including a chart on impressions of the status of injured athletes, which lists an overview of interventions suitable for injured athletes. This chapter concludes by suggesting how to evaluate the effectiveness of interventions instituted (i.e., outcomes).

DECISIONS TO MAKE ABOUT THE ASSESSMENT INTERVIEW

To conduct an effective assessment interview, the sports medicine professional must make several important decisions before the actual interview. These include clearly identifying the purposes of the interview, determining which athletes would benefit from an interview, and structuring the who, when, and where of the actual interview setting in order to enhance the **counseling environment**.

counseling environment—The milieu or gestalt of the setting in which the counseling interview is conducted. It pertains to the feeling generated by both personnel and the physical surroundings. The counseling environment for injured athletes should be comfortable and nonthreatening. The athlete should feel respected and valued in the ideal counseling environment.

Purpose of the Interview

The major purpose of an assessment interview with an injured athlete is to gain insight into the meaning of the injury to the athlete. The assessment interview provides the sports medicine professional or sport psychology counselor with an understanding of the athlete's dreams, preferred sports, motivation for participation, perceived athleticism, cognition about the injury, sport goals, sources of pressure, social support, and emotional response to injury. During the interview, the person conducting the assessment can also query concerns tangential to the injury, which may have prompted the interview or referral (e.g., drug use, eating patterns, etc.) Based on the assessment interview, the sports medicine professional can arrange for necessary consultation or initiate appropriate interventions to help the athlete cope with injury.

Which Injured Athletes to Interview

In our practice at the Mayo Clinic Sports Medicine Center, physicians are the sports medicine professionals who conduct the initial physical examination and obtain the athlete's medical history and the history of the injury. If obvious emotional distress (such as feelings of anger, depression, frustration, fear of reinjury, a sense of violation, lack of compliance to the rehabilitation program, drug or alcohol abuse, a history of sexual abuse, an eating disorder, or exercise addiction) is suspected, the athlete is referred to the sport psychology counselor. In other sports medicine settings, the athletic trainer or physical therapist may conduct these examinations and is observant of emotional distress symptoms.

Who Should Conduct the Interview

Sports medicine professionals who work in settings where they perform the initial evaluation should conduct the assessment interview with athletes about whom they are concerned for reasons such as those previously mentioned. In practices where a sport psychology counselor is available (such as sports medicine clinics or university settings), the athlete can be referred to the sport psychology counselor for a screening evaluation.

When to Conduct the Interview

The assessment interview should be conducted after the injured athlete is examined physically, the diagnosis has been established, and initial treatment and comfort measures have been instituted. Injured athletes should be interviewed when they are relatively comfortable physically and, ideally, cognizant of the injury and its consequences.

Where to Conduct the Interview

Unlike the history and physical examination conducted by the sports medicine professional, which is often performed in the presence of significant others, the sport psychology assessment interview is most effective when only the injured athlete and interviewer are present.

Although subject to time constraints, I usually use the Emotional Responses of Athletes to Injury Questionnaire (**ERAIQ**, developed after open-ended interview with hundreds of injured athletes) by asking the questions and recording the answers. I thus can also depart from the structured questionnaire to query areas of concern that might affect the athlete's rehabilitation. The questionnaire, however, can also be completed by the athlete, and then the sports medicine professional can review the responses and form an impression (see ERAIQ-SMP Form, figure 5.1).

COUNSELING STYLES USED DURING THE ASSESSMENT INTERVIEW PROCESS

ERAIQ—The Emotional Responses of Athletes to Injury Questionnaire serves as a guide for the psychosocial assessment of an injured athlete. It has been used in several research projects and in a sports medicine practice.

As in general counseling psychology, most sport psychology counselors rely on a few counseling theories and methods in which they have developed expertise. For example, counselors may use either a humanistic, rational emotive, developmental, psychodynamic, social-learning, or behavioral-therapy orientation in the counseling situation. A brief comment on the emphasis inherent in each of these counseling theories is helpful in understanding the role of the counselor.

- *Humanistic psychology* counselors emphasize that the individual has the capacity to choose his or her life pattern and to reach greater fulfillment and maturity. This theory seeks to understand behavior in terms of its meaning to the individual.

- *Cognitive psychology* counseling theory emphasizes the processes of thinking (remembering and knowing). Counseling helps the athlete think through the meaning of the injury, its consequences, and its conclusions.

- *Rational emotive therapy (RET)* is based in the theoretical belief that people are born with the potential to be both rational and irrational. It is the tendency to be irrational that causes problems. RET is cognitive, action directed, and disciplined; involves homework; and is often hardheaded or confrontational. Nevertheless, it is often most effective in accomplishing its goals in less time and in fewer sessions than many other counseling methods.

- *Developmental psychology* counseling focuses on the physical cognition and social changes that occur across maturation or throughout the life cycle. For example, consideration of the influence of adolescence on a 14-year-old's response to injury might use developmental counseling.

Emotional Responses of Athletes to Injury Questionnaire:

Sports Medicine Professional Form

Name _____ Age _____ Date ___/___/___

Address _____ Phone _____

City _____ State _____ Zip _____

Sport _____ Position _____

Level of participation _____

---

1. What you want to do or be in life _____

_____

2. List your preferred sports and activities _____

   1. _____ 2. _____ 3. _____ 4. _____

3. Why do you participate in sports?

   Rank order of all that apply in descending order of importance (#1 is your most important reason)

   ___ Stress management   ___ Fun   ___ Earn scholarship

   ___ Weight management   ___ Fitness   ___ Socialization

   ___ Personal improvement   ___ Competition   ___ Livelihood

   ___ Pursue excellence   ___ Other   ___ Keep scholarship

4. Would you describe yourself as an athlete? (circle one)

   1   2   3   4   5   6   7   8   9   10

   Absolutely not   Somewhat so   Absolutely yes

5. When did your injury occur?

   ___ Off-season   ___ Pre-season   ___ Mid-season   ___ End of season

   Date of injury ___/___/___

6. What type of injury did you have? _____

7. What sport were you injured in? _____

   What do you think was the major cause of your injury? _____

8. What goals do you have in sports? _____

9. Who exerts most of the pressure on you in sports?

   ___ Self ___ Coach ___ Mother ___ Father ___ No one

10. Do you have a support system of persons who know about your injury?

   ___ Yes ___ No

   If yes, who can you count on for support?

   ___ Coach ___ Friends ___ Teammates ___ Family ___ Other

(continued)

11. Is your injury the major source of stress in your life right now?

___ Yes ___ No

If no, what is?

12. List the emotions you have been feeling since the injury:
    1. _____ 2. _____ 3. _____ 4. _____

13. If 0% is no recovery and 100% is fully recovered, what percentage of physical recovery have you made relative to your preinjury physical status?

    0%   10%   20%   30%   40%   50%   60%   70%   80%   90%   100%

14. Are you a motivated person for rehabilitation exercises?

    1   2   3   4   5   6   7   8   9   10

    Not at all   Moderately   Extremely

15. Would you like to see a professional sports counselor to assist you with the emotional or psychological aspects of your injury or return to sport competition?

    ___ Yes ___ No

If yes, would you like assistance with a referral to an appropriate counselor?

    ___ Yes ___ No

Figure 5.1 Emotional Responses of Athletes to Injury Questionnaire: Sports Medicine Professional Form.

Modified with permission from *Sports Medicine,* December, 1996, p. 403. © Adis International Limited.

- *Psychodynamic counseling* is based on Freud's idea that behavior arises from unconscious drives and conflicts from childhood. This theory is usually better suited to long-term problems that require psychoanalysis and is less appropriate for problems that can likely be resolved in two or three counseling sessions (a goal for most counselors).

- *Social-learning* counselors work on the premise that most behaviors are learned, modeled, and reinforced by significant others. Therefore social-learning counselors might work with the coach, family, or teammates to alter behaviors.

- *Behavioral psychology* counselors are concerned about how behaviors are learned, reinforced, or extinguished. These counselors are concerned about motivation and often use goals and reinforcement for changing behaviors.

Frequently, counselors combine aspects or properties from several theories in what is known as an eclectic style. For example, in my practice during the assessment phase I generally use a humanistic (Rogerian) approach, which is based on nonjudgmental, unconditional positive regard. Within that counseling style, I also use behavioral contingencies and RET. I refer injured athletes most often to a psychodynamically oriented psychiatrist when their problem surpasses my expertise or counseling skills. Generally, these injured athletes are very depressed and often need short-term antidepressant therapy or in-depth psychotherapy. Although the psychiatrist has a psychodynamic background, clinically he is a gifted doctor who is usually able to make a very accurate, expedient diagnosis and to guide interventions appropriately.

FACTORS THAT PROMOTE AN EFFECTIVE ASSESSMENT INTERVIEW

Both the professional and personal characteristics of sports medicine professionals influence the quality of their counseling relationships with athletes. Recognizing that individual sports medicine professionals have various strengths and styles, the subsequent sections identify some of the characteristics thought most related to initiating and maintaining an effective relationship.

Personal Characteristics of the Counselor

A sport psychology counselor or a sports medicine professional who conducts assessment interviews of injured athletes appreciates that psychology is the science of behavior and mental processes. The art of psychology is the ability to establish a therapeutic relationship and depends greatly on being accepting and nonjudgmental. Sports medicine professionals are effective at conducting assessment interviews if they are truly interested in the injured athlete, are good listeners, and recognize that it is important to understand the meaning of injury to the athlete. Developing a reputation for maintaining confidentiality and objectivity are essential to a successful relationship.

Professional Characteristics of the Counselor

All sports medicine professionals should have a foundation in anatomy, physiology, biomechanics, epidemiology of injury, mechanism of injury, and pathophysiology. Although not all sports medicine professionals are physicians, physical therapists, or athletic trainers, it is essential to be knowledgeable about treatment options, potential outcomes, the healing process, and general rehabilitation procedures. Because most sports medicine professionals understand the nature of injury, the optimal outcome, and the likelihood of the athlete returning to his or her sport or position, they also have insight into whether the athlete's psychological response to injury is realistic, overly optimistic, or pessimistic. By having a realistic understanding of an injured athlete's potential to return to highly demanding or recreational sport and of the possible fears associated with returning to specific sport situations, the sports medicine professional will be able to intervene effectively or make referrals as necessary.

All sports medicine professionals should be positive, cohesive members of a sports medicine team. Most injured athletes are cared for either in a medical center or in an athletic training room. Either way, most athletes have a physician, a physical therapist, an athletic trainer, or all three involved in their care. It is imperative that sports medicine professionals who counsel athletes have a genuine respect for the contributions that other members of the team make to the process of rehabilitation from injury. A positive relationship among members on the team fosters the confidence that injured athletes have in all members of the sports medicine team.

Establishing the Counseling Relationship Before the Assessment Interview

To establish a counseling relationship, it is important to shake hands and make eye contact when introducing yourself to the injured athlete and to explain your role as a sports medicine professional. Briefly mention your affiliation with the team or academic institution, credentials, strengths, and limitations, and explain the purpose of the counseling interview. Usually, the first priority is to explore the psychosocial impact of the injury and to determine how these factors affected or may affect injury occurrence and rehabilitation. A second purpose of the interview is to help provide coping strategies that will optimize the athlete's recovery from injury. It is necessary to clarify that the discussion can be either confidential if the athlete prefers or, at the athlete's discretion, shared with other physicians, athletic trainers, physical therapists, or mental health practitioners on the sports medicine team. The only situations or exceptions to this general rule of confidentiality are thoughts and feelings experienced by the injured athlete that have the potential to harm the injured athlete or others.

Privacy

The assessment interview should take place when the injured athlete has the interviewer's individual attention during the session. Background noise, distractions, frequent interruptions, and threats to privacy are barriers to a meaningful interview and are troubling to the injured athlete.

It is therefore ideal if the sports medicine professional conducts the interview away from other injured athletes or training room personnel who might overhear the conversation. When no empty office is available, the sports medicine professional can take the injured athlete to a nearby examining room or a cafeteria to interview. Ideally, injured athletes should be interviewed alone. Occasionally—due to the teaching responsibilities of the sports medicine professional—the injured athlete may be asked to grant permission to include in the interview a qualified observer, such as a student athletic trainer, physical therapist, or medical student.

I rarely ask an injured athlete to grant permission to include an observer if I anticipate a need to question the athlete about sensitive issues (e.g., suspected alcohol or drug use, sexual abuse, suicidal ideation). Injured athletes may not answer questions honestly if they fear they are being judged by a stranger in the observer's chair. Furthermore, if an observer is present during an interview and I suspect a need to query a sensitive topic, I might gently excuse the observer, to create an atmosphere of total acceptance or unconditional positive regard.

Counseling Atmosphere

In an ideal counseling situation the chairs are the same size, with no "power seats." If possible, avoid a room where a large, ominous desk separates you from the injured athlete. To convey the sense that the injured athlete and the sports medicine professional are on the same team, they should each occupy the same space in the room, share a work table, and both have pens. It is important to ensure that the injured athlete is comfortable (offer to elevate an injured knee or foot or get an ice bag) so that both can concentrate on the interview.

A third person granted permission to witness the interview must be instructed on confidentiality and advised to be a quiet observer. In my practice I explain to the observer that I will angle my chair and body away from the observer and toward the injured athlete to exclude the observer and more effectively include the athlete in the one-on-one interview process. If the observer is drawn into the interview process, it becomes distracting, and issues important to the injured athlete and the sports medicine professional may not get addressed.

Demonstrating Respect

It is advisable that phone calls be held and pagers be turned off to avoid disruptions during the interview, as both are annoying to the injured athlete and distracting to the sports medicine professional. Furthermore, disruptions interrupt the flow of the interview. For practical reasons, a clock should be visible so that there is no need to look at a watch during the interview. Also, if the sports medicine professional plans to use questionnaires, forms, or handouts, they should be ready. This courtesy conveys organization and respect for the injured athlete and the interview process.

Generally, it is helpful at the end of the interview to ask the injured athlete whether subjects or concerns were discussed that should not be shared with the coaches or with other members of the sports medicine team. By giving the athlete control over what information should be shared, you convey to injured athletes the importance of their role as captain of their own sports medicine team. It is critical to avoid value-laden responses such as "bad," "good," "right," or "wrong" during the interview. Maintaining a professional, unbiased demeanor projects to the athlete your willingness to accept any thoughts or feelings that the athlete is experiencing, which enhances the likelihood that the athlete will be honest and direct.

After completing the assessment interview, depending on my clinical judgment, I might opt to use the **Profile of Mood States** (POMS) to quantify the magnitude of the injury's impact in greater depth (McNair, Lorr, & Droppleman, 1971). The POMS has subscales for measuring tension, depression, anger, vigor, fatigue, and confusion. If I choose to use the POMS, I graph the results and discuss them with the injured athlete in terms of the degree of mood disturbance and what methods or therapeutic strategies would best serve the athlete.

Profile of Mood States (POMS)— A psychological inventory that assesses six individual moods states (tension, depression, anxiety, vigor, fatigue, and confusion). These may be combined to create a total mood disturbance (TMD) score.

FACTORS THAT IMPEDE AN EFFECTIVE ASSESSMENT INTERVIEW

The previous section identified some of the factors most critical to an effective counseling relationship, but it is also important to recognize some of the potential barriers to a successful working relationship. These include the athlete's circumstances, the sports medicine professional's circumstances, and environmental circumstances. Some of these barriers are identified and discussed next.

Athlete's Circumstances

therapeutic counseling relationship—The interaction or relationship between two people in which the goal is to provide assistance to the client. This relationship may be directed at helping the client solve problems, understand feelings, or become motivated for a rehabilitation program.

There are several circumstances or personality characteristics of injured athletes that have the potential to make a **therapeutic counseling relationship** between the athlete and the sports medicine professional difficult. For example, if there is pending litigation relating to the athlete's present injury, the injured athlete's conscious or unconscious secondary gains may prevent the athlete from giving 100 percent effort to the rehabilitation regimen. Unfortunately, even though such athletes may express sincerity in wanting a full recovery, they may be financially rewarded by the courts for lasting sequelae or physical damage from which they are "unable" to recover. This situation is becoming more frequent and is too often the explanation for malingering that occurs when athletes achieve less than the anticipated recovery.

Injured athletes may have obsessive-compulsive disorders, exercise addiction, drug addiction, eating disorders, steroid abuse difficulties, or other psychological or psychiatric problems. Although some of these athletes can be assisted to optimal recovery, establishing an effective therapeutic relationship with them usually requires a highly skilled, experienced counselor. In most cases, these injured athletes will benefit from a referral to a clinical sport psychologist, a clinical psychologist, or a psychiatrist (see chapter 8).

Injured athletes suspected of malingering for reasons such as rationalizing the loss of starting status, offsetting realizations of insufficient ability, offsetting expectations of others, or attracting attention (Rotella and Heyman, 1993) may resist the efforts of the sports medicine professionals who are dedicated to promoting their optimal rehabilitation and return to sport. Often these athletes may need a sport psychologist to help them understand that their behavior is indeed malingering. Once the athlete understands what is happening and why, he or she may be counseled successfully on disengagement from sport.

Sports Medicine Professional's Circumstances

When the sports medicine professional is employed by the same institution that granted the athlete a scholarship or employs the injured athlete, conflicts of interest may arise to impede a therapeutic counseling relationship. For example, owners, coaches, and management might pressure the sports medicine professional to "get the athlete back to competition fast" for reasons of gate receipts, play-offs, or championship games. The implication is that the sports medicine professional's job is on the line if the injured athlete is not rehabilitated promptly. In these circumstances, the sports medicine professional may have difficulty maintaining confidentiality or earning the trust of the injured athlete. Understandably, the injured athlete in this situation will have difficulty being honest about fears of reinjury, burnout, or performance anxiety. The sports medicine professional may need to refer the athlete to an objective mental health professional.

Another difficult circumstance or impediment to a counseling relationship occurs when the sports medicine professional does not respect or like the injured athlete, or vice versa. Although this occurs rarely, if the injured athlete senses disapproval, it is unlikely that a therapeutic relationship will develop. In this situation sports medicine professionals must recognize their feelings and refer the athlete when appropriate.

Environmental Considerations

The physical environment of the interview can prove to be an enhancement to the counseling process or a barrier if not carefully attended to. Thus it is important for the sports medicine professional to pay careful consideration to establishing an environment conducive to an effective interview with the injured athlete.

USING THE ERAIQ-SMP FORM TO GUIDE THE ASSESSMENT INTERVIEW

Unless there are unusual circumstances (e.g., major time constraints), the ERAIQ-SMP might best be used in a semistructured interview format: Ask the athlete questions while observing his or her affect, interest, and verbal energy, and jot down the answers on the form. Additional questions can be asked that build on issues that you detect as important to the injured athlete. The injured athlete can also complete the form and review the answers with the sports medicine professional if time does not permit the interview to be conducted in the preferred manner. If depression is observed or offered on question 12 of the ERAIQ-SMP form, the Profile of Mood States (POMS) might be administered by a sport psychology counselor, if available. Some sport psychology counselors administer the Beck Depression Inventory (BDI). The choice of which objective measure of depression to use depends on the counselor's preference, training, and experience.

The ERAIQ (Smith, Scott, & Wiese, 1990) queries critical components of the Wiese-Bjornstal and Smith model (Wiese-Bjornstal & Smith, 1993; Wiese-Bjornstal, Smith, & LaMott, 1995). The ERAIQ is used clinically in our sports medicine practice to assess the emotional responses of athletes to injury. Research on the responses of athletes to injury has been integrated into the response-to-injury model (see figure 2.3 on p. 32). Although the original form was developed to assess the injured athlete more comprehensively in relation to the Wiese-Bjornstal et al. (1995) model, a short form—labeled the Emotional Responses of Athletes to Injury Questionnaire: Sports Medicine Professional Form (ERAIQ-SMP; see figure 5.1)—is suggested for use by sports medicine professionals because of their time-management challenges. The short form is an appropriate guide for a relevant yet expedient interview.

Characteristics of the ERAIQ-SMP

The questions are designed so that some are open ended, some are closed, and some involve ranking or rating. The questions purposely progress from relatively impersonal to more personal; the more personal questions are comfortably addressed later in the interview process. The questions apply generically to all athletes and provide a starting place for most interviews, regardless of the athlete's specific injury, level of participation, sport, or position on the team.

The general content areas addressed by the ERAIQ-SMP are the preinjury factors—such as personality, coping resources, and history of stress (Andersen & Williams, 1988)—and personal and situational characteristics—such as motivational orientation or time in season—that moderate athlete responses (Wiese-Bjornstal & Smith, 1993; Wiese-Bjornstal et al. 1995). The ERAIQ-SMP assesses the response-to-injury components of the model (see figure 2.3 on p. 32), which are designated cognitive appraisal, emotional response, and behavioral response.

The sports medicine professional must be familiar with the strengths and weaknesses of this assessment tool (Smith, 1996; Wiese-Bjornstal & Smith, 1993). At the end of the interview the information gathered must be assimilated into a working hypothesis or a general impression of the injured athlete's status so that decisions for future recommendations can be made.

Content Assessed by Specific Questions

Answers to the first question can provide the sports medicine professional with insight into the injured athlete's dreams, values, and priorities. An athlete who feels manipulated or pressured in sport frequently can be identified from the answer to the first question. Pressure from others may be evident if the response provided differs markedly from what was anticipated.

Case Example: Response to Question 1

A 13-year-old gymnast trained in three cities in three years with different coaches. She acknowledged that gymnastics at the Olympic level had been a dream when she was six, but it was not her dream any longer. For the past few years it was the dream of her mother and coach only. She felt trapped. Her dream now was to be a lawyer.

The second question assesses the athlete's sport and activity preferences. When the content of the answer to question 2 is viewed with the answers to questions 5 and 7, the sports medicine professional can see how the injured athlete prioritizes specific sports and activities and whether the injury occurred during the on- or off-season of the athlete's most-preferred activity. Knowing, for example, that football is a favorite (question 2) and knowing the injury was sustained in midseason (question 5), the sports medicine professional can appreciate not only the time in the season, but also that the injury occurred during the athlete's most-preferred activity. The following example illustrates how important it is to understand the value the injured athlete assigns to a specific sport.

Case Example: Response to Question 2

A high school junior was experiencing severe low-back pain. Although the injury occurred to this fine athlete during basketball season, his preferred activities were fly fishing, playing guitar, and skiing. Basketball was at the end of his list of interests. Because he was tall, skilled, strong, fast, and a success in basketball, it was expected that he participate. Actually, he hated basketball, and the stress he experienced from participating aggravated his already tight, sore back muscles. On his second visit, the sports medicine professional counseled him to disengage from basketball and provided strategies to help him tell his parents and coach. Specifically, relaxation and imagery of his meeting with his coach and parents were paired to desensitize him before these confrontations. He role played the senario in the presence of the counselor and gradually gained a sense of control.

The third question provides the sports medicine professional with insight into why the athlete participates in sport and addresses the athlete's motivation. Earning a scholarship, maintaining a scholarship, or earning one's livelihood were added to the ERAIQ-SMP form for those sports medicine professionals who work with college or professional athletes. The astute sports medicine professional must be aware that information is also gleaned by recognizing omissions from anticipated responses. For example, athletes with eating disorders often rank weight management as the least important of their concerns when, in fact, they are plagued incessantly with thoughts of food and worry obsessively about self-esteem, body size, and shape.

Case Example: Response to Question 3

A college cross-country runner referred by a sports physician because of stress fractures, obvious low body fat, and admitted amenorrhea ranked her reasons for running in the following manner: pursuit of excellence (10), personal improvement (9), fitness (8), competition (7), self-discipline (6), socialization (5), fun (4), outlet of aggression (3), stress management (2), and weight management (1). Clearly, weight management issues were dominating her eating and exercise patterns despite her attempt to deny its importance.

The fourth question assesses the degree to which athletes identify with sport or rate themselves in terms of perceived athleticism. It is not intended to assess how they feel that their coach or significant others view them as athletes. It assesses the degree to which the athlete's personal identity is intertwined with sport. This is important, as Brewer (1993) determined that self-identity in sport can influence **postinjury depression**. Morrey (1997) identified clear differences in rehabilitation progress related to whether athletes were recreational or competitive. Competitive athletes had greater range-of-motion gains and obtained higher physician ratings in the early postoperative period.

Case Example: Response to Question 4

An elite figure skater rated herself as a 4-5 on athleticism. She reminded the counselor that she was also an excellent student, was on the student council, and was very interested in friends and family. These interests and maintaining a balance in her life were important to her.

Question 5 asks when during the season the injury occurred, which assesses the sport-specific situational factor of time in the season, an important moderator of response to injury.

Question 6 assesses the nature of the injury, which addresses the cognitive appraisal aspects of the response-to-injury section of the global model (see figure 2.3 on p. 32). It is important that injured athletes understand pertinent details of their injuries so that they can appreciate what healing has to take place and the principles of their rehabilitation program.

By asking about the sport in which the athlete was injured and how it happened (question 7), the sports medicine professional obtains information about sport situ-

postinjury depression—Feelings such as despondency, discouragement, lack of motivation, and fatigue frequently experienced by athletes who have sustained a serious injury. This postinjury emotional disturbance often parallels the athlete's perceived recovery and frequently subsides approximately four weeks after injury.

ational factors, such as the injury context. Answers to this question provide information about the athlete's response to injury and may help identify potential fears that may be associated with the athlete's return to sport.

Case Example: Response to Question 7

An accomplished soccer player had played the game since he was a child. Soccer was a main source of friendships (socialization needs), stress management, fun, and fitness. He sustained a serious knee injury when an opponent aggressively ran at him deliberately intending to injure him. He did not anticipate returning to play after the rehabilitation, which augmented his sense of anger, loss, and depression. Therefore the perceived cause or context of injury greatly affected the young athlete's life and future play.

Question 8 asks about the athlete's specific goals in sport and alerts the sports medicine professional to the athlete's aspirations and plans in sport. It also may reflect the goal adjustment necessary as a consequence of the type and severity of the injury. The degree of goal adjustment necessary may have a significant impact on the athlete's emotional response to the injury.

Case Example: Response to Question 8

A senior in high school had a goal of playing professional hockey. He opted, after much deliberation, to go out for football. As a defensive end, he helped his team to the state finals. In the sectional play-offs he sustained a bad fracture to his leg, which required surgery and months of rest and rehabilitation. The injury occurred one week before he was to start captain's practices for hockey. He was the captain on a team that was in the final four of the state championship the year before. He felt guilty and depressed as he anticipated missing most of his final high school year—the year most players are scouted for a scholarship.

Case Example: Response to Question 8

A high school softball player tore her anterior cruciate ligament in her sophomore year and understood both the nature of the injury and the potential for joint laxity and further meniscal damage. She decided to have her knee reconstructed and set a realistic goal to return to softball as a senior and to play well enough to earn a college scholarship. This was an appropriate, rational cognitive response and a goal that she achieved after much hard work.

The answer to question 8 provides the sports medicine professional with an opportunity to assess the appropriateness of the athlete's appraisal of the type of injury sustained and the potential consequences. It is important to ensure congruency between the athlete's perception of the injury and the perception of the rest of the sports medicine team about the injury. In the soccer and football examples above, both injuries are classified as serious or severe and as such have the potential for marked postinjury depression (Leddy, Lambert, & Ogles, 1994; McDonald & Hardy, 1990; Smith, Scott, O'Fallon, & Young, 1990; Smith et al. 1993). While the softball injury was as serious, the athlete has responded in a healthy manner.

Question 9 helps the sports medicine professional understand the athlete's level of comfort in the sport and to determine to what extent significant others influence the athlete's choice or decision to participate.

Question 10 assesses the athlete's perception of having a social support network. It also permits the sports medicine professional to differentiate between a sport-related support system and the support extended by friends and family (Bianco & Orlick, 1996).

Question 11 gives the sports medicine professional insight into how athletes report on the stressors in their lives. For some injured athletes the injury is their major concern, whereas for others coaching pressure, finances, school work, or a personal relationship causes more stress than the injury.

An important question on the ERAIQ-SMP is question 12, the open-ended question about the athlete's emotional response to injury. This question is deliberately placed well into the interview so that a trusting relationship has been established and a candid response to this question can be anticipated. It is important to remember that a greater degree of depression is expected in athletes with more serious injuries because emotional responses to injury often parallel the athlete's perceived rating of recovery (McDonald & Hardy, 1990; Smith, Scott, O'Fallon, & Young, 1990). When depressed, discouraged, sad, blue, or a synonym is offered first or second, the sports medicine professional conducting the interview should assess in more depth the degree of depression experienced.

The sports medicine professional can gather additional information by noting the nonverbal cues emitted by the injured athlete, including facial expression, body language, posture, walk, and hand shake (see chapter 4 on nonverbal communication). It is also helpful to ask the injured athlete to take the word offered first or second, such as depression, sad, frustrated, or angry, and start a sentence with that word (e.g., "I am depressed because . . . " or "I am angry that . . . "). This allows athletes the opportunity to express the thought uppermost in their minds, which is often not the answer the sports medicine professional expects to hear.

Case Example: Response to Question 12

A young football player spent the off-season running, lifting weights, and cross-training. In the final scrimmage before the season opener he experienced a season-ending injury. During the interview he was very open in expressing his feelings of depression. When asked to start a sentence with depression, he said he was depressed that he had been "robbed" or "cheated" of the chance to perform, an opportunity he felt he deserved.

Case Example: Response to Question 12

Another young athlete acknowledged depression when his magnetic resonance image (MRI) did not show the ligament disruption anticipated. Because he hated his coach and was lonely at college, in his mind he felt that injury was a socially acceptable way out of sport.

Injured athletes who identify depression as the most bothersome emotion should be asked about symptoms of depression that relate to their eating habits, quality of sleep, exercise patterns, adherence to rehabilitation (exercise and program), recent changes in decision-making skills, and changes in social interactions.

Question 13 pertains to the percentage of recovery made. The athlete is asked to state the percentage of recovery, from 0 to 100 percent, that the athlete believes he or she has made. If the injury affects an arm, leg, or shoulder, the athlete can be asked, "What percentage of recovery has been made in comparison to your unaffected side?" This question addresses the cognitive appraisal and response section of the global model (see figure 2.3 on p. 32), specifically asking for the injured athlete's rating of perceived recovery.

Question 14 assesses the athlete's self-appraisal of his or her motivation to give priority and adhere to the rehabilitation regimen. This is important because the majority of sport injuries require a high degree of commitment by the athlete to achieve total recovery. Athletes who are not highly motivated perhaps can be assisted by a sport psychologist to increase both the priority of and energy allocated to rehabilitation.

The final question (question 15) provides the sports medicine professional with an opportunity to offer additional counseling to the injured athlete and to do so in a manner that is easily declined if the injured athlete perceives that he or she is doing well.

Evaluating the Risk for Suicide

It is important to determine whether seriously injured athletes are at risk for suicide (Smith & Milliner, 1995). Those athletes at risk for suicide usually have acknowledged depression and have a flat affect or other signs and symptoms of depression. With these athletes the line of questioning depicted in table 5.1 is often appropriate.

Table 5.1 concludes with a request that significant others be notified and a prompt referral be made. Referral should be to a clinical psychologist or psychiatrist who has the authority to order medication and who has admitting privileges to a hospital. Suicidal precautions include a behavioral contract to keep the athlete at risk for suicide in an environment free from the means to commit suicide (e.g., medications, open windows, glass, bedsheets). Professional staff try to maintain surveillance until the crisis has passed and the depressed mood has improved. Most sports medicine professionals are not qualified to enter into contract setting, nor should they be in a position of living with the consequences if an injured athlete (frequently a volatile adolescent) acts on his or her ideation (Smith & Milliner, 1995).

Case Example: Suicide Risk

One basketball player acknowledged feeling very depressed but adamantly denied suicidal ideation and denied having a plan or the means. Sadly, he missed his next appointment. I learned he had been admitted to a psychiatric unit following a suicide attempt (an over-the-counter drug overdose).

As this case example illustrates, our questions unfortunately do not always result in honest answers for a wide variety of reasons. Despite our good intentions, we need to be careful that our lines of questioning do not trigger negative ideas in the minds of athletes. This example also illustrates a limitation of a questionnaire and the interview process, both of which depend on honesty.

Table 5.1   Screening for Suicide Ideation

1. Is this the worst depression you have experienced?
2. Has this depression prompted you to think life is not worth living?
3. Is life worth living?
4. If not, have you thought of a plan as to how you might end it?

   (Note: To this point, the athlete is not necessarily suicidal.)
5. Have you secured the means that you would use?

If the athlete answers yes to the preceding questions, acknowledges a plan, and has possession of the means to execute the plan, the interviewer is obligated to seek professional help for the injured athlete by consulting a clinical psychologist or psychiatrist. It is imperative to notify a significant other who can be in close contact with the injured athlete until the crisis is resolved and the depression treated (Smith & Milliner, 1995). Unfortunately, our questions do not always result in honest answers.

Overall Impressions of Injured Athlete's Status

On completion of the interview the sports medicine professional must summarize, or assimilate, the objective and subjective findings and form an impression of the injured athlete's status. The injured athlete's status can usually be expressed by one of the following descriptions:

1. The injury is minor, there are few psychosocial consequences, and the athlete has strong social support and adequate coping skills.

2. The injury is severe and has major consequences, but the injured athlete has strong social support and excellent coping skills.

3. The injury is minor, but the athlete has exaggerated the consequences and has little social support and poor coping skills. In this case you may wish to seek a referral to a mental health professional or recommend some initial interventions (see chapter 8).

4. The injury is severe, and the consequences are grave. Despite strong social support and good coping skills, the athlete is seriously depressed and may need a prompt referral to a psychologist or psychiatrist. In addition to your referral, some injured athletes will benefit from seeing you again for follow-up. Although it requires sound professional judgment to avoid duplication of services, it is equally important to avoid dropping the injured athlete and fragmenting the services provided.

Figure 5.2 offers a flowchart to guide the sports medicine professional through forming an impression based on the interview to the appropriate initial intervention phase of counseling.

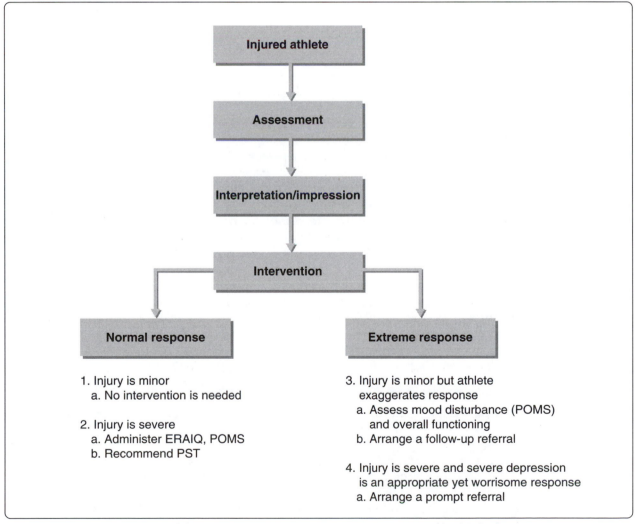

Figure 5.2 A flowchart from interview to impression to appropriate intervention for injured athletes.

AFTER THE ASSESSMENT INTERVIEW

An effective assessment interview sets the stage for a therapeutic counseling relationship between sports medicine professionals and athletes, which is essential to maximizing both physical and psychological recovery from sport injury. After the assessment interview, the sports medicine professional is able to form an impression about the physical and psychosocial consequences of the injury to the athlete. Although there are some exceptions, the flowchart in figure 5.2 guides sports medicine professionals toward appropriate initial interventions such as consultation and referral.

If possible, the sports medicine professional and the injured athlete should agree on the sports psychology interventions indicated, set a deadline by which to accomplish appropriate goals, and agree on a method for outcome evaluation. Then, as equal members of the sports medicine team, they can begin the mutually agreed upon physical and psychological therapeutic processes.

CASE STUDY

Wayne was a 19-year-old ice hockey player (right wing) who sustained a fractured lateral malleolus when he blocked a 95 mile per hour (153 kilometer per hour) slap shot. The injury occurred in a U.S. Hockey League (USHL) game on December 3. After receiving the necessary medical care—physical examination, PRICE (protection, rest, ice, compression, and elevation), X ray, physician consultation, and casting—Wayne and his sports medicine professional learned it would be six to eight weeks before Wayne could return to full on-ice participation. A few days after the injury they sat down to discuss the impact of injury using the adapted ERAIQ-SMP as an interview guide.

As a second-year USHL player, Wayne's dream was eventually to play in the National Hockey League, but of pressing importance was earning a Division I college scholarship. Hockey was his preferred sport, and he usually participated for reasons of fun, competition, personal improvement, and socialization. He needed to obtain a Division I hockey scholarship this year, or he would not be able to attend college or continue hockey. He planned to study kinesiology and obtain a coaching certificate. He understood the nature of his injury and that he would be on crutches for four to six weeks. The fracture occurred on December 3, so the earliest scrimmage or game in which he could participate was January 15.

Pressure on Wayne was largely self-imposed. He felt social support from his family, but unfortunately, they were over a thousand miles away. He felt "replaced" on the team as the coach and linemates, of necessity, quickly adjusted to his inability to play. When asked about life stress, he acknowledged that the injury and such consequences as "not being scouted" and "not being offered a scholarship" were his primary concerns. When asked which words described the emotions he was experiencing, he offered "robbed, shocked, frustrated, and depressed" as emotions descriptive of his present mood state. He felt that he was about 15 percent recovered because the swelling had decreased, but he understood the healing, regaining range of motion, and strengthening that would be a lengthy and necessary aspect of rehabilitation before his return to sport.

He was highly motivated to do whatever was necessary to obtain effective rehabilitation. Although clearly discouraged, Wayne's affect was not flat. He made good eye contact, and he was open and eager to learn about strategies that might facilitate his rehabilitation. Wayne understood that he would need to stay sharp and on top of his game mentally if he were to have a chance to break back into his team's lineup as soon as he was cleared medically to return to competition.

Wayne was instructed in the Psychological Skills Strategies of goal setting, relaxation, imagery, attribution theory, positive self-talk, and cognitive structuring, which applied to his rehabilitation and to his return to sport. He was also given inspirational, sport-specific reading assignments, and an alternative conditioning program was implemented. All strategies were instituted to complement and enhance his rehabilitation program.

QUESTIONS FOR ANALYSIS

1. How would you have established a conducive environment in which to interview Wayne?

2. To which impression category would you assign Wayne, based on the assessment interview?

3. What additional assessment questions would you have posed to Wayne to elicit more information?

4. Would you recommend referral to a counselor for Wayne? Why or why not?

5. What physical and psychosocial interventions would you recommend for Wayne during his rehabilitation period?

SUMMARY

An effective assessment interview sets the stage for a therapeutic counseling relationship between sports medicine professionals and athletes, which is essential to maximizing both physical and psychological recovery from sport injury. After the assessment interview, the sports medicine professional will be able to form an impression about the physical and psychosocial consequences of the injury to the athlete. Although there will be some exceptions, the flow chart will guide sports medicine professionals toward appropriate initial interventions such as consultations and referrals.

If possible, the sports medicine professional and the injured athlete should agree on the sports psychology interventions indicated and set a time limit by which to accomplish appropriate goals and agree upon a method to evaluate outcome. Then, as equal members of the sports medicine team, they can begin the mutually agreed upon physical and psychological therapeutic process.

I would like to thank my colleagues, Dr. Michael Stuart and Dr. Edward Laskowski, co-directors of the Mayo Clinic Sports Medicine Center for the opportunity to participate on the Sports Medicine team. Appreciation is also expressed to Johannson-Gund scholar, Mr. Steve Ginnie, MEd, for his assistance in proofreading the chapter.

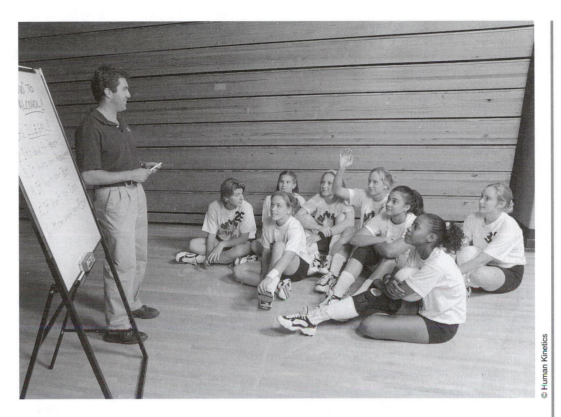

© Human Kinetics

Effective Group Health Education Counseling

Frances Flint, PhD, ATC, CAT(C), *York University, Ontario*

CHAPTER OBJECTIVES

Understand the external and internal forces inherent in sport groups and their impact on team behavior

Understand the dynamics of counseling sport groups as compared with counseling individual athletes

Understand the types of health-related issues associated with sport groups

Understand the qualities and skills needed to be a counselor with sport groups

Learn how to use various techniques and tools when counseling sport groups

Often sports medicine professionals are called on to provide health-related information to sport groups or to counsel groups on healthy approaches to lifestyle and sport performance. Most frequently, the request for a sports medicine professional to address groups on health issues is initiated because of incidents of health-threatening behavior, such as drug or alcohol abuse. The ideal scenario, however, for providing health education counseling is in a preventive mode rather than as a reaction to an event. Encouraging and educating members of sport groups to adopt healthy approaches to lifestyle and sport performance before they have adopted potentially harmful habits is more productive than attempting to change established behavior.

CONCEPTUAL MODEL FOR COUNSELING WITH SPORT GROUPS

intervention—A deliberate intercession between a practitioner and a target individual or group. It can take the form of counselor–individual or counselor–group sessions.

modus operandus—A way of operating or working.

Health education counseling with athletes in sport groups presents a unique challenge because of the array of confounding factors that may affect the counseling **intervention**. For example, when dealing with an individual athlete, the counselor can usually expect to interact with coaches, parents, teachers, and perhaps friends of the athlete. However, it is more complicated to provide health education counseling to athletes in sport groups because of the added interaction with teammates. The increased opportunities for interaction (i.e., teammate to teammate) create the potential for many more scenarios to unfold, which must be considered when providing counseling services. The purpose of this chapter is to help you gain insight into the various ways of determining a group's needs and the possible avenues open for addressing the health education counseling needs of sport groups.

Within the conceptual model for health education counseling with sport groups, a multitude of spheres of influence become evident (see figure 6.1). Before a **modus operandus** for the counseling intervention can be developed, all the influencing factors must be considered along with the attributes of the counselor or counseling team. First, the unique aspects of a sport must be considered in order to comprehend the full impact of competing in that sport. Second, the group's needs and characteristics should be reviewed to discern any idiosyncrasies that may have a bearing on the type of intervention or on the qualities and skills required of the counselor. Last, the kind of health-related problem must be appraised to determine what particular knowledge base the sports medicine professional must have and what specific intervention may be effective.

The three spheres of influence in the conceptual model for counseling—sport characteristics, the group's needs and characteristics, and the nature of the health concern—interact with each other within the design of the modus operandus. Thus an interactionist approach is beneficial in group counseling because it allows the counselor to understand why one group or sport may have different health-related problems and that they may deal with those problems in vastly different ways. Before actually initiating an intervention, all the available information must be appraised. This approach to the counseling intervention is no different from the preparation a good coach makes before an upcoming competition. If the "scouting" is poorly conducted and all available information is not assimilated into the "game plan," the outcome may be disastrous. A good coach never goes into a game blind, and neither should the person counseling a sport group.

Sport Characteristics

The area of sport characteristics includes several different factors that may influence health education counseling: the type of sport, the level of play, the social status accorded this sport and group, and the organizational relationships influencing the team. External factors and the demands of sport can affect the functioning of a group and may impose certain behavioral expectations and codes of conduct (see figure 6.2). A perceptive sports medicine professional will tune in to the nuances of each sport and will integrate these subtleties into the counseling process.

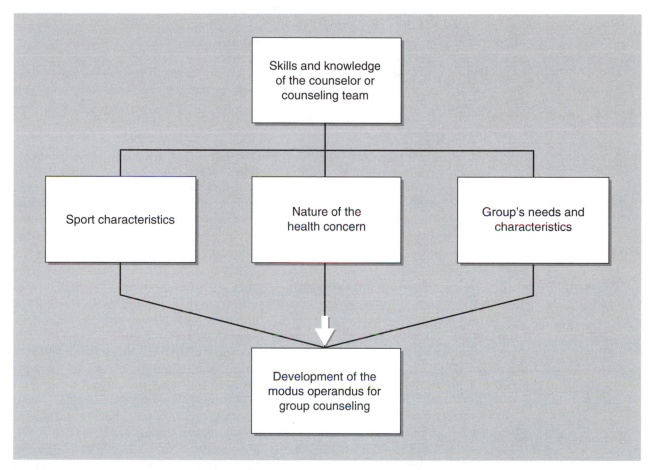

Figure 6.1   Factors influencing the development of a modus operandus for group health education counseling.

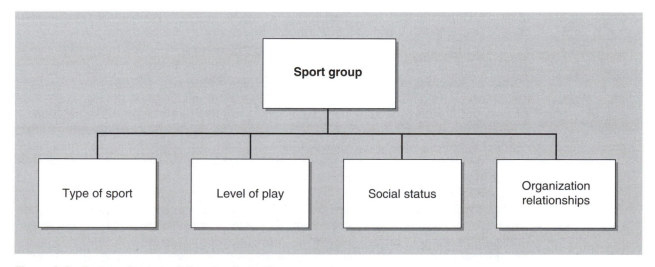

Figure 6.2   Factors that help define the distinctive nature of a team.

Type of Sport

Those who provide health education counseling to athletic teams will find it valuable to have an understanding of sport in general and the uniqueness of each sport in particular. Each sport carries certain implicit and explicit expectations with respect to player conduct, dealing with injuries, and tactics (Taylor, 1995). For example, a stark contrast in the expression of pain is seen between rugby and soccer. In rugby the expectation is that players will not wear protective equipment nor express pain when injured. In soccer, however, there is demonstrable expression of pain and injury. The expectation that pain and injury should be accepted without reservation is also seen in football at the professional level. There is an assumption that important players will play in the big games even if hurt. In comparison, other team sports, such as rowing, base health-related conduct on different premises. Dissimilar presumptions were evident when a Canadian rower voluntarily made the decision to remove herself from the crew of four's competition at the Barcelona Olympics because she felt she might jeopardize the team's chances of a medal. Because these rowers were the current world champions, they were virtually assured of a medal. These kinds of sport behavioral expectations often dictate how groups deal with specific health-related issues, and an understanding of the implied behavioral standards and guiding principles of each sport is essential for those providing counseling services.

Level of Play

Health education counseling with professional teams is based on different foundational criteria than those of varsity or recreational leagues. In most cases the level of play helps to determine how the counseling intervention is viewed and implemented. In the case of professional athletics, with respect to winning games or spectator interest, a player's monetary value may influence how health education counseling is managed. Unfortunately, the pressure to win in professional sport outweighs concern for athletes' health. In some sports, health-related concerns are not dealt with unless they affect the ability of the player to perform. As long as the athlete's or team's health behavior is not detrimental to sport entertainment, the health issue is tolerated. Thus, lifestyle and health-related issues are disregarded until they reach a crisis and affect the athlete's and team's performance. This was demonstrated by statements that were made after Magic Johnson's announcement that he had tested positive for human immunodeficiency virus (HIV). Much subsequent discussion and bragging centered around the exceptionally high levels of sexual promiscuity evident in professional basketball. Only recently have professional sports begun to provide health education counseling for its own sake and not just because of the monetary value of team members.

Within the educational framework of varsity team sports, we have seen teams dealing with health-related issues on a more proactive basis than in professional team sports (Petruzzello, Landers, Linder, & Robinson, 1987; Salmela, 1989; Zimmerman, Protinsky, & Zimmerman, 1994). Perhaps the best example of proactive examination and management of a health-related issue in college and Olympic sports is the legislation against ergogenic aids. Much research, many educational seminars, and many counseling sessions have been conducted by educational institutions to produce a change in the attitudes of athletes toward this health concern. Unfortunately, professional sports have lagged far behind in addressing the issue of ergogenic aids.

The level of play may also affect other health and safety issues, such as the equipment that is worn by athletes. For many years amateur ice hockey players have been required to wear approved protective helmets and face guards (shields or cages). Research for the past 40 years into eye injuries in ice hockey has demonstrated the benefit of head and face protection. Legislation mandating helmets in the National

Hockey League (NHL) lagged far behind amateur sport and was met with considerable resistance from professional players. One reason given for not wearing helmets was that players want to be recognizable to their fans. Wayne Gretsky of the Los Angeles Kings announced that he should not have to wear the same kind of approved helmet as amateurs because he is a professional and knows how to play the game. Less stringent professional NHL team rules allow this double standard.

Social Status

"Values taught in sport can be incongruent with the values necessary to achieve in society outside of sport" (Lopiano & Zotos, 1992, p. 180). In the case of high-visibility sports in which fans accord a special status to athletes, decisions are often made or expectations are held that can be detrimental to the health of athletes. Decisions relating to health matters in the public sector usually take precedence over occupations and work commitments. This incongruence is evident when athletes are encouraged to return from injury too quickly in order to help the team win an important game. In this case the athlete is taught that his or her value as a person is related only to the performance of a task.

The high profile and social status that many athletes enjoy carry with them certain responsibilities, especially in professional team sports. Wayne Gretsky, for example, is a model for young ice hockey players and his behavior, lifestyle, and equipment become the standard for these players. Media coverage and the idolizing of popular professional athletes has made them highly visible to the public. Thus, when a professional athlete endorses equipment or has a lifestyle visible to the public, both social and sport standards are influenced. This modeling force has a profound impact on young athletes and parents. Health education counseling dilemmas are created when the public witnesses poor health practices by athletes in high social positions. Demonstrating to athletes that their role models are unhealthy is difficult and often met with resistance. In these instances the best health education counseling approach may be to depict the correct approach to the health behavior and not to deride the behavior that the sport role model is demonstrating.

Organizational Relationships

The value placed on winning and entertainment by owners and managers of high-profile sports teams often outweighs beneficial health-related decisions and practices for athletes. In such cases sport becomes an industry, and the athlete is a disposable resource. If management is perceived by athletes as sympathetic and caring in its health-related policies and practices, then athletes feel valued as people as well as for their sport skills. When there is a sense that management and owner decisions are based solely on economics, however, athletes may resort to self-protective actions. This has been illustrated in professional sports in which some groups of athletes have felt they must hire their own medical practitioners and refuse to use management-employed sports medicine professionals in order to ensure unbiased health care. Sports medicine professionals working with groups must be cognizant of the existing contractual and organizational relationships between athletes and management to achieve effective interventions.

Group's Needs and Characteristics

The goal of establishing effective working relationships with groups requires a recognition of the many factors such as the group's chemistry and social structure that affect the functioning of the group (see figure 6.3). How athletes and staff perceive leadership, group strengths and weaknesses, the sanctity of private lives, and common goals influences how receptive the group may be to outside health care interventions. This aspect of group counseling is paramount and plays an important role in determining what kind of intervention would be effective with a group. The counselor's observational skills and intuition must be utilized to "read" the group in order to determine the most productive approach to the group issues and members.

Internal Power Structure

Zimmerman and colleagues (1994, p. 104) suggest that athletic teams may function in the same manner as families where "the hierarchy of the coaches and seniors resembled the hierarchy of parents and older siblings in a family." The premise is that "all groups organize whether they are related by blood or not" (p. 102) and that clear lines of power are established. The seniors and the coaches may be designated the role of parents while the other group members vie to gain favor or position with the dominant role members. It is important that the sports medicine professional recognize the hierarchy within the group and work to have the dominant group members accept or "buy into" the counseling intervention. To be completely integrated into the group process, the central figures in the group (i.e., coaches, seniors) must be both physically present and philosophically in consonance with the theme of the counseling intervention. Health education counseling cannot be effective if the principal members of the group are uncooperative.

Problems within groups often remain covert since group members want to avoid confrontation that might upset the performance of the group. Viewing the group structure like a family may provide the opportunity to understand some of the dynamics of communication, social support, rivalry, and hierarchy. New or young members of the group may require extra backing by the health education counselor to be heard and understood.

Team Chemistry and Character

The chemistry of a group is often described by terms such as *cohesive, united,* or *divided.* Carron (1982) describes cohesion as "a dynamic process which is reflected in the tendency for a group to stick together and remain united in the pursuit of its goals and objectives." Cohesive groups are more likely to identify the strengths and weaknesses of the group members and find ways to capitalize on these areas. This cohesiveness may relate to specific tasks through which a group strives to achieve recognized goals or to social aspects in which friendship, camaraderie, and social support are emphasized. The receptiveness of a group to health education counseling can be influenced by task or socially aligned cohesiveness. For example, if a task-oriented group (e.g., a team that wants to win) perceives nutritional counseling as

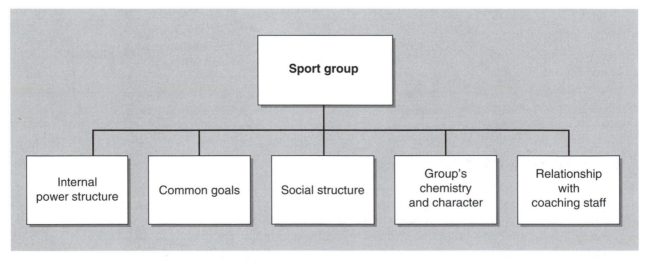

Figure 6.3 The needs and characteristics of teams.

beneficial to achieving its goals, the members of the group are much more likely to adhere to suggested nutritional guidelines. Identifying the level of cohesiveness in a group can aid the sports medicine professional in determining how an intervention can be initiated.

Sports medicine professionals should realize that there may need to be an intervention to increase group cohesion before any health education counseling will be effective. It is often difficult to be effective in encouraging healthy behavior patterns with groups that are too dissimilar in nature or not cohesive. **Initiative tasks** focusing on group dynamics and team building may be instrumental in fostering more group cohesion and thus creating a united approach to the health behavior.

Social Structure

The social structure of a group may contribute to the foundation on which the group makes health-related decisions. Additionally, this social structure may determine the receptiveness of the group to discussions concerning health issues. If, for example, the group wishes to deal only with performance-related issues (e.g., winning), then group members may not be open minded when it comes to dealing with health issues. For example, an athlete's personal life may be in disarray, but fellow team members extol her athletic prowess with the comment, "Her life is a mess, but she always comes to play." In these cases, the group is interested only in the ability of the athlete to perform, and any health-related action is not considered to be within its purview. In these situations it may be difficult for the sports medicine professional to convince the group that issues unrelated to athletic performance are of importance to the group.

Social structures may also be displayed via the cliques that form within groups. Recognizing the circles of influence is important for the sports medicine professional because receptiveness to counseling depends on these small, intragroup cliques. It may be that membership in the cliques is related to experience within the group (i.e., seniors, rookies), but it may also be correlated with health behavior (i.e., drugs, alcohol). In either case, the sports medicine professional in conjunction with staff and group members must use open lines of communication and intuitive observational skills to discern any obstructive or uncooperative cliques within the group.

initiative tasks—Group-related activities that create situations requiring group interaction, communication, and initiative to solve.

Common Goals

Expectations, objectives, and goals of the group are important factors to consider in designing a health education counseling intervention. If the group's goals and objectives are not related to health issues and group members see no value in counseling, nothing will be accomplished through the intervention. It is important that the group's goals be known and that a link be made between the health education counseling and what the group wants to accomplish. Much more will be accomplished with the group if the group's goals and the health counseling share a common purpose.

Relationship With Coaching Staff

The relationship between the coaching staff and the group is important, particularly if the coaches are perceived as being in and using strong power positions when making group-related decisions. As Zimmerman et al. (1994) have pointed out, the coaches may be viewed as parents within the group structure and, depending on their use of this power position, may be treated in the same manner as parents by the group members. If the coaches initiate or endorse health education counseling sessions and these sessions are successful or popular, the group is much more likely to be enthusiastic about future counseling. Obviously, then, the reverse is true, and thus it is important that the first health education counseling session organized by the coaching staff be successful.

Along with the potential for parentlike relationships between coaches and groups is another component when the coach and the group are of opposite sexes. This added dynamic of sexual relationships presents unique concerns, particularly in light of the incidence of sexual harassment and assault charges that have been made against coaches within the last several years. Over half of all the coaches of women's teams are male, and the number of female coaches has decreased since 1980 (Lopiano & Zotos, 1992). Parents, coaches, individual athletes, and groups have all expressed concern about the potential for sexual impropriety in sport, and this has resulted in an increase in the number of health education counseling sessions dedicated to the topic of athlete–coach relationships.

Nature of Health Concerns

Health-related concerns can be magnified within groups by the potential for physical intimacy of group membership, privacy issues, and conceivable disruption of the group's cohesiveness. When an athlete in an individual sport encounters a health-related problem, typically only the athlete, the family of the athlete, and possibly the coach are affected. This is not the situation in team sports when groups of athletes are involved, which contributes to the need for special attention to health concerns in groups. Some examples of health concerns that may implicate more than one athlete include stress management, infectious diseases, alcohol and drug abuse, and sexual relationships (see figure 6.4). Surveying groups for health-related concerns (e.g., by using questionnaires), particularly if anonymity is ensured, can provide valuable information about topics that are pertinent to the group.

Stress Management

With groups it is particularly important to pay attention to the unique stress-reaction tendencies of each member of the group because of their potential to affect other group members. Each person within a group deals with imposed psychological stress in a different manner, and often these idiosyncrasies have a bearing on how other

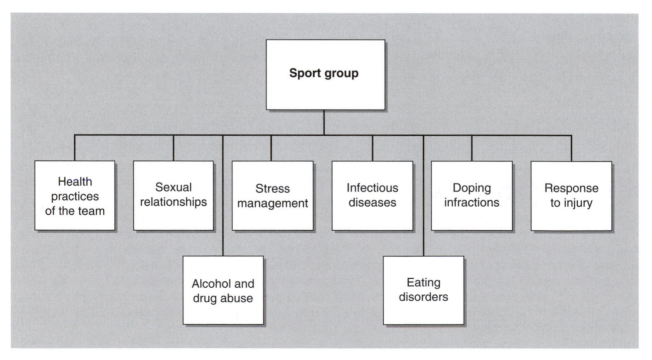

Figure 6.4 Common themes for group health education counseling of sport teams.

individuals in the group and the group as a whole cope with pressure. An athlete who exhibits nervousness by excessive talking can aggravate other group members and may spread this nervousness throughout the group like an infectious disease. Within a group setting, individual dispositions need to be recognized and tolerance for uniqueness developed.

Infectious Diseases

Groups are particularly vulnerable to concerns associated with infectious diseases because of close working relationships and interaction among athletes. If a member of a group has an infection, especially one that is embarrassing, threatening to others, or highly communicable, then everyone in the group is influenced. Sports medicine professionals should establish privacy policies and practices that alleviate concerns of group members and encourage open lines of communication while at the same time protecting others from infection. This is particularly important in "blood sports" such as rugby and wrestling where protocols for body fluid management must be in place and known by all participants.

Eating Disorders

The expectations required by the sport and held by the team can have an influence on diet, eating habits, and the prevalence of eating disorders. Athletes in body-image activities (e.g., gymnastics, dance) are particularly susceptible to performance pressure based on a pleasing visual image of beauty, proportion, or strength. Eating disorders, such as **anorexia nervosa** and **bulimia nervosa**, can become systemic in certain groups (e.g., adolescents) and cannot be dealt with effectively within groups nor with general health education counseling except in the preventive sense. This particular health concern requires the attention of specially trained practitioners who recognize the inherent dangers associated with these conditions. Establishing a referral process as part of the health education counseling process is beneficial for groups, especially because parents and coaches may not be aware of existing support groups and health care professionals within the community who deal specifically with eating disorders.

anorexia nervosa and *bulimia nervosa*— *Personality disorders that manifest in disruptions in eating patterns and behavioral responses— sometimes very severe—to food.*

Sexual Relationships

Presentations concerning sexual relationships can be very effective in group settings because many of the misconceptions and exaggerations concerning the topic are often created and fostered within groups of friends or teams. The aggrandizement of sexual exploits by leaders of a group sets the tone for other group members to follow. Misinformation about sex proliferates quickly in group settings. In addition, because this is a topic about which many athletes are nervous, the group presentation allows them the comfort and security of numbers. Even though unspoken by most athletes, concern about health care in sexual relationships is prevalent.

Responses to Injury

The social structure of groups can be conducive to assuaging injury and can provide incentive for increased compliance with injury-recovery programs. The injured athlete, however, may feel external or internal pressure to return too soon after injury because of the close relationships apparent within the group. This is particularly evident in professional sport, where it is seen as a demotion and an embarrassment to go down to the minors for play-related recovery after injury, even when this represents the best possible course of action for the athlete. The group can be a major source of encouragement and social support for injured group members when used well. The sports medicine professional should provide information on the impact injuries can have on a group and how the group's social structure can be helpful in injury situations.

Health Practices of the Group

Each sport, and indeed each group, deals with health practices in a different way. For example, the timing of water breaks and the sharing of common water bottles by several team members varies with each group. Unnecessary illness can be prevented by providing health education counseling about the need for proper hydration under training conditions and the high risk of spreading infectious diseases through common drinking sources. Other examples of group health practices include the use of smokeless tobacco, uniform cleanliness, and personal hygiene. Not washing a uniform after a win and while a winning streak continues is a common group-influenced behavior, even though group members are aware of healthy hygiene habits. Influencing health practices within groups is a challenge because of the close interrelationships within the group and the traditional habits of specific groups.

Alcohol and Drug Abuse

Social pressure within groups and the common need to feel included often dictate alcohol and social drug practices in groups of athletes. In many cases, the family structure suggested by Zimmerman and Protinsky (1993), in which senior members of a group set the standards for the group, has a strong influence on new members. Health education counseling often fails to place alcohol and drug abuse in the proper context, especially for teenagers who see drinking and drug use as an entry into the adult world. In particular, alcohol advertising associated with sport implies that the two activities are linked and thus that sport affiliation implies alcohol affiliation.

With alcohol and drug experimentation occurring at very young ages, it is important that preventive health education counseling be initiated well before the teenage years. In addition, because many children are exposed to alcohol and drug abuse within their homes, health education counseling can be expanded to include parent groups, community groups, teachers, and coaching associations. The health education counseling should provide an awareness of the health concerns related to alcohol and drug abuse, education about its prevalence, signs and symptoms of abuse, and sources of support within the community.

Doping Infractions

*ergogenic aids—
Pharmacological,
physical, or
psychological
techniques or
substances used
to enhance
performance.
Some of these
substances and
techniques are
banned by sport
governing bodies.*

The use of **ergogenic aids** and practices has become a common topic in health education counseling within the group setting. Again, the social relationships of a group often influence group members to engage in activities that the group has implicitly endorsed. The norms established within a group may be very difficult to change, especially if the counselor uses a purely health-related focus. Little change is seen when health counseling emphasizes only the health problems of ergogenic aids. The "that won't happen to me" attitude proliferates within groups. It is important within the context of groups to discuss several aspects of the use of ergogenic aids, including ethics, impact on the group, dependence, and the pressure to excel. Health education counseling must also include ways to alleviate some of the stressors (i.e., stress management) that create the sense that ergogenic aids are required and necessary.

DEVELOPING A MODUS OPERANDUS FOR COUNSELING SPORT GROUPS

The interactive nature of group health education counseling must be considered when designing the modus operandi. Interaction involves attending to the nature of the health concern, the characteristics of a specific sport or sports, and the group's needs and character. If any of these factors is neglected, health education counseling may be deficient and may not serve the needs of the group. In addition, the skills and knowledge of the sports medicine professional must be sufficiently comprehensive to fulfill the requirements of group health education counseling.

Skills and Knowledge of the Counselor

The attributes of the counselor or counseling team are a vital component in the establishment of health education counseling programs. The message will not be attended to nor adhered to if the messenger is lacking either communication skills or health knowledge. Bull (1995) has suggested that it is vital to the establishment of a sound working relationship with a group that the counselor be seen as part of the group or part of the support staff. Although Bull was talking about sport psychology consultants, this premise can be extended to anyone providing health education counseling to a group.

Regardless of who provides health education counseling programs to groups, the counselor must exhibit specific skills and knowledge. Of particular importance in counseling is the ability to communicate well and to gain the attention of athletes in a group setting. Communicating effectively and designing attractive presentations are learned skills that are a prerequisite of all counseling situations. Listening skills are also a part of communications and allow the establishment of two-way dialogue and the sharing of information. Unfortunately, in most cases communication and listening skills are not taught within university programs, and the assumption is that it is easy to acquire these skills through experiential learning. Very often effective listening skills and keys to communication must be explicitly taught and practiced.

Another aspect of health education counseling involves the establishment of a working relationship between the sports medicine professional and the group. No longer are dominant/subservient roles valid for coaching and counseling athletes. More effort is being placed on forming partnerships within sport. Karl Mohr (University of California, Berkeley) and Tom Fay (Vanderbilt University) developed "The Ten Commandments" for coaches in an attempt to foster positive feelings between swimmers and coaches. Even though these guidelines were established for coach–athlete relationships, they provide a foundation on which counseling services can be formulated.

The Ten Commandments for Coaches*

1. I am committed to your well-being and fulfilment.

2. I will not hurt you.

3. I will not judge you.

4. I will support you.

5. I will accept you.

6. I will listen.

7. I will not make you wrong or make you lose, dominate or invalidate you.

8. I will expand my reality to include and respect you.

9. I will not take it personally.

10. I will be honest, straightforward and open.

* And in every case I am worthy of the same from you!

Mohr & Fay, quoted in Pate, McClenaghan, & Rotella, 1984, p. 62

It may seem obvious, but it is also important in group health education counseling that the sports medicine professional have knowledge of health-related issues. Thus group health education counseling requires someone with health knowledge, communication skills, and a counseling background. This is an unusual combination, but one that may become more prevalent as more sports medicine professionals acquire skills in sport or counseling psychology.

Who Should Provide Group Health Education Counseling?

Since athletes often subject themselves to unreasonable physical, physiological, and psychological demands in the name of performance, those who provide health counseling must be unbiased voices of reason. Thus the question about who should provide health education counseling is a valid one. Those with implicit (if not explicit) responsibilities for health counseling include certified athletic trainers, coaches, expert practitioners in health care or counseling, and sport psychologists. Team physicians and sport physical therapists are also important members of the health counseling team.

Coaches

Since coaches understand the intricacies of sport and play such an integral role with athletes, it could be argued that they should be responsible for health education counseling. There are some important concerns about the delegation of this function to coaches, however, which relate primarily to coaches' roles. The coach has overall responsibility for the athletes under his or her care; however, the coach is also charged with the improvement of performance and in most cases is required to be successful in either winning or producing outstanding athletes. This means that there may be some overriding influences on coaches that make the dual functions of health care counseling and coaching mutually exclusive. This has been demonstrated through research into health-related decisions with high school and university basketball coaches. Flint and Weiss (1992) investigated how coaches made decisions regarding the return of players to competition after injury. They found that coaches made decisions based on the player's status (how good an athlete he or she was) and the game situation (winning, losing, or a close game). "The pressure on the head coach from administration, parents, and eager players often, if only subliminally, creates an inappropriate scenario for reasonably prudent decisions with respect to athlete health care" (Flint & Weiss, 1992, p. 35). Pressure to win or maintain employment as a coach often places coaches in a position of ethical and moral dilemma when it comes to the health care of athletes.

Certified Athletic Trainers

It is clearly stated within the National Athletic Trainers Association's scope of practice that education and counseling are responsibilities inherent in the role of athletic trainer. Certified athletic trainers traditionally counsel and advise athletes regarding rehabilitation and treatment of specific injuries. Their guidance has also extended to any other health matter that might affect athletes. Counseling is not the primary focus of the athletic trainer's work, but they do perceive it to be an important part of the job. This was demonstrated quite clearly in a study by Furney and Patton (1985), in which 89.8 percent of athletic trainers indicated that they felt counseling on health-related topics was an important aspect of their work. In reality, however, only a small percentage of athletic trainers actually did perform a significant amount of health counseling, and this was primarily about injury prevention and injury therapy. Furney and Patton (1985) also found that 50 percent of athletic trainers felt that their college training had prepared them either adequately or very adequately for this counseling role. In most cases, the knowledge base for health education counseling is acquired through accredited athletic training education programs. Of concern, however, are the skills and knowledge of counseling techniques and educational presentation. This kind of training is not evident within educational programs for athletic trainers, and it cannot be assumed that this knowledge and skill are innate.

Counseling or Sport Psychologists

The professionals with the best background and education in counseling and intervention are psychologists (clinical, sport, or educational psychologists). Generally, programs involving clinical and sport psychology have intervention components that emphasize the interaction between the psychologist and the individual or group. These professionals therefore have the requisite knowledge of intervention and techniques; however, unless they have a concomitant background in health or physical education, they may be untrained in the specifics of health education counseling.

Organizations such as the Association for the Advancement of Applied Sport Psychology (AAASP) specifically emphasize intervention, performance enhancement, and health psychology. Within the Health Psychology section of AAASP the focus is the role of psychological factors in sport and exercise. Psychological factors relating to disease development and remediation, coping with stress, and health promotion are particularly emphasized. Another major focus of AAASP involves the close relationship between mental health and physical health, and thus this group of professionals would appear to be especially suited to health education counseling. Sport or clinical psychologists who have a background in physical or health education appear to have the necessary combination of skills, knowledge, and background to provide effective health education counseling services to groups.

When an Intervention Should Occur

In most cases, health education counseling and interventions do not occur until a need is recognized or a crisis has occurred. A good example of this is teaching relaxation skills or stress management techniques to groups that are already experiencing stressful situations. This method of imparting knowledge and teaching skills is the antithesis of sound teaching practice and philosophy. Teachers and coaches should not teach a new skill under stressful situations. The technique or skill should be taught without any pressure and then with gradually escalated stress so that the skill is ingrained through increasingly stressful scenarios. In this manner the athlete gains confidence in his or her skill and ability to adapt to imposed demands. In short, we should not wait for a crisis to deal with potentially threatening conditions. We know enough about unhealthy tendencies and practices in sport to be proactive in preventive actions rather than reactive when a predicament occurs.

The early season is an opportune time to present health education counseling to groups because acceptable practices and policies are established at this stage. Using this window of opportunity sets the tone for the season ahead and lays the foundation for subsequent interventions. If openness is established at a group presentation, individual athletes within the group may feel secure seeking advice as a consequence of the presentation. This kind of a presentation early in the season also demonstrates to the group that managers and coaches are concerned with conveying knowledge about health care.

How to Initiate an Intervention

There are a number of ways to present health education information in group settings, including single-sport group meetings, multisport meetings, guest speakers, group role playing, health-related interest groups or clubs, and initiative tasks for groups. Other resources, such as video and audiotapes, are also useful. In addition, a group meeting at which specific topics are covered can establish the opportunity for later individual meetings.

Single-Sport and Multisport Meetings

Group presentations can be offered to single- or multisport groups. The single-sport approach offers the opportunity to have various age groups or leagues in attendance so that sport-specific health issues can be presented. In a multiple-sport presentation, health education counseling can focus on general health issues for all participants regardless of their sport. When role models are the presenters (e.g., well-known former athletes), it may be more effective to use a single-sport format unless the presenter is well known to multiple sport groups.

Guest Speakers

Guest speakers, either as individuals or in panels, can be an effective and informative way of providing health education counseling to groups. A dynamic presentation by a few experts followed by a group discussion ensures that specific information is transmitted and allows interaction. With this method, athletes have the opportunity to learn new information and also can gain the answers to questions they may have about the topic.

Group Role Playing

Group role playing can be an effective, fun way to deal with health-related issues, but only if the group "buys into" the process. Often people are self-conscious in settings outside their spheres of expertise, and athletes are no exception. Role playing can create social and psychological discomfort, which may negatively affect role playing and render this an ineffective intervention. Effective role playing requires timely presentation and only to groups that are receptive. You must remember that group role playing is only a medium or method for transmitting a message. If the method is poorly presented or received, the message may be lost.

Group Membership

Group membership can be the defining characteristic that determines who receives specific health education counseling. For example, varsity athletes at one Canadian university are invited to become members of the "ACL Club." Membership in this group depends on having surgery for a torn anterior cruciate ligament. By having a club, the injured athletes gain an identity, have meaningful social interaction, are provided with coping models, and can obtain specific health education counseling. Health education counseling sessions can be established for the members of a group who share a specific health concern and can address problems that are likely to be encountered during rehabilitation (i.e., psychological and physical concerns).

Initiative Tasks

Initiative tasks are group-related activities that create situations requiring group interaction, communication, and initiative to solve. The tasks can be designed in such a way as to create dilemmas or obstacles that can be solved and overcome only if the group works collectively. For example, a group is charged with getting every member over a 12-foot-high (4-meter-high) wall without using any props, ropes, or ladders. The group members must work collectively to help each member over the wall, keeping in mind the problem of the last group member left on the other side. If the group analyzes the problem, establishes a working relationship, and deals with all the inherent obstacles, it can be successful. Through this initiative task, the group can learn about leadership, group dynamics, group strengths and weaknesses, and the most productive ways of dealing with problems it may encounter.

Initiative tasks generally include a briefing at the beginning of the task to define the parameters of the problem and a debriefing at the conclusion of the task. This debriefing allows for a discussion of the problem and the way the group sought to solve the dilemma. It also provides the opportunity for further investigation into all aspects of the problem and other potential solutions not considered by the group. This kind of intervention can be effective because it engages the group in a challenge that can be fun and yet deals with a specific health-related dilemma.

Evaluating the Effectiveness of Health Education Counseling Interventions

Evaluating health education counseling can be a difficult task, especially since personal health habits are often private and not open to public or group scrutiny. A number of techniques can be used to evaluate an intervention's effectiveness on health-related behavior, including goal setting for group performance and outcome, observational studies by the coaching or sports medicine staff, acknowledged and anonymous questionnaires of group members, and follow-up discussions or debriefings. Any form of evaluation of the effectiveness of the counseling should be decided beforehand so that specific, measurable knowledge or behavioral changes can be noted and recorded throughout the counseling sessions. It is also important to discuss the concerns, goals, and objectives of those who have requested the health education counseling session. A format for designing and evaluating a counseling session includes (1) discussion of group's needs, (2) goals and objectives of the session or sessions, (3) content and methods of presentation, (4) means of measuring the goals and objectives, and (5) follow-up and contingency plans based on the outcome of the evaluation.

KEYS TO PROVIDING GROUP-ORIENTED COUNSELING SERVICES

Effective group health education counseling is a challenging but important role that sports medicine professionals are well suited to take on. Adhering to the following 10 guidelines should help you improve this aspect of your professional practice:

1. Develop a working relationship with the athletes and the coaching staff, which involves open lines of communication.
2. Observe the interrelationships of the group so that you can identify group leadership, social structure, and cohesiveness.
3. Ensure that you are not viewed as a "management" person and that you are there for the good of the athletes and the group as a whole.
4. Ensure confidentiality so that group members can feel comfortable opening up to you.
5. Learn about the sport and the dynamics of group relationships so that you can understand the sport-specific nuances.
6. Remember that what is acceptable health-related behavior in one sport may not be acceptable in another.
7. Understand the pressures placed on the athletes by group membership and by the specific sport.
8. Be flexible so that you can fit into the group's structure and timetable; do not make the group adapt to you.
9. Understand the power relationships among players and staff in the group.
10. Develop your own counseling skills in many different sport situations so that you can adapt to changes.

CASE STUDY

About midseason, it became known that four members of the defensive line on a varsity football team were taking anabolic steroids. They had evidently discussed the use of these drugs during the previous off-season when they met to talk about the results of last year's play and the year ahead. These athletes had felt a considerable amount of pressure from other team members, family and friends, and the press to improve their performance. They all felt that they had let the team and fans down and desperately wanted to improve to ensure a winning season. They were all aware of the health risks associated with the drugs but felt that they knew all about these dangers and could "keep an eye on things" so that they would not experience any harm. They also knew that these drugs were banned and that being caught meant severe penalties. They felt the risk was worth it.

Two other members of the team have found out about the drug use but are unsure how to proceed. They know that neither the medical nor the coaching staff would endorse the use of these banned substances. These two players are under pressure from their teammates not to tell anyone, but they are angry that these players would jeopardize the whole team's eligibility through the use of the banned substances. They are also worried because of the random drug testing that is being done, especially if one of the players tests positive and it becomes known that they were aware of the infractions but did nothing to expose the problem. In addition, since the team has been winning and the four defensive linemen have been performing well, they do not want to cause problems that might upset the team and the chances for a championship.

QUESTIONS FOR ANALYSIS

1. What are the health-related implications of the use of performance-enhancing drugs?

2. The violating team members have created a predicament for the two team members who are now aware of the use of the banned substances. What are the implications of this illegal drug use for both the violating team members and the two team members who are aware of the violations?

3. What are the undue stresses placed on the players to improve performances?

4. If the two team members decide to discuss the steroid violations with the team's athletic trainer, how should the athletic trainer proceed? If the athletic trainer asks another sports medicine professional to intervene, what approach should that professional take with the team as a whole, the four players involved in the drug use, and the two players who were aware of the problem?

5. What responsibilities do teammates have for other team members?

6. Suppose that the four violators claim that their opponents are using steroids to enhance their performance. What ethical, moral, and legal implications does this supposition create?

7. Assign roles to the members of the group (i.e., coach, athletic trainer, athletes, sport psychologist, parents). Give each role player guidelines about the dilemma being faced in the role he or she is playing (e.g., coach being told of doping infractions). Allow time for the complete scenario to be enacted, then initiate discussion and comments.

SUMMARY

Sports medicine professionals are particularly well suited to provide counseling in group health education settings. A group intervention should ideally be a form of prevention rather than a reaction to health-related events on a team. Athletes on a team are influenced by the characteristics of the sport, the needs of the group, and the nature of their health concern. The methods of group health education counseling should be determined only after considering the skills and knowledge of the sports medicine professional. Sports medicine professionals, along with coaches and sport psychologists, can be effective in the role of group health counselor. The early part of the season is a good time to begin interventions of this type. Many methods of group health education counseling are available, including single- and multisport meetings, guest speakers, group role playing, membership in a support group, and initiative tasks. Sports medicine professionals should establish in advance the methods they will use to determine the effectiveness of their group health education counseling efforts. They should follow the 10 important guidelines for effective group health education counseling.

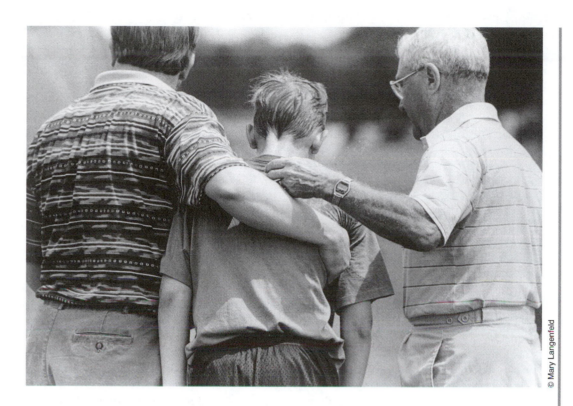

© Mary Langenfeld

Using Family Systems Theory to Counsel the Injured Athlete

Toni Schindler Zimmerman, PhD, *Colorado State University*

CHAPTER OBJECTIVES

Understand the importance of social support in healing the injured athlete

Recognize the similarities between teams and families

Identify how family therapy techniques can be applied to athletics to increase social support

Describe family systems theory and how it relates to athletic injuries and social support

Identify and map cycles of interaction that involve members of the athlete's social support systems

Learn how to acquire techniques that serve to break cycles that interfere with social support

OPENING CASE STUDY

Midseason in her junior year of high school, Misha led the nation in assists. She and her basketball teammates had acquired a large fan following after completing two winning seasons. The team was expected to win the state championship this year. Misha was recognized on campus and in the community as the Tigers' star point guard. She loved playing basketball and felt especially close to her teammates. When she needed advice or support, she likely would rely on one of her coaches. In the second quarter of a midseason game, her left knee went out during a scramble for the ball, resulting in a serious injury. The team physician told Misha, "Chances are that you are out for the season."

Misha, like many athletes, has built an identity in sports. With her injured knee, Misha faces the end of her basketball season and has to come to grips with the loss of recognition as a key player. Furthermore, she must deal with the loss of a portion of her identity, her future dreams, and a means for staying in shape and having fun (Lanning & Toye, 1993). While this is occurring for Misha, all the people to whom she would be likely to turn for support go on with their lives playing and coaching basketball. When injury occurs and throughout the recovery process, athletes often find themselves in a similar situation. They lack the needed social support that is critical to the healing process, both emotionally and physically (Brewer, Jeffers, Petitpas, & Van Raalte, 1994; Hardy, 1992; Larivaara, Vaisanen, & Kiuttu, 1994; Sachs & Ellenberg, 1994).

In this chapter you will learn about the role of social support in the healing of an injured athlete and how to encourage support from those who are most important to the athlete. Family systems theory, which involves learning a variety of techniques that will help the injured athlete cope with the loss, is introduced. These techniques, which emerge from the field of family therapy, are applicable and valuable to sport situations (Zimmerman, 1993; Zimmerman & Protinsky, 1993; Zimmerman, Protinsky, & Zimmerman, 1994).

THE ROLE OF SOCIAL SUPPORT IN COUNSELING ATHLETES

The people who give individuals encouragement, advice, or a helping hand when they are down and those who join them in enjoying the good times in their lives constitute their social support system. Family and friends most often fill that role (Larivaara et al., 1994). This social support system has been recognized as a key factor in both prevention and treatment of athletic injuries (Brewer et al., 1994; Hardy, 1992; Larivaara et al., 1994; Petrie, 1992; Sachs & Ellenberg, 1994). Athletes who report low social support or high life-events stress are more likely to suffer injuries (Hardy, 1992; Petrie, 1992). Once an injury occurs, the reactions of others influence the athlete's recovery time (Nideffer, 1989; Patterson, 1991). Research on individuals suffering from a variety of illnesses or injuries has found social support to be a powerful variable in how well patients comply with medical instructions and rehabilitation procedures. Compliance is higher when families expect them to comply and have a positive attitude about the process (Becker, 1989). Athletic trainers have reported that athletes who cope most successfully with injury rehabilitation have high social support (Wiese, Weiss, & Yukelson, 1991). With social support playing such an essential role in the healing process, knowing how to encourage social support of the injured athlete is a critical skill for an athletic trainer, coach, or other sports medicine professional.

Research indicates that athletes often feel a sense of loss with injury, reacting with grief to the incident and often experiencing feelings such as guilt, anger, or depression (Grove, Hanrahan, & Stewart, 1990; Hardy, 1992; Lanning & Toye, 1993; Lynch, 1988; Nideffer, 1989). These intense emotions can actually aggravate an injury by creating anxiety and muscular tension (Lynch, 1988). Throughout the literature on grief, social support is emphasized as a key factor in emotional healing (Cook & Dworkin, 1992). It is important for people who experience a major loss to know that significant others will still be there for them as they reshape their lives (Cook & Dworkin, 1992). Faced with an uncertain future, these support systems can provide the injured athlete with a sense of stability.

Supportive others can aid healing in many ways, such as by offering encouragement, listening, or helping the athlete to take his or her mind off the loss for a while. Parents might join the injured athlete at doctor's appointments to offer support and ask questions about the injury and the process of rehabilitation. A coach could leave an encouraging note in the athlete's locker, or a teammate might take the athlete out to a movie as a distraction from the injury. Not only an athlete's family, but also the coach and the team are recognized as a part of the athlete's social support system. In many ways the athlete's team is similar to a family. This is especially true if the athlete has chosen to compete at a college or university that is far from home. Because an athletic team can be viewed as an extended family by the athlete, many of the theories of family systems can be applied and provide useful information on how to encourage and increase social support for athletes.

Similarities of Teams and Families in Providing Social Support

While family is the most common source of social support, teammates, coaches, and athletic trainers frequently become a part of the athlete's social support system. In fact, in a survey of athletic trainers, social support from coaches was found to be more important than that received from family and friends (Wiese et al., 1991).

The social support by a team is significant because athletic teams look and function much like families. Members of athletic teams have a history and future together and have developed organized ways of behaving with one another (Lanning & Toye, 1993; Zimmerman, 1993; Zimmerman & Protinsky, 1993; Zimmerman et al., 1994). The coaching staff, especially at the university level, assumes a surrogate parent role. The coach often sets the curfew, awards the traveling and scholarship money, provides the rules for acceptable behavior, sets nutritional guidelines, and acts as a disciplinarian. The veteran athletes take on the role of older siblings, teaching the new recruits "the ropes" and assuming an increased amount of team responsibility. The freshmen, who are generally less experienced, look up to the older players for support and guidance as a younger sibling might turn to an older brother or sister for support. Viewing a team in the context of a family is based on a psychotherapeutic framework referred to as **family systems theory** (Zimmerman, 1993; Zimmerman & Protinsky, 1993; Zimmerman et al., 1994).

APPLYING FAMILY SYSTEMS THEORY

Although many theoretical orientations are possible and useful when working with injured athletes, to increase social support, family systems theory is recommended in this chapter for the following reasons. First, family systems therapy was developed to work briefly with people (in 1 to 10 sessions). Sports medicine professionals are likely to have brief relationships with injured athletes rather than years of interaction. Second, family systems focuses on the "what" (i.e., behavior) not the "why" (i.e., insight) in situations. Trained therapists can hypothesize why certain behaviors exist within individuals. It is not recommended, however, that sports medicine professionals engage in this activity. Instead they can track down what (i.e., behav-

family systems theory—A psychological theory that focuses on the relationships and interactions among members of a group rather than on the individuals.

ior) happened in a given situation. Third, family systems therapy focuses on the "here and now" instead of a historical perspective about problems. This is a good fit with the immediacy of injury and the brief relationship between athlete and sports medicine professional. Fourth, family systems is based on a health model rather than a pathology model of mental health. Therefore, it is more appropriate for a normal population—such as the majority of injured athletes—versus a clinical population. Interventions encourage searching for strength and change rather than searching for appropriate mental health diagnosis and assessments.

In family systems theory the family or team is seen as a single dynamic system made up of interacting parts, its members (Nichols & Schwartz, 1995). The theory focuses on the relationships between members rather than on the individuals. When one member experiences change, such as an injury, its effects are felt throughout the system (Larivaara et al., 1994; Patterson, 1991). An analogy that is commonly used is to compare the family or team to a mobile hanging from the ceiling. When one part of the mobile is moved, the other parts are influenced and forced to shift positions, some more than others. This phenomenon can be seen by returning to the basketball case study of Misha injuring her knee. This injury affected Misha, but it also affected the lives of those in the system around her. Her parents could no longer come to the games to watch her play. Her coaches had to determine a new game plan without their star point guard, and her teammates had to adjust to a different person playing in Misha's position. The injury also made it awkward for her friends because they did not know what to say to help her feel better and had to find topics other than basketball to talk about. Misha's injury affected many people throughout several systems, such as her team, family, and friends. Conversely, how the members of those systems react influences how well Misha will cope with losses related to the injury (Larivaara et al., 1994). A basic tenet of systems theory is that patterns are created by the actions and reactions to change within a system. These patterns are called **cycles of interaction** or **feedback loops** (Nichols & Schwartz, 1995).

cycles of interaction (feedback loops)—A basic tenet of systems theory referring to the patterns that are created by the actions and reactions to change within a system.

Cycles of Interaction

Change occurs as a result of an injury; the reactions from the athlete and others that emerge as a result of the change form cycles of interaction. Traditional psychology views problems in a linear fashion. In a simplified version of a linear model, the injury to Misha's knee causes her to be depressed (see figure 7.1). A linear model is more appropriate when dealing with an individual issue than a situation that involves others. For example, if a player is anxious, a psychologist might teach the player relaxation or biofeedback or look for interpersonal causes of anxiety (e.g., biomedical reasons). A systems model (see figure 7.2), however, would look at how others react and respond to the anxious person, how the anxious person responds back, and whether this cycle is helpful or not.

The focus of treatment in the traditional psychological model is on how Misha can change her feelings about the injury and thereby experience less depression. From a family systems perspective, however, cause and effect are interdependent and circular (Larivaara et al. 1994; Murray, Sullivan, Brophy, & Mailhot, 1991; Nichols &

Figure 7.1
Linear model of reaction.

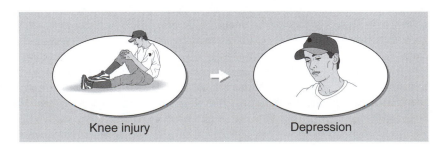

Knee injury   Depression

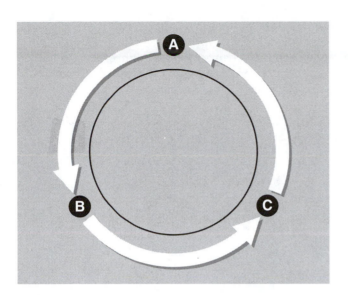

Figure 7.2 Cycles of interaction.

Schwartz, 1995). For example, when Misha is feeling depressed about her injury, she calls her teammate for support. Misha's teammate responds by telling Misha to be tough and that the situation is not as bad as it seems. These comments anger Misha because she feels that her teammate is implying that Misha is exaggerating the severity of the injury. As a result, Misha pulls away from the team, attempts to train on her own, and increasingly aggravates the injury. Through her attempts at training she becomes more discouraged because she cannot perform as she did in the past. A mapping of this cycle of interaction is shown in figure 7.3.

Cycles of interaction can be found in all of Misha's support systems. Another example is an interaction between Misha and her coach (see figure 7.4). Misha seems down because of her injury, therefore, her coach avoids talking with her about her progress because her coach does not want to dwell on the injury. Instead the coach asks Misha about school, her family, or her friends. Misha feels as though the coach

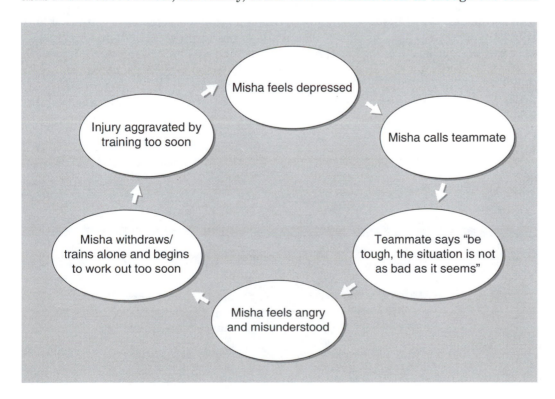

Figure 7.3
Problem cycle I: Misha and teammate.

has given up on her and that her chances of playing again with the team are over. Without the hope of playing she gives her rehabilitation program minimal effort. Her progress slows, and she becomes even more frustrated and depressed. As can be seen in this example, an individual with good intentions often can actually contribute to the problem.

Figure 7.4
Problem cycle II: Misha and coach.

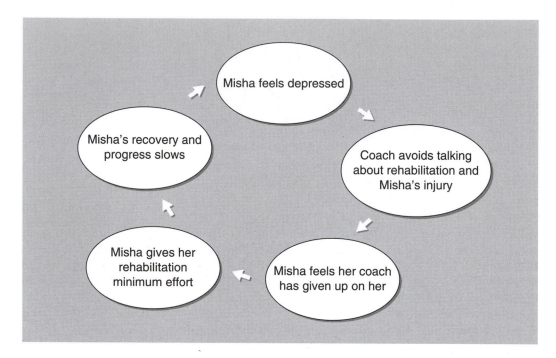

Because of their importance in the injured athlete's support system, sports medicine professionals can also play a role in the cycles of interaction (Larivaara et al., 1994; Lynch, 1988; Thompson, Hershman, & Nicholas, 1990; Wiese & Weiss, 1987). One of Misha's athletic trainers was known for her enthusiasm and positive attitude. Knowing that Misha was having a difficult time with her injury, this athletic trainer was always sure to offer Misha a smile and some words of encouragement. Misha was appreciative but felt the athletic trainer was not taking her injury seriously. Misha did not feel that she could complain or be honest about her emotions and feelings in this "happy" environment. The athletic trainer's enthusiasm only made Misha more depressed, leading her to spend less time in rehabilitation. This cycle is shown in figure 7.5.

Figure 7.5
Problem cycle III: Misha and athletic trainer.

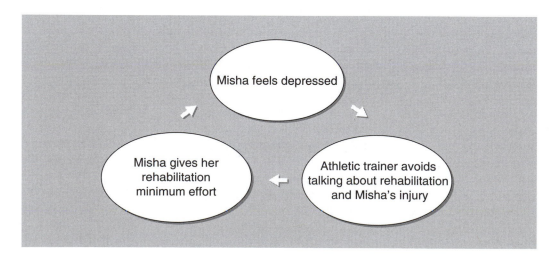

The diagrams in figures 7.3 through 7.5 illustrate **problem cycles**. Even though her teammate, coach, and athletic trainer are attempting to help Misha feel better, their behaviors actually maintain the problem (Fisch, Weakland, & Segal, 1982; Zimmerman, 1993; Zimmerman & Protinsky, 1993; Zimmerman et al., 1994). Not all cycles, however, are negative. Interactions are often effective in decreasing the problem and encouraging a solution.

A positive cycle of interactions is called a **solution cycle** (de Schazer, 1988). Sometimes the reactions of the athlete and their support system are built on positive interactions. Misha was asked to help her position replacement learn a new offensive play. This interaction helped Misha feel as if she was still part of the team. She spent extra hours after practice working with the player and came home feeling enthused rather than depressed about basketball. With a more positive attitude, Misha was able to be patient with her rehabilitation exercises, and her hopes about playing with the team next season increased.

problem cycles—
A cycle of interaction in which the behaviors of the members of a social support system maintain or encourage problems.

solution cycle—
The reactions of an individual and support system that are built on positive interactions.

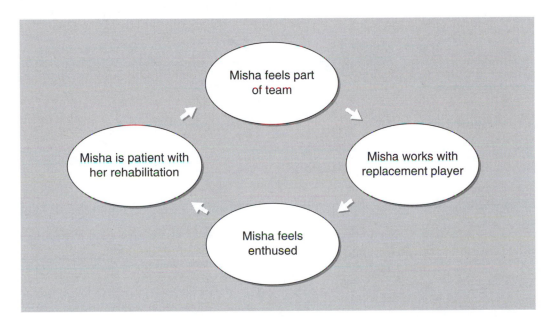

Figure 7.6
Solution cycle I: Misha and her replacement.

Another solution cycle involving a minor interaction between Misha and her coach had great results. One day Misha's coach decided to leave a message on Misha's answering machine, just to let her know that she was proud of how hard Misha was working and that the team missed her. The encouragement helped Misha feel more hopeful about her progress. She had great workouts that week and was very patient with her rehabilitation exercises. She began to feel stronger and noticed some improvement in her ability to perform.

Because everyone is different, actions that may result in a problem cycle for one athlete could actually be part of a solution cycle for a different athlete. While enthusiasm and a positive attitude from the athletic trainer were not helpful to Misha, the same approach could be very encouraging to another injured athlete.

Evaluating when your cycles of interaction are effective and when they are not is important if you desire to be successful in helping efforts. You can evaluate your effectiveness with others in several ways. First, you can watch for cues that your comments or actions are helpful. These cues can be as subtle as facial expressions or as overt as the athlete saying, "Thanks, that was helpful." Second, you can evaluate effectiveness by being attentive to what follows the initial interaction. For example, does the athlete's disposition, symptoms, or mental attitude improve? These are all cues that the interactions were helpful. In addition, it is a good idea to directly ask

Figure 7.7
Solution cycle II:
Misha and
coach.

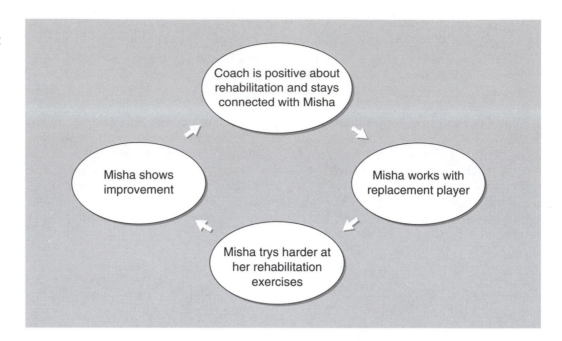

Figure 7.8
Solution
cycle III

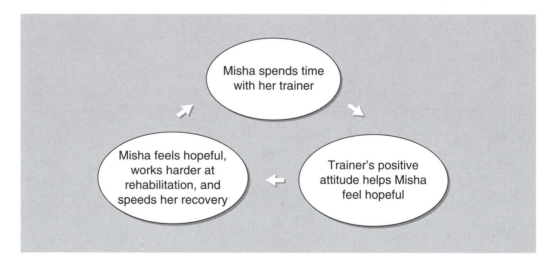

the athlete questions such as "Does it help when I . . . ?" Discussing your intention and asking what is more effective allow you to evaluate effectiveness. Furthermore, it lets athletes know that sports medicine professionals care enough to sensitively evaluate their interactions with the athletes. Additionally, asking directly encourages the athlete to take some responsibility in the cycle by telling others whether their actions are effective or ineffective.

Using Cycles of Interaction

The systems perspective of cycles of interaction is useful because it offers many opportunities for change or intervention. Because interactions within a cycle depend on one another, taking a different action at any point will result in a completely different cycle and outcome, whereas taking the same actions allows the cycle to continue (Murray et al., 1991).

Problem cycles present the opportunity for change. The problem pattern continues until something different happens to break the cycle. A change necessary to break the cycle can take place anywhere within that cycle. Instead of concentrating only on

Misha's feelings about the injury, the counseling focus could be on changing what she does when she is feeling depressed or when she is angry at a teammate. For example, if a teammate attends a doctor's appointment with Misha to be supportive and learn about her injury, the implementation of this new action could result in a different response and thus a breakdown of the problem cycle.

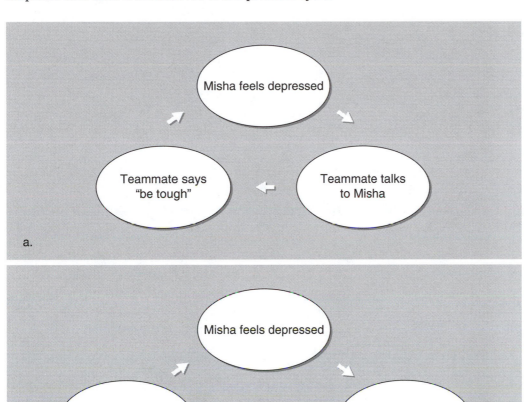

Figure 7.9
Creation of a new cycle I: Misha and teammate. (*a*) Ineffective cycle; (*b*) effective cycle.

When a cycle of interaction is working (a solution cycle), every attempt should be made to repeat and build upon the interaction that is eliminating the problem. For example, if Misha feels more positive when she is able to help other players, then every effort should be made to allow an opportunity for Misha to do that. If just a small amount of encouragement from the coach helps Misha to be more hopeful, then the coach should provide encouragement as much as possible.

As one of the people who deals most directly with an athlete's injury, the sports medicine professional has a unique opportunity to be a supportive other within the team system. Following are a variety of techniques that can help the sports medicine professional to identify and break cycles of interaction that may be hindering (problem cycles) or reinforce those that are helping (solution cycles) the athlete's progress. Sports medicine professionals can also use the techniques to guide others, such as coaches, teammates, parents, and friends, in their efforts to be supportive.

Figure 7.10
Creation of a new cycle II: Misha and parents. (*a*) Ineffective cycle; (*b*) effective cycle.

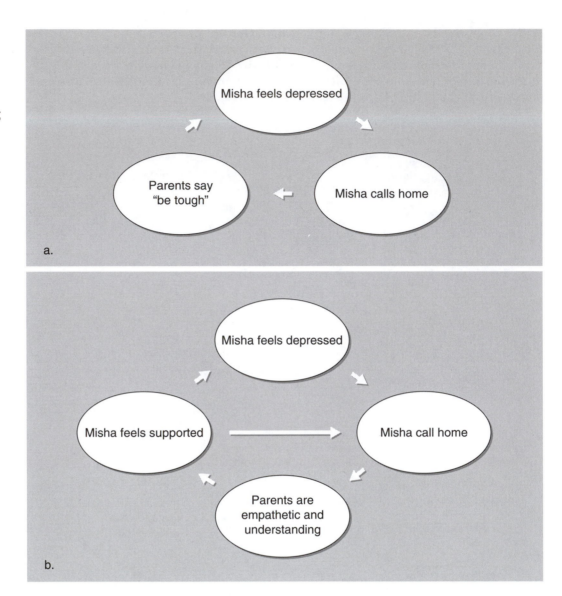

Mapping the Cycle

The drawings of problem and solution cycles are referred to as *maps*. Creating a visual image helps you identify the behaviors that are maintaining a cycle and determine where opportunities exist to break or reinforce the behavior. As you ask questions about the injury, begin to gather information about the athlete's social support system. Who does the athlete turn to for support? When the athlete is feeling down, begin to ask simple questions that help clarify the cycles of interaction that affect the athlete's feelings, such as "What seems to help?" or "When do you feel less depressed or more motivated?" This questioning is one way to assess problem and solution cycles. Another way to assess the athlete's feelings is through observation of the athlete's signs of discouragement or improvement. You can build a more complete picture of the cycles you discover by asking, "After that happened [the actions that made them feel better or worse], what did you do?" "Then what happened?" "What happened next?" Using this information, create a map (either on paper or in your mind), and look for ways to break or reinforce the pattern. You may choose to draw the cycle with the athlete and brainstorm ideas together. It may be empowering for the athlete to see that interactions and cycles can be self-influenced and changed.

Reinforcing Solution Cycles

As you map cycles of interaction, you will discover times when the athlete feels more positive than at other times. You can encourage the athlete to continue to build on these types of interactions. Discuss ways the athlete can make the positive interaction occur more frequently and how the action could be transferred to other situations. For example, when Misha was allowed to help coach another player, she felt better about herself. To build on this cycle, the athletic trainer could encourage Misha to tell the coach directly that she would like to continue this activity and help other players as well. Misha could ask to be involved in planning team strategies or conducting a portion of the practice. The more time she spends in activities that encourage her and support her solution cycles, the less time she will have to involve herself in problem cycles.

Cycle-Breaking Techniques

A key concept in systems theory is that even the smallest action can have a large impact. While the following techniques are simple, they are also very powerful tools for eliminating problem cycles.

Acknowledging, Normalizing, and Predicting

In addition to physical discomfort, an injured athlete feels emotional pain about the losses caused by injury. Friends, family, coaches, teammates, and even the athlete often fail to understand the pain or discount such feelings (Lanning & Toye, 1993). One way to break cycles that are created by this misunderstanding is to speak openly about the athlete's emotional pain. Specifically, sports medicine professionals can acknowledge, normalize, and predict the athlete's difficult feelings in order to have a positive interaction with the athlete.

1. **Acknowledging** involves simply recognizing the variety of emotions that the athlete may be experiencing. When an athlete describes the anger felt at not being able to play, the sports medicine professional might say, "It sounds like that is very frustrating to you." When the athlete describes the throbbing in an ankle, the sports medicine professional could respond, "That must really hurt." Acknowledgment helps the athlete to feel heard and understood.

2. In addition to being understood, injured athletes need to know that they are not alone. Letting the athlete know that the expressed emotions are common in other athletes with similar problems is called **normalizing**. Examples of normalizing statements include "It is common to feel depressed when you are dealing with injury and temporarily have to give up your training," "I once knew an athlete who felt very much as you do," or "It is okay to feel angry about your injury."

3. You can help athletes prepare for the variety of emotional responses they may experience by **predicting** that these responses will occur (Wiese et al., 1991). You can do this through such comments as "You may begin to feel depressed and angry," "Some athletes feel alone and left out when they are injured," or "You might experience some good days and some bad days throughout your recovery." Another way to predict and normalize an athlete's feelings is to provide the opportunity for the athlete to talk with other athletes who have been injured and can relate their own similar experiences (Wiese et al., 1991).

To illustrate the process of acknowledging, normalizing, and predicting, we return to the problem cycle with Misha and her enthusiastic athletic trainer. Misha was feeling down and needed to be permitted to experience those feelings. The ath-

acknowledging—
Recognizing the variety of emotions that someone may be experiencing and expressing that recognition.

normalizing—
Letting a person know that his or her emotions or feelings are common among individuals with similar problems.

predicting—
Hypothesizing a possible emotional response that another individual may be experiencing or may experience in the future.

letic trainer's optimism, while well intended, left Misha feeling that her emotions were invalid and not understood. The athletic trainer could have combated this by saying, "You must be feeling really sad about not being able to play" (acknowledging) or "You will probably have a lot of these feelings for a while" (predicting). The athletic trainer could then arrange for Misha to talk to another athlete who had experienced the same feelings of depression and discouragement after an injury (normalizing; Wiese et al., 1991). Using these techniques can break the problem cycle and leave Misha feeling more positive about spending time with her athletic trainer in her rehabilitation.

Figure 7.11 Creation of a new cycle III: Misha and athletic trainer. (*a*) Ineffective cycle; (*b*) effective cycle.

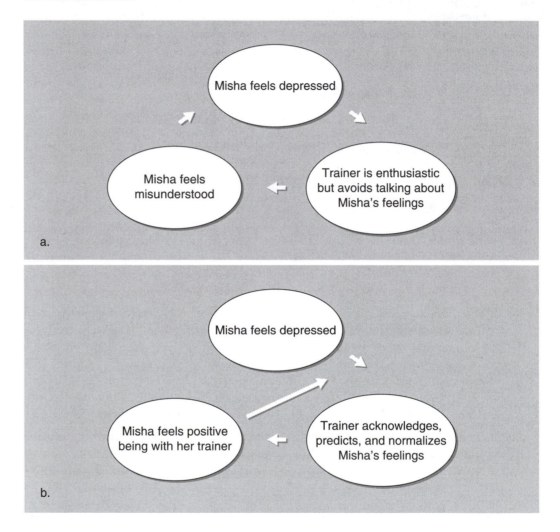

Using Metaphor

Using metaphors to address a problem can help people to talk about uncomfortable issues or to understand situations in a different context. A **metaphor** is a story or an analogy that addresses an issue using an object or situation different from the current scenario. Common metaphors include such phrases as "It's raining cats and dogs" or "He's sawing logs." Sporting events and sports commentary are typically filled with expressions that provide metaphors for life experiences. Some examples are "We've got two strikes against us," "Come out swinging," or "That's just the way the ball bounces." The following examples show how metaphor can be used to encourage an injured athlete who is growing impatient with rehabilitation and recovery.

When building a bonfire, if you toss a match on a pile of logs, chances are the match will just fizzle out. To create a bonfire, you have to start by lighting small pieces of kindling, then slowly and carefully fan the sparks until the larger wood catches fire. As the night progresses, you'll need to continue to fan the flames to keep them burning. Like a fire, an injured athlete must begin small to avoid "burning out." The athlete must build slowly and carefully, continuing to "fan the flames" to keep from becoming reinjured.

Most of us are familiar with the story of the "Three Little Pigs" and the building of their homes. The three little pigs each made a choice about how they were going to construct their homes and how much effort they wanted to put into the construction. One little pig chose straw, another chose sticks, and the last chose bricks and mortar. When the wolf came along and "huffed and puffed," he successfully blew down the straw house and the stick house because the first two pigs had been careless and lazy in the construction of their homes. The third pig who took the time and effort, carefully constructing a home with bricks and mortar, defeated the wolf and was left with a strong home that could withstand the worst of conditions. The pigs in this story can be compared to injured athletes: Athletes who take the time and have the patience to rebuild slowly have a strong basis on which to rely and are thereby less likely to be reinjured or to collapse under pressure and stress. Those who rush the process of rehabilitation, building with weak material and little patience, will be more likely to reinjure themselves in future performances.

Using metaphor and story moves the issue of the athlete's injury a step away from the personal level and allows a more objective understanding of the situation. Additionally, good metaphors create visual pictures that inspire athletes to proceed forward even when faced with feelings of frustration and impatience.

Reframing

Another way to break problem cycles is to change the meaning that is attached to a situation without changing the facts (Zimmerman & Protinsky, 1993). This technique is called **reframing**. Every action within a cycle has advantages and disadvantages. The goal of reframing is to help injured athletes accept an attitude that focuses on the advantages of the situation and the positive intentions of others. Through reframing, sports medicine professionals can help athletes view their injuries differently (Lynch, 1988). Perhaps the injury allows the athlete to catch up on studies, friendships that have been neglected, or activities that have been passed by due to a demanding practice schedule. Maybe a right-handed volleyball player with a shoulder injury has the opportunity to strengthen the movements of her left arm. Returning to the example of Misha and her teammate, the athletic trainer could help Misha reframe the teammate's response to Misha's depression. Rather than seeing her behavior as discounting Misha's injury, she could be described as having confidence that Misha will get through the situation and as trying to focus on how strong and capable Misha is because she hates to see Misha depressed and discouraged. By reframing the situation, Misha is able to see the good intentions in the teammate's behavior and is therefore less likely to respond with anger, thus breaking the problem cycle.

Focusing on Strengths

An injury can be overwhelming. With constant discomfort and long hours spent in rehabilitation, athletes may get caught in a variety of cycles that make them feel as

metaphor—A story or analogy that addresses an issue using an object or situation different from the current scenario.

reframing— Changing the meaning that is attached to a situation without changing the facts.

focusing on strengths—Looking at the positive aspects of a situation to avoid concentrating on a specific problem.

though the injury has become the focus of their life. Like reframing, **focusing on strengths** helps motivate athletes by creating positive attitudes and breaking problem cycles that are centered around negative perceptions. Every time you work with the athlete, spend some time focusing on an aspect of the athlete's body or character that is functioning well. For example, the sports medicine professional might want to talk to Misha about the strength she is developing through the extra time she is able to spend in the weight room. The therapist could compliment her on how dedicated she is to the rehabilitation process or let her know how much her help with the other team players is appreciated.

Sharing Your Skills With Members of the Athlete's Social Support System

As discussed earlier in the chapter, social support is a crucial aspect of recovery. Therefore, by spending some time focusing on the important people in the athlete's life, a sports medicine professional can help facilitate the athlete's recovery. Any of the techniques presented can be used to help the members of the athlete's social support system cope with the injury and act in a supportive way toward the athlete.

These techniques can be used with athletes, coaches, teammates, family, or friends. For example, the sports medicine professional could acknowledge the frustration that a teammate is feeling about her friend's injury. Speaking with an athlete's father using metaphor to help him to understand the emotional pain his son or daughter is facing can be helpful. Reframing could help a discouraged coach cope with the loss of a star player.

The sports medicine professional can also suggest ways that these significant others can use the techniques themselves. Periodic calls to an athlete's family and friends and discussions with coaches and teammates can keep them up to date on the injury and give the sports medicine professional a chance to suggest ways for them to break or reinforce cycles of interaction (Nideffer, 1989). Let people in the athlete's support system know what they are doing that contributes to solution cycles and encourage them to do more of it (Larivaara et al., 1994). For example, tell the coach how much Misha appreciated the encouraging phone call and suggest that she leave notes in Misha's locker for an additional boost of encouragement.

Address problem cycles with ideas about cycle-breaking techniques. For example, the sports medicine professional could predict the negative feelings that Misha will experience to a close friend and explain ways in which the friend can acknowledge those feelings. The sports medicine professional could talk to a family member about the balance between focusing on strengths and allowing the athlete to experience the realistic emotions that accompany an injury. The sports medicine professional could draw a problem cycle for a coach and explain how any small change could break the cycle.

The impact of significant others on an injured athlete can be immense. By using some of these very simple techniques, social support systems can serve the athlete in a very positive manner and aid in the process of recovery.

CASE STUDY

Sage grew up playing volleyball. She was the star player and captain in high school and is currently a key player on an athletic scholarship at a major university. During the last preseason practice Sage broke her wrist. Consequently, she was "red shirted" her junior year. Her family was a very positive source of support for her. They enjoyed doing many activities together, such as board games and hiking. The more they did together that was not related to volleyball, the better Sage felt mentally. Yet her friendships centered around volleyball. She now felt isolated from her friends and missed having something in common with them.

The more isolated she felt, the more uncomfortable her teammates and friends felt around her. The sports medicine professional who was treating her injury realized her feelings of isolation and tried to intervene.

QUESTIONS FOR ANALYSIS

1. Map a possible problem cycle between Sage and her teammates.

2. Map a solution cycle between Sage and her family.

3. What might a sports medicine professional learn from the solution cycle to break or intervene in the problem cycle?

4. Based on the techniques described in this chapter, what minor changes can make major differences? Which of these changes might a sports medicine professional try?

SUMMARY

The role of social support in the healing of injured athletes and how to encourage support from those people most important to the athlete are key areas for athletic trainers, coaches, and other sports medicine personnel. A person's social support system is made up of those who give him or her encouragement, advice, and a friendly ear in times of trouble or despair. Usually, family and friends make up an individual's support system, which is recognized as a key factor in both prevention and treatment of athletic injuries. Athletes who report low social support or high stress are more likely to suffer injuries; if an injury occurs, social support also influences recovery time. Research has found that social support plays a key role in how well patients comply with medical instructions and rehabilitation procedures. Specifically, compliance is highest when an athlete's family expects compliance and has a positive attitude about the process. While family is the most common source of social support, teammates, coaches, and athletic trainers also frequently become a part of an athlete's social support system. With social support being such a significant element in the healing process, knowing how to encourage social support of the injured athlete is a critical skill for an athletic trainer, coach, and other sports medicine professionals.

Many theoretical orientations are useful when working with injured athletes, but when the objective is to increase social support, family systems theory has been recommended in this chapter. Sports medicine professionals are likely to have brief relationships with injured athletes rather than years of interaction, and family systems therapy has been developed to work briefly with people (in 1 to 10 sessions). Also, family systems focuses on behavior rather than on situations and on the "here and now" instead of from an historical perspective. This system fits well with the immediacy of injury and the short-term relationship between athlete and sports medicine professional. Family systems is based on a health model rather than a pathology model of mental health—it is more appropriate for a "normal" population rather than a clinical population. Interventions encourage searching for strength and change rather than searching for appropriate mental health diagnosis and assessments.

When a cycle of interaction is working (a solution cycle), every attempt should be made to repeat and build upon the interaction that is eliminating the problem. We looked at several scenarios in which cycles of interaction broke down and several others where they led to a solution, and we compared and contrasted the cycles to find the common threads of success along with the common patterns of failure. Because everyone is different, actions that may result in a problem cycle for one athlete could actually be part of a solution cycle for a different athlete. While enthusiasm and a positive attitude from an athletic trainer or coach might not be helpful for some athletes, the same approach could be very encouraging to another.

chapter

8

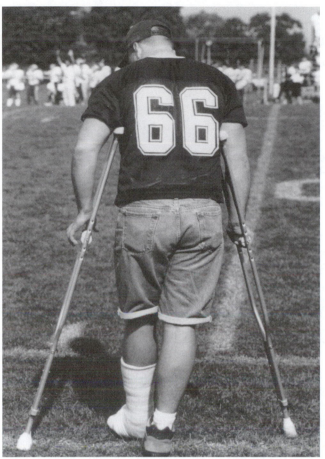

© Terry Wild Studio

Referral of Injured Athletes for Counseling and Psychotherapy

Britton W. Brewer, PhD
Albert J. Petitpas, PhD
Judy L. Van Raalte, PhD
Springfield College, Springfield, Massachusetts

CHAPTER OBJECTIVES

Identify common reasons for referring injured athletes for counseling and psychotherapy

Describe factors affecting the timing of referrals for counseling and psychotherapy

Explain the process of referring injured athletes for counseling and psychotherapy

Outline key considerations in developing a referral network

In addition to the obvious ramifications for physical functioning, there are psychological consequences of sport injury. Sustaining a sport injury can be a significant source of stress (Brewer & Petrie, 1995) and can adversely affect emotional functioning (Brewer & Petrie, 1995; Chan & Grossman, 1988; Leddy, Lambert, & Ogles, 1994; Pearson & Jones, 1992; Smith et al., 1993), as described in greater detail in chapter 2. Counseling may be useful in assisting injured athletes to adjust psychologically to their injuries. Because of the primacy and frequency of sports medicine professionals' involvement in the rehabilitation process, they are in a unique position to provide counseling to injured athletes. In some circumstances, however, it may be appropriate for sports medicine professionals to refer injured athletes to mental health professionals for counseling services (Henderson & Carroll, 1993; Kane, 1982; Wiese-Bjornstal & Smith, 1993).

The purpose of this chapter is to address issues central to the referral of injured athletes for counseling and psychotherapy. We first present a rationale for referral and identify specific reasons for referral. Next, we discuss factors affecting the timing of referral, elements of the referral process, and aspects of referral networks. The chapter concludes with a case study that illustrates key points in the referral of an injured athlete for psychological treatment from a mental health professional.

RATIONALE FOR REFERRAL

In athletic therapy the act of referring an injured athlete for counseling or psychotherapy is consistent with the guiding principle of attempting to enhance the physical and psychological well-being of injured athletes. Referral not only addresses the psychological needs of injured athletes, but also may indirectly influence physical outcomes of interest due to the interrelationships between psychological and physiological processes (Ievleva & Orlick, 1991; Wise, Jackson, & Rocchio, 1979). Moreover, in situations where referral of an injured athlete for counseling or psychotherapy is mandated, it is the professional responsibility, ethical obligation, and, in some cases, legal duty of the sports medicine professional to provide a referral (Kane, 1984; Makarowski & Rickell, 1993; National Athletic Trainers Association, 1992). Thus there is a compelling rationale for sports medicine professionals to become familiar with and proficient in referral for counseling and psychotherapy.

REASONS FOR REFERRAL

Sports medicine professionals may encounter a number of situations that warrant referral of an injured athlete to a mental health practitioner. Most of these situations involve circumstances outside the limits of the training, competence, and comfort of the sports medicine professional.

Perhaps the most obvious situation warranting referral is when the injured athlete requests a referral for counseling or psychotherapy. Although this occurs infrequently, it can happen when the injured athlete has identified a personal concern that he or she deems appropriate for psychological consultation. The injured athlete may or may not be comfortable with disclosing the exact nature of the concern to the sports medicine professional.

Another reason for referral to a mental health professional is that the injured athlete displays overt signs of psychological disturbance (Heil, 1993a; Henderson & Carroll, 1993; Makarowski & Rickell, 1993). If the injured athlete shows symptoms of anxiety, depression, eating disorders, substance abuse, or other patterns of disordered behavior, referral is clearly indicated. Psychological disturbance may signify a poor psychological adjustment to injury or may reflect the exacerbation of a preexisting condition. Regardless of the source, it is essential for sports medicine professionals to recognize **psychopathology** in injured athletes and refer appropriately (National Athletic Trainers Association, 1992). Highlighting the need for competency in this area, preliminary research suggests that approximately 5 to 13 percent of injured athletes experience clinically significant levels of psychological distress (Brewer, Linder, & Phelps, 1995; Brewer, Petitpas, Van Raalte, Sklar, & Ditmar, 1995; Leddy et al., 1994) and that emotional disturbance is associated with poor adherence to sport injury rehabilitation regimens (Daly, Brewer, Van Raalte, Petitpas, & Sklar, 1995). Further, one study found that sports medicine professionals' observations did not correspond well with injured athletes' self-reports of psychological distress (Brewer, Petitpas, et al., 1995), indicating a possible need for additional training in the recognition of disordered behavior for sports medicine professionals.

psychopathology—The presence of a psychological disorder; also, the scientific study of abnormal behavior and mental processes.

Referral is also appropriate when the injured athlete reports or exhibits adjustment difficulties in important life domains, such as social relationships, school, work, and other areas of social and personal functioning (Henderson & Carroll, 1993; Makarowski & Rickell, 1993). These difficulties may be symptomatic of an underlying psychological disorder or, more likely, may simply indicate that the injured athlete is having a hard time coping with his or her injury and the associated treatment demands. An example of a situation where a referral might be made for the reason of adjustment problems would be an injured college athlete who, although typically a top-notch scholar, remarks that she is "doing lousy in school and failing a few classes" because she "just can't concentrate."

Sometimes injured athletes display no apparent signs of distress or impaired functioning but instead convey problems in adjustment through more subtle means. For example, an injured student athlete might spend an inordinate amount of time "hanging around" the athletic training room. Such behavior may reflect dependence on the sports medicine professional or the rehabilitation environment (Henderson & Carroll, 1993; Makarowski & Rickell, 1993; Petitpas & Danish, 1995). Other cues to which sports medicine professionals should be attuned include excessive preoccupation with when a return to sport is possible, extreme denial of any adverse consequences associated with injury, statements regarding guilty feelings about not being able to help the team, boastful comments about past performances, and social withdrawal (Petitpas & Danish, 1995). Presence of these behaviors warrants further inquiry by sports medicine professionals and possible referral should investigation reveal more profound difficulties in adjustment.

Rehabilitation difficulties are an additional set of circumstances for which referral may be appropriate. At first glance, this may seem counterintuitive, as sports medicine professionals are trained and competent in physical rehabilitation practices. However, some potential aspects of rehabilitation have a distinct psychological component, such as major rehabilitation setbacks, nonadherence, chronic pain, overcompliance, somatizing, and bothering athletic therapy personnel. Accordingly, referral for counseling or psychotherapy may be indicated if any of these behaviors or circumstances are encountered (Heil, 1993b; Kane, 1984; Petitpas & Danish, 1995). Similarly, suspicions of intentional injury or malingering should be investigated carefully, with referral as a possible outcome (Heil, 1993b; Kane, 1984).

This list of reasons for referral of injured athletes to a mental health practitioner is not exhaustive. In general, sports medicine professionals should refer injured athletes for counseling or psychotherapy if they encounter circumstances that exceed their training, competence, or comfort or represent a conflict between the interests of the athletic organization and those of the injured athlete (i.e., if disclosure of the information discussed in sports medicine professional–injured athlete interactions could be detrimental to the injured athlete; Makarowski & Rickell, 1993). The decision of whether to refer an injured athlete for counseling or psychotherapy can have important ethical or legal ramifications for sports medicine professionals. Practicing outside their competencies or failing to act in the best interests of injured athletes may violate ethical codes and leave sports medicine professionals open to criminal penalties and civil suits where applicable (Makarowski & Rickell, 1993).

TIMING OF REFERRAL

Once a reason for referral has been identified, the point in time at which referral to a mental health professional is introduced to the injured athlete may influence the ultimate success of the referral. A variety of factors should be taken into account when determining the optimal timing of referral. As displayed in figure 8.1, these factors include the severity of psychological symptoms, the coping resources available to the injured athlete, the sports medicine professional's skills and training, the nature of the relationship between the sports medicine professional and the injured athlete, the nature of the relationship between the sports medicine professional and the professional to whom the injured athlete is referred, and immediate environmental and situational factors.

Severity of Symptoms

As previously noted, injured athletes who display signs of psychological disorders or social or personal adjustment problems may need to be referred to a mental health professional. In general, the more severe the symptoms of psychological difficulties, the more promptly a referral should be made (Heil, 1993a). Referral is particularly urgent when suicide attempts are a likely possibility (Smith & Milliner, 1994). Warning signs for suicide include depression, withdrawal, diminished self-esteem, decreased concern with personal hygiene, loss of interest in school or work, and veiled communications of extreme distress (Carson, Butcher, & Mineka, 1996). Case study research has shown that common factors among injured athletes who have attempted suicide include sustaining a serious time-loss injury, experiencing a notable decrement in sport skills, and having been replaced in their position on the team as a consequence of their injury (Smith & Milliner, 1994).

Coping Resources

The strength of the coping resources available to the injured athlete may influence the timing of referral for counseling or psychotherapy. Coping resources include not

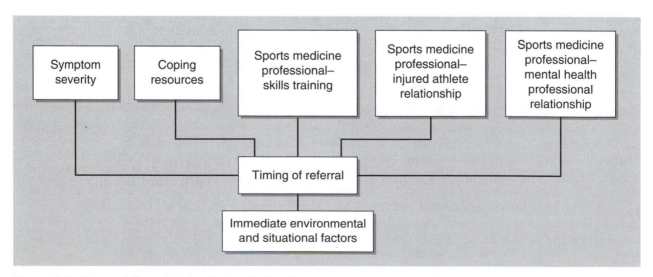

Figure 8.1 Factors influencing the timing of referral.

only the athlete's personal attitudes (e.g., "I will get better"), beliefs (e.g., perceived control over recovery), and attributes (e.g., hardiness), but also those of the injured athlete's social support system, which consists of coaches, teammates, friends, parents, and family members (Petitpas & Danish, 1995). A strong arsenal of coping resources available to the injured athlete may offset adverse circumstances and delay, at least temporarily, the need for referral.

Sports Medicine Professional's Skills and Training

The extent to which the sports medicine professional has developed counseling skills and competencies in identifying situations in which referral is appropriate may affect the timing of the referral. Sports medicine professionals who are able to listen effectively to their patients, ask the kinds of questions that elicit pertinent information from their patients, and recognize the warning signs of poor adjustment to injury are in a better position to make a referral to a mental health professional before their patients' problems have reached a critical stage. Likewise, sports medicine professionals with a solid background in counseling and psychology may feel more comfortable in broaching the subject of referral with injured athletes.

Relationship Between the Sports Medicine Professional and Injured Athlete

A primary influence on the timing of referral is the nature of the relationship between the sports medicine professional and the injured athlete. Once a sports medicine professional has established rapport with the injured athlete and has earned the injured athlete's trust, he or she is more likely to be privy to the kind of information that may lead to referral. Injured athletes may be reluctant to disclose personal information to their sports medicine professional until they know and feel sufficiently comfortable with him or her. Introducing the idea of referral to a mental health professional before a relationship of trust has developed may alienate the injured athlete. Clearly, the importance of the relationship between the sports medicine professional and the injured athlete must not be underestimated.

Relationship Between the Sports Medicine Professional and Mental Health Professional

The relationship between the sports medicine professional and the mental health professional to whom the injured athlete is referred may play a role in determining the timing of referral. When the mental health practitioner is someone with whom the sports medicine professional is well acquainted, the sports medicine professional may be less hesitant to consult the practitioner for advice or to make a referral. This is most likely to be the case when the mental health professional is an official member of the sports medicine team. An established professional relationship between the sports medicine professional and the mental health practitioner can facilitate a proactive approach in which the psychological needs of injured athletes are addressed early in treatment, before significant problems develop.

Immediate Environmental and Situational Factors

The factors identified to this point that affect the timing of referral provide general guidance as to when referral may be most appropriate but do not pinpoint an exact moment to bring up referral with injured athletes. Features of the immediate clinical environment and situation can prove quite influential in determining the timing of referral. For example, if the clinical setting (e.g., an athletic training room) is crowded with other injured athletes and sports medicine professionals, discussion of referral may have to wait until the setting clears or until a private location can be found. Similarly, if an injured athlete is especially angry and is complaining vehemently to the sports medicine professional, it may be best to delay referral until the athlete is calmer and more receptive to what the sports medicine professional has to say. Attending to aspects of the immediate environment and situation can enable sports medicine professionals to time their referrals more effectively.

THE REFERRAL PROCESS

Although referring injured athletes for counseling or psychotherapy is commonplace among sports physicians (Brewer, Van Raalte, & Linder, 1991) and is recognized as an important skill for sports medicine professionals to possess (National Athletic Trainers Association, 1992), recent research indicates that few sports medicine professionals make psychological referrals. Indeed, national surveys have revealed that most athletic trainers have never referred an athlete for injury-related counseling (Larson, Starkey, & Zaichowsky, 1996) and that most athletic trainers and sports medicine clinics do not have standard procedures for referring injured athletes for counseling or psychotherapy (Gipson et al., 1989; Larson et al., 1996). Therefore, it is essential for sports medicine professionals to become familiar with the referral process, which can be divided into the following five phases (see figure 8.2): (1) assessment, (2) consultation, (3) trial intervention, (4) referral, and (5) follow-up.

Assessment

assessment—*The initial phase of the referral process in which the sports medicine professional observes and evaluates an injured athlete's psychological status.*

As depicted in figure 8.2, the initial phase of the referral process is **assessment**. This phase occurs naturally during the course of rehabilitation, from the time the injured athlete begins treatment to discharge. Assessment consists of observing and evaluating the athlete's psychological responses to injury. Listening to what injured athletes have to say (and, conversely, listening for topics that injured athletes avoid), asking injured athletes how they are getting along, and watching for signs of poor adjustment to injury are important assessment skills. Given the wide range of possible responses to injury, it is necessary to monitor the thoughts, feelings, and behaviors of injured athletes (Brewer, 1994; Wiese-Bjornstal, Smith, & LaMott, 1995) while performing the more traditional tasks of athletic therapy.

Figure 8.2
The referral process.

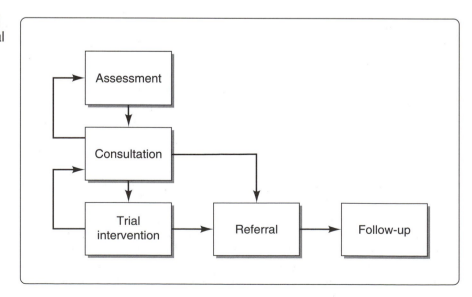

Consultation

The next phase of the referral process, **consultation**, occurs once the sports medicine professional has identified a potential reason for referral. Consultation consists of contacting a mental health professional, describing the injured athlete's circumstances, and soliciting an opinion on a logical course of action. If a sport psychologist or other mental health practitioner is a member of the sports medicine team, then consultation can occur informally or at a staff meeting. However, if there is no mental health professional on the treatment team, as is likely to be the case (Cerny, Patton, Whieldon, & Roehrig, 1992; Larson et al., 1996), the sports medicine professional contacts an outside practitioner for consultation. In such situations, it is helpful if the sports medicine professional has discussed the possibility of consultation and referral before the need arises. As a result of consultation, the mental health professional may advise immediate referral (in urgent situations), recommend additional assessment, or suggest a trial intervention to be carried out by the sports medicine professional.

consultation—
The phase of the referral process in which the sports medicine professional contacts a mental health professional to discuss the status of an injured athlete.

Trial Intervention

The nature of the trial intervention suggested by the mental health professional depends on the injured athlete's circumstances. Regardless of the particular situation, the intervention is likely to be easy for the sports medicine professional to carry out and simple for the injured athlete to follow. If, for example, the injured athlete reports having difficulty sleeping, the mental health professional may recommend that the sports medicine professional assist the injured athlete in acquiring relaxation skills and may suggest a few specific relaxation exercises for the sports medicine professional to teach. The purpose of the trial intervention is to provide the injured athlete with an alternative coping mechanism (Heil, 1993a) and to further evaluate the need for referral. If the intervention works, no further action may be necessary, although it is a professional courtesy to inform the mental health practitioner of the intervention's success. If the intervention does not appear to be successful, referral or additional consultation are likely next steps.

Referral

Once a decision to refer an injured athlete for counseling or psychotherapy has been reached, it is time for the most delicate part of the referral process: referral itself. How a referral is presented to an injured athlete may influence the success of the referral and, ultimately, the athlete's physical and psychological well-being. Because athletes who seek psychological assistance may be derogated by others (Linder, Brewer, Van Raalte, & DeLange, 1991; Linder, Pillow, & Reno, 1989; Van Raalte, Brewer, Brewer, & Linder, 1992), some injured athletes may be resistant to or even insulted by the idea of referral for counseling or psychotherapy (Brewer, Jeffers, Petitpas, & Van Raalte, 1994). Therefore, it is crucial to be sensitive to potential concerns that injured athletes may have about the referral process (Andersen, Denson, Brewer, & Van Raalte, 1994; Van Raalte & Andersen, 1996). Sports medicine professionals should prepare injured athletes for referral by explaining in plain language the reason for referral and describing what is generally involved in working with the mental health professional to whom they have been referred, perhaps noting the success of similar referrals in the past. Injured athletes may be more receptive to referral if the stresses of injury rehabilitation and the mind–body connection (i.e., psychological factors may influence recovery of physical functioning) are emphasized (Heil, 1993a). This reassures injured athletes that they are not "head cases" (Heil, 1993a) and normalizes referral without discounting its importance. Table 8.1 offers tips for suggesting referral to injured athletes.

Table 8.1 Presenting Referral to an Injured Athlete

KEY TIPS

1. Establish rapport with the athlete.

2. Gather information about the athlete.

3. Be sensitive to the athlete's possible concerns about being referred. Allow the athlete to maintain dignity and to save face.

MAKING THE REFERRAL

1. Describe observed behaviors using "I" statements and tentative language.

   "I'm concerned about you and need your help in understanding how things are going for you. On one hand, it seems as if you have been making good progress in rehabilitation and have been working hard. On the other hand, you seem more distracted and upset about things than when you started. Can you help me to understand what's going on?"

2. Seek clarification.

   "Are there other things going on in your life that are making things tough for you now? Is there anything else?"

3. Assess the athlete's coping and support resources.

   "It seems that you have a lot of things that you are dealing with. How have you been handling the all this? How has that approach been working for you?"

4. Suggest referral.

   "It sounds as if you are working hard to manage everything. Maybe speaking to someone about this could help you get back on track more easily. I remember another athlete who was going through some of the same things you are who talked to a mental health professional, Dr. X. That athlete told me that he learned some new ways of dealing with things and that it was pretty helpful. How would it be if I were to arrange a meeting for the three of us—you, me, and Dr. X— to sit down and talk about this together?"

For an injured athlete who is a minor (i.e., younger than 18 years of age), discussion of referral should include the athlete's parent(s) or guardian(s). As is the case with medical interventions, the mental health practitioner needs to obtain consent to treat from the minor athlete's parent or guardian before the commencement of counseling or psychotherapy. Sports medicine professionals should provide parents and guardians with a clear rationale for referral without revealing potentially sensitive information that injured athletes have disclosed in confidence. Conveying general concern for an injured athlete's physical and emotional well-being is helpful in convincing parents and guardians of the necessity for referral.

If the injured athlete accepts the referral for counseling or psychotherapy, sports medicine professionals can facilitate follow-through on the referral by helping the injured athlete schedule an appointment with the mental health professional (Heil, 1993a). When the mental health practitioner is an on-site member of the sports medicine team, the sports medicine professional may be able to introduce the injured athlete and the practitioner. Sports medicine professionals may even want to consider bringing a mental health practitioner into the sports medicine setting for the first visit with the athlete. Having the sports medicine professional, mental health practitioner, and athlete all sit down together even once can help the referral process go more smoothly. Sports medicine professionals should obtain written consent to provide the mental health practitioner with pertinent information about the injured athlete (Strein & Hershenson, 1991). To reduce the likelihood that the injured athlete will feel abandoned or rejected by the sports medicine professional, the sports medicine professional should reassure the athlete that their work together on physical rehabilitation will continue without interruption (Heil, 1993a). If the injured athlete does not accept the referral, the sports medicine professional can reimplement a trial intervention and should not hesitate to reintroduce the idea of referral at a later date (Heil, 1993a).

Follow-Up

The final phase of the referral process, **follow-up**, comes after the injured athlete has been referred to the mental health professional. Follow-up consists of communication between the sports medicine professional and the mental health practitioner and between the sports medicine professional and the injured athlete. Upon meeting with the injured athlete, the mental health professional may obtain a waiver of confidentiality from the athlete to share general information regarding the injured athlete's progress in counseling with the sports medicine professional (Strein & Hershenson, 1991). This does not mean that the mental health practitioner will provide all details pertaining to the injured athlete's involvement in counseling or psychotherapy to the sports medicine professional. Instead, the practitioner is likely to furnish the sports medicine professional with a courtesy letter acknowledging the referral, a written consultation report, and possibly informal dialogue, with information about the injured athlete disclosed at the practitioner's discretion (Meyer, Fink, & Carey, 1988; Strein & Hershenson, 1991). Again, in situations where the mental health professional is an active part of the sports medicine team, the communication between the sports medicine professional and the mental health professional may be of a more informal variety.

During the follow-up phase, communication between the sports medicine professional and the injured athlete regarding the referral is less structured than that between the sports medicine professional and the mental health professional. Some injured athletes may inform their sports medicine professional about their progress in counseling or psychotherapy. Other injured athletes, however, may make no mention of the consequences of the referral. With these athletes, the sports medicine professional can ask "How's it going with Dr. X?" or can return to an assessment mode to evaluate indirectly the success of the referral. Periodically, the sports medicine professional and the mental health professional may want to confer in order to ensure that the referral process is working smoothly for both parties. Sports medicine professionals should document the occurrence of these consultations without divulging confidential information that is potentially damaging to injured athletes. A sample notation might consist of a statement that the sports medicine professional "Conferred with Dr. X about the psychological status of [injured athlete]. Agreed to follow up in two weeks."

follow-up—The final phase of the referral process in which the sports medicine professional communicates with the mental health practitioner and the injured athlete following referral.

REFERRAL NETWORKS

Most sports medicine professionals, who do not have a mental health professional available to them as a member of the sports medicine team (Cerny et al., 1992; Larson et al., 1996), find it necessary to develop a referral network of outside mental health practitioners to help meet the psychological needs of their injured athletes. We describe various types of mental health professionals and discuss considerations in developing a referral network in the following sections.

Mental Health Professionals

There are many types of mental health practitioners, who differ in terms of training, theoretical orientation, interest in working with injured athletes, and availability for referral. Several types of mental health practitioners and their specialty areas are presented in table 8.2.

Types of Mental Health Practitioners

The training that mental health practitioners receive varies greatly depending on the individual practitioner's area of specialization. Clinical and counseling psychologists, psychiatrists, psychiatric social workers, academic athletic counselors, and alcohol- or drug-abuse counselors are some of the mental health practitioners who are likely to work with injured athletes. These practitioners may have experience working in such areas as compliance, pain management, eating disorders, substance abuse, interpersonal relationships, and career counseling. It is important to note that experience working with injured athletes is not required for any of these specialties.

Clinical and counseling psychologists have strong backgrounds in psychology and typically have earned a PhD (doctor of philosophy), a PsyD (doctor of psychology), or an EdD (doctor of education) degree. Their professional preparation generally includes a minimum of four or five years training beyond the bachelor's degree in the areas of psychological assessment, psychotherapy, and mental health research. Nearly all states require that psychologists also pass a licensing or certification exam. Clinical and counseling psychologists work with clients ranging from those who have adjustment problems to those who suffer from mental disorders.

Psychiatrists have earned an MD (medical doctor) degree followed by at least a three-year residency working with patients in a mental health setting. Many psychiatrists take a psychiatry examination and become board certified. Currently, psychiatrists are the only mental health professionals who can prescribe medication and administer treatments such as electroconvulsive therapy. Therefore, psychiatrists often see clients with more serious mental disorders.

Psychiatric social workers typically hold an MSW (master of social work) degree from a school of social work. Their two-year post-bachelor's degree training typically includes development of skills in interviewing, family evaluation, psychotherapy, and treatment. Like psychiatrists, psychiatric social workers typically see clients with more serious mental disorders.

Academic athletic counselors typically hold a master's degree in counseling, education, sport psychology, or a related field. National training standards for academic

---

Table 8.2 Degrees and Specialty Areas of Various Mental Health Practitioners

Title	Degree	Areas of specialty
Psychologist (clinical, counseling)	PhD, PsyD, or EdD	Adjustment problems, psychological disorders
Psychiatrist	MD	Psychological disorders
Psychiatric social worker	MSW	Broad-based mental health services
Academic athletic counselor	MA, MS, or MEd	Academic, career, and personal counseling
Alcohol- or drug-abuse counselor	Varies	Substance abuse

athletic advisors do not currently exist, but most academic athletic advisors have experience in working with college student athletes on academic concerns and career issues. Academic athletic counselors may also have other areas of specialization.

Alcohol- and drug-abuse counselors are typically paraprofessionals whose training has focused specifically on the evaluation and management of people with alcohol and drug addictions. Because the government neither licenses the skills nor controls the activities of alcohol- and drug-abuse counselors, training of alcohol- and drug-abuse counselors can vary greatly. Many alcohol- and drug-abuse counselors work as part of a team with other mental health practitioners.

Theoretical Orientation

Each individual mental health practitioner brings his or her academic training, applied experience, and personal skills to the therapeutic relationship. Some mental health practitioners focus on current feelings, others focus on behaviors, and still others focus on the unconscious mind. Different theoretical orientations may be appropriate for different athletes. Research has indicated that the outcome of a therapeutic relationship depends strongly on the match between the therapist's and client's expectations, personal qualities, and feelings of free choice about the relationship (Kazdin, 1979). Thus there is no single "correct" theoretical approach. Accordingly, what is important is for the athlete to feel comfortable with the particular therapeutic approach selected.

Financial Considerations

Generally, the more training that mental health practitioners have, the higher their fees. Thus psychiatrists typically charge the highest fees, followed by psychologists, psychiatric social workers, and various paraprofessionals. It is important to note that higher fees do not guarantee higher-quality services. Many mental health practitioners allow some of their patients to pay what they can afford on a sliding-scale basis. Most health insurance policies offer at least limited coverage of mental health services. It should be noted, however, that assignment of a formal psychiatric diagnosis that becomes part of the athlete's permanent insurance record is typically required for insurance reimbursement. Some athletes, when informed of this fact, may elect to pursue payment options other than insurance reimbursement. Sports medicine professionals should not hesitate to discuss issues pertaining to payment for counseling or psychotherapy with injured athletes. Insurance coverage, mental health practitioner fees, and payment options should be clarified before referral.

There is a great deal of variability in the training, areas of expertise, and costs of mental health practitioners. The best mental health practitioner is one who meets the specific needs of the injured athlete. These needs include a mental health practitioner with expertise relevant to the injured athlete's problem, with time to meet with the injured athlete, with a fee scale that the injured athlete can afford (or that insurance will cover), and with whom the athlete feels comfortable. Finally, the mental health practitioner should be someone whom the sports medicine professional knows, trusts, and can work with as part of a referral network.

Developing a Referral Network

For sports medicine professionals who work with injured athletes, a **referral network** consists of a group of mental health practitioners to whom injured athletes can be referred. The referral network should include practitioners with expertise in treating the range of problems likely to be encountered by injured athletes (e.g., emotional disturbances, eating disorders, substance abuse, grief, pain). Ideally, the mental health professionals selected should have experience working with injured

referral network—A group of mental health practitioners to whom sports medicine professionals can refer injured athletes.

athletes. At the least, they should be interested and open to working with an injured athletic population (Van Raalte & Andersen, 1996).

Developing a referral network takes time and motivation on the part of the sports medicine professional. The sports medicine professional needs to identify practitioners who are appropriate for the referral network, contact the identified practitioners to determine whether they are interested in receiving referrals, develop relationships with the practitioners, and modify the referral list on an ongoing basis (Heyman, 1993; Van Raalte & Andersen, 1996).

There are several ways that a sports medicine professional can identify mental health practitioners for a referral network. One of the simplest ways to begin the referral list is to obtain suggestions of interested and capable mental health practitioners from other sports medicine professionals and members of the sports medicine team. For sports medicine professionals who work in academic settings (e.g., high schools, colleges, universities), likely on-campus candidates for the referral network are guidance counselors, counseling center staff members, and academic counselors within the athletic department (Andersen & Brewer, 1995; Misasi, Davis, Morin, & Stockman, 1996). People in the community who are knowledgeable about mental health practitioners can also provide assistance in the development of a referral list. Ideas for potential referral targets can also be found by exploring mental health resources available in the community. Telephone book yellow pages have a section devoted to mental health care providers. The local community United Way may publish a *First Call Community Service Directory,* which lists nonprofit social service agencies and programs. One or all of these sources can provide sports medicine professionals with a pool of practitioner names to be considered for a referral list.

After creating the pool of names, the sports medicine professional should contact the identified practitioners to determine whether they are interested in receiving referrals. Mental health practitioners who express interest in receiving referrals should be willing to consult with the sports medicine professional about their patients and should also be willing to accept referrals as necessary. The mental health professionals selected should be practitioners with whom the sports medicine professional feels comfortable speaking and consulting. Selecting an ethnically diverse group of both male and female mental health practitioners with various professional backgrounds and theoretical orientations may be useful. Because many athletes have limited time and funds, the sports medicine professional may want to include some local mental health practitioners who provide services on a sliding-scale basis (Van Raalte & Andersen, 1996).

Once interested mental health practitioners have been identified, the sports medicine professional should begin to develop working relationships with them. The sports medicine professional can telephone the mental health practitioner or schedule a meeting to learn the specifics of the mental health practitioner's expertise and approach. If the sports medicine professional is interested in working with the mental health practitioner, a consultation and referral plan should be developed. For consultation, it is important for the sports medicine professional to be able to reach the mental health practitioner to discuss particular patients. A communication plan that respects athletes' privacy but allows an effective working relationship between the sports medicine professional and mental health practitioner is ideal. For referral, it is important for the sports medicine professional to be familiar with the mental health practitioner's typical procedures (e.g., how sessions are scheduled, what sessions are like, how many sessions are typically scheduled, what payment procedures are used) and preferred referral process (Bobele & Conran, 1988). This information can enable the sports medicine professional to reduce an injured athlete's anxiety by clearly explaining what working with the mental health practitioner will be like and to enhance the likelihood of a successful working relationship between the athlete and the mental health practitioner (Heil, 1993a).

Once a referral network has been created, practitioners' areas of expertise, types, names, addresses, and phone numbers can be typed so that the referral list is easy to access and use (Kane, 1984). Sports medicine professionals can use the referral list themselves and may also want to make copies (of at least a subset of the information) available to their athlete patients. A referral list is not a static document; it should be modified on an ongoing basis (Kane, 1984). Sports medicine professionals may find it useful to touch base periodically with the members of the referral network to maintain the relationship. The mental health practitioners who move, with whom the sports medicine professional does not work well, and with whom injured athletes are dissatisfied should be deleted from the referral list. New practitioners can also be added to the referral list, particularly in areas of specialty without representation on the list.

Development and use of a referral network can greatly enhance the outcome of the referral process. Judicious use of referrals can help to keep problems from developing into crises and can provide necessary support to injured athletes in crisis situations.

Chris is a talented, 19-year-old college sophomore who became a starting forward for a nationally ranked Division II basketball program as a freshman. The oldest of six children, Chris grew up in a tough neighborhood in a major metropolitan area. His parents, who have had an "on again, off again" relationship for as long as Chris can remember, often struggled to make ends meet. Chris frequently found himself in the caretaker role, responsible for his younger siblings while his mother worked. Nevertheless, he somehow managed to find the time and energy to excel both on the court and in the classroom.	**CASE STUDY** *Part I*

Although Chris was an exceptional athlete, he lacked the height to play forward and the ball-handling ability to play guard at a major Division I school. Fortunately, he received a scholarship from a fine Division II college that was located several hundred miles from his home. At first he did not want to be that far away from home, but his mother insisted that it was time that he started to look after himself. As it worked out, Chris quickly made the adjustment to college and had a fine freshman year both academically and athletically.

Chris began his sophomore year with high expectations. Unfortunately, just two days before basketball practice was to begin, Chris incurred a serious knee injury while playing touch football with several of his teammates. This was the first major injury that Chris had experienced, and he found himself alternating between being angry at himself for being "so stupid to get injured" and a "little afraid" of what was going to happen.

Although his surgery went well and his physician told him that he would be as good as new in a matter of weeks, Chris still had his doubts. He kept questioning: Would his knee come back strong enough for him to play? Would he lose his starting position? Would he really be as good as new? Chris had a lot of questions and a lot of strong emotions, but he was not sure where to go for answers. He thought about home, but his father was gone again, and he did not want to upset his mother. His teammates and coaches told him not to worry about anything, but this did not seem to help very much, and Chris often found it easier to be alone than to be there when his teammates were talking about practice or scrimmage games. To make matters worse, Chris's moodiness apparently caused a big blowup with his girlfriend. It was clear that Chris had a lot of emotional stuff going on, but he kept it bottled up inside him.

It was during the first week of rehabilitation that Chris's sports medicine professional began to suspect that Chris perhaps was having some problems coping with his injury. To begin with, Chris was frustrated with the pace of his physical therapy, even though he was progressing as expected. This seemed to be magnified by Chris's obsession with the question, "When can I play again?" In addition, Chris would continually ask if his range of motion or strength had improved. Ironically, when Chris was asked about his level of pain, he would always report it at the highest level.

By chance, Chris's sports medicine professional learned that Chris was ignoring her recommendations and spending several hours at the fitness center each evening doing additional exercises for his knee. When she confronted Chris about this situation, he became enraged and told her to mind her own business. She persistently tried to communicate the dangers of overdoing the exercises and prolonging rehabilitation, but he wanted to hear none of it. As a result of this incident, the sports medicine professional decided to get some additional information about Chris and soon discovered from one of his teammates that Chris seemed to be avoiding his friends and had missed two of his midterm exams.

QUESTIONS FOR ANALYSIS

1. What are some of the interpersonal and intrapersonal warning signs of a potentially difficult psychological adjustment to injury found in Chris's case?

2. Should injured athletes such as Chris be encouraged to maintain contact with their teammates?

3. Based on the information presented, what should Chris's sports medicine professional do?

Part II

Chris's sports medicine professional contacted a psychologist who served as the liaison between the college counseling center and the athletic department. Without identifying Chris by name, the sports medicine professional described her concerns about the situation. After concluding that there were enough warning signs of possible psychological disturbance present, the psychologist agreed to work with the sports medicine professional to help her evaluate the situation more closely and, if required, make an appropriate referral.

Chris's sports medicine professional called Chris and scheduled a meeting "to work through the problems of the other day." Chris eventually agreed to the meeting, which the sports medicine professional used as an opportunity to try to understand what Chris was going through, being particularly sensitive to his emotional reactions and his withdrawal from sources of support. As it turned out, Chris was able to voice some of his fears and doubts for the first time. As the sports medicine professional patiently listened to and paraphrased his concerns, Chris began to open up and disclose that his father is "an alcoholic and a loser." By being successful at sports and graduating from college, Chris could prove to everybody that he wasn't like his father. Unfortunately, the injury had threatened everything that Chris had worked for and filled him with all the old doubts and fears that he had growing up.

At the end of the meeting, Chris agreed to go with the sports medicine professional to meet with a counselor who specialized in working with people who grow up in alcoholic families. The sports medicine professional was able to identify an appropriate referral through the counseling center liaison and joined Chris for the first appointment. During this meeting Chris gave the sports medicine professional and counselor written permission to consult about his case.

Chris continued to work with the counselor and also joined an off-campus support group for adult children of alcoholics. These activities appeared to give Chris an outlet to express his feelings and concerns. In any event, he seemed to be in better control of his injury situation and was able to return to his typical academic and social routines. The sports medicine professional and the counselor consulted weekly on Chris's situation, and by all accounts, he seemed to be back on track. His physical rehabilitation progressed as expected, and he was able to reenter competition by midseason, both physically and mentally ready to play.

QUESTIONS FOR ANALYSIS

1. Why did the sports medicine professional decide to refer Chris to the psychologist even though Chris did not display any overt signs of psychopathology?

2. Who are the primary support people described in this case, and what were their roles in facilitating Chris's successful return to competition?

3. What proactive steps can sports medicine professionals take to build comprehensive referral networks?

SUMMARY

In the course of treating injured athletes, sports medicine professionals may encounter situations in which referral for counseling or psychotherapy is appropriate and, in some cases, ethically mandated. Common reasons for referral of injured athletes for counseling or psychotherapy include patient requests for referral, overt displays of psychological disturbance, adjustment difficulties in important life domains, subtle displays of distress, and rehabilitation difficulties. Factors affecting the timing of psychological referrals include the severity of psychological disturbance, the injured athlete's coping resources, the sports medicine professional's competencies and background, and the nature of the sports medicine professional's relationships with the injured athlete and with the mental health professional.

The referral process consists of assessment, consultation, trial intervention, referral, and follow-up phases. A variety of mental health professionals are likely referral targets, including clinical and counseling psychologists, psychiatrists, psychiatric social workers, academic athletic counselors, and alcohol- or drug-abuse counselors. A mental health practitioner's areas of expertise, theoretical orientation, and fee scale should be taken into account when making a psychological referral. In developing a referral network, sports medicine professionals need to identify, contact, and develop relationships with a wide range of appropriate mental health practitioners. Judicious use of referral for counseling or psychotherapy can enhance the psychological and physical well-being of injured athletes.

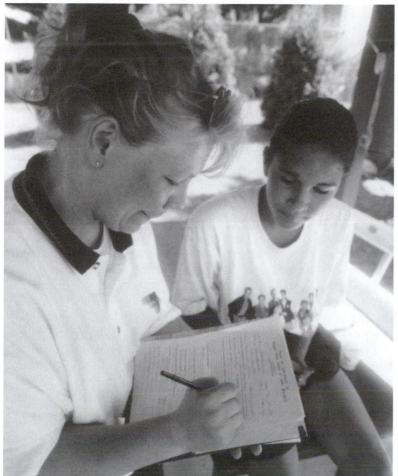

© Mary Langenfeld

Documentation in Counseling

Richard Ray, EdD, ATC, *Hope College, Holland, Michigan*

CHAPTER OBJECTIVES

Understand the importance of proper counseling documentation to the athlete, the sports medicine professional, and the institution

Understand the different methods of documenting counseling, including the strengths and weaknesses of each

Understand the common errors made in documentation and how to avoid them

Understand the common elements of counseling documentation in sports medicine

Understand the legal and ethical responsibilities of the sports medicine professional in documentation of counseling

Sports medicine professionals are usually taught a healthy appreciation for the importance of the medical record. Unfortunately, this appreciation usually extends only to the documentation of our athletes' physical complaints. The counseling we provide to our patients often goes undocumented. When documentation is attempted, the result is usually a record that provides little basis to reconstruct the facts associated with the counseling. This chapter is intended to help sports medicine professionals—athletic trainers, physical therapists, and team physicians—understand the importance of counseling documentation, some of the issues related to mental health record keeping, and various techniques for documenting counseling in sports medicine settings.

Record management is just as important as any other counseling skill we use with athletes. It may be the most important evidence in assessing the practitioner's counseling professionalism (Holmes & Karst, 1989). The poorly managed counseling record often reflects a poorly managed case. Yet even mental health professionals tend to do a substandard job in this area. Perlman and his colleagues (1982) found that mental health professionals fail to document some important information in as many as 70 percent of the cases they treat. Of this group, physicians tended to be the most delinquent record keepers. This may be the result of poor training in mental health documentation. Fewer than half of the mental health professionals in Reynolds's (1992) study reported receiving "a great deal of emphasis" on this aspect of their work during their professional education. Of these mental health professionals, physicians received the least training. A critical number of health care professionals simply do not appreciate the importance of appropriate and comprehensive documentation of counseling. Indeed, British counselors are not even required to document their interaction with their clients (Bond, 1993). An increased awareness of the importance and various methods of documenting counseling will help sports medicine professionals improve this critical component of their practice.

WHY DOCUMENT?

Record keeping can be a time-consuming task. It is almost universally viewed as drudgery. Why should busy sports medicine professionals take the time to document the counseling they provide to their patients? Isn't it enough to simply record physical interventions? Good record keeping, including documentation of counseling activity, helps sports medicine professionals address the following important concerns (Ray, 1994; see figure 9.1).

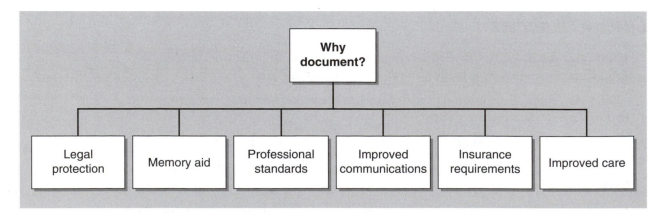

Figure 9.1 Reasons to document counseling activities in sports medicine.

Legal Protection

Record keeping is one of the five highest areas of exposure to legal liability for counselors (Piazza & Baruth, 1990). Record keeping helps protect the rights of both the athlete and the practitioner by documenting the athlete's problem, the intervention, and the response to treatment or advice. Without adequate records, disputes between aggrieved athletes and sports medicine professionals are reduced to "your word against mine." A properly constructed record of the counseling relationship provides evidence of the care taken by the sports medicine professional to meet the needs of the athlete (Bond, 1993). Athletic trainers or physical therapists who fail to adequately document counseling may actually expose their supervising physicians to legal liability, especially where the physician employs them directly (Walzer, 1989). Finally, sports medicine professionals have a duty to refer patients with mental health problems to practitioners trained and licensed to work with these problems. Failure to document such a referral or an athlete's response to the referral (Iyer & Camp, 1991) could pose legal difficulties for the sports medicine professional.

Memory Aid

Busy health care professionals who treat scores of patients every week often forget the details of their patients' problems and their responses to those problems. "Did I teach Jim how to do these exercises last week?" "Mary was concerned about something at home when I last saw her. What was it again?" Sports medicine professionals should be able to refer to the patient's records for the answers to these and similar questions. In addition, the written record should provide sports medicine professionals with written rationale for the treatment decisions they make (Holmes & Karst, 1989).

Professional Standards

Several professional groups require that all patient care be thoroughly documented. The standards of practice of the National Athletic Trainers Association (NATA, 1985), although not explicit on the subject of counseling documentation, require athletic trainers to keep records of every aspect of the athlete's care. The *Criteria for Standards of Practice for Physical Therapy* of the American Physical Therapy Association (APTA, 1995) requires physical therapists to document patient care, including the counseling that constitutes the basis for informed consent for treatment. In addition, it requires physical therapists to adhere to a code of ethics that explicitly cites the psychological well-being of the patient as falling within the purview of the physical therapist. Documentation of the care taken to preserve the patient's psychological health, although stated implicitly rather than explicitly, is presumed to fall within the standard. Finally, the Joint Commission on Accreditation of Healthcare Organizations mandates the documentation of psychosocial elements of patient care (Iyer & Camp, 1991). Since many sports medicine professionals are employed in hospitals accredited by this body, they too are subject to this standard.

Improved Communications

Sports medicine professionals should refer athletes with serious mental health problems to professionals specifically trained and licensed to deal with these problems. The quality of the counseling record should be of significant value to mental health professionals in accepting these referrals and making treatment decisions. Obviously, great care must be taken to obtain the athlete's informed consent to release these records to the mental health professional. Assuming such consent is granted, the well-written counseling record should be very useful. The sports medicine professional is in a better position than the mental health professional to determine certain aspects of the athlete's behavior, especially those related to athletic performance. This information will be helpful to the mental health professional.

Insurance Requirements

Although sports medicine professionals do not usually bill third-party payers for "counseling," they often bill for services related to "patient education." Since patient education is frequently a significant component of the counseling process, the argument can be made that sports medicine professionals get paid, in part, for counseling their patients. Documentation of patient outcomes to treatment and education are a critical element in the ability to get paid in sports medicine. The degree to which a practitioner can document the patient's mastery of educational interventions often determines the insurance company's willingness to pay for the service.

Improved Care

Documentation of our counseling efforts should result in better care for our athletes (Bond, 1993). Documentation of counseling requires sports medicine professionals to organize and reflect on their thoughts regarding the particular aspects of their athletes' well-being. This reflection should result in improved care for the athlete.

DRAWBACKS OF DOCUMENTING COUNSELING

Is counseling documentation the answer to all our counseling-related problems? Is it always logical? Even though I have tried to make a convincing argument in favor of documenting counseling in sports medicine, it should be noted that such documentation can create problems, both for the athlete and the practitioner.

Interference With Communication

Counseling should be characterized by attentive, active listening. The sports medicine professional's attention should be focused on the athlete and what he or she is communicating—verbally and nonverbally—including his or her affect or mood and noticeable, perhaps even incongruent, behaviors. Record keeping, especially note taking, can interfere with the communication process by drawing the practitioner's focus away from the athlete and toward the notebook.

Damage to the Athlete

Even though sports medicine professionals may agree to protect the confidentiality of the athlete's counseling records, this should not be—and often is not—viewed as an ironclad promise or agreement. Courts of law can order the release of medical records, even if they contain confidential counseling information. In many legal jurisdictions the content of the mental health record is privileged only in the context of a relationship between a patient and a licensed psychologist or psychiatrist (although this privilege may not exist if the athlete is under 18). The release of sensitive information may damage the athlete's reputation or standing in the community. If athletes know that sports medicine professionals are documenting the content of counseling sessions, it may be difficult to establish the trust so important for successful resolution of their problems. This problem may be especially difficult to overcome when the sports medicine professional works for a university or professional team that has technical ownership of athletes' medical records.

None of these problems are good enough reasons to avoid documentation of counseling altogether. They are included to point out where some of the pitfalls of documentation may be found. Creative sports medicine professionals will still manage to document their counseling efforts, even in the face of these difficulties. Suggestions for how to do this can be found later in this chapter.

WHAT TO DOCUMENT

A comparison of the same athlete's records—one prepared by the sports medicine professional and the other by a mental health professional—would certainly reveal differences in the detail with which counseling and other psychological interventions are recorded. The mental health professional, by virtue of his or her training and license, will likely record a much more detailed psychological examination, assessment, plan for treatment, and response to treatment. The sports medicine professional, except for the most minor or temporary cases, will not actually "treat" the athlete's psychological condition and will therefore not generate the same level of detail in the counseling record. The sports medicine professional should, however, document in the athlete's record any information pertaining to the athlete's psychological condition and the steps taken to intervene in any problems (Piazza & Baruth, 1990). The following elements of the athlete's counseling record may be appropriate for some or all sports medicine professionals to document.

Physical Exam

Many psychological problems have their roots in physical ailments. The sports medicine professional should be sure to document the details of the patient's past history and present physical status as part of any psychological record keeping (Piazza & Baruth, 1990).

Mental Status Exam

Although athletic trainers and physical therapists have only rudimentary training in psychological assessment, several characteristics of a troubled athlete's mental status may become evident during the course of a routine interpersonal contact. Physicians should be more adept at assessing the athlete's mental status (see figure 9.2). Iyer and Camp (1991, p. 13) recommend that the following elements of the mental status assessment be documented:

- General behavior and appearance
- Characteristics of speech
- Emotional state
- Content of thought
- Orientation to time, place, and person
- Memory
- General intellectual level
- Abstract thinking (interpretation of simple proverbs)
- Insight evaluation (whether the athlete recognizes the significance of the situation and feels the need for psychological intervention)

Mental Status Record

General appearance (note posture, ease, poise, anxiousness, etc.)

Behavior and psychomotor activity (note mannerisms, gestures, twitches, agility, rigidity, etc.)

Speech (note speed, degree of hesitancy, emotional content, etc.)

Attitude toward interviewer (examples: cooperative, attentive, frank, defensive, hostile, guarded)

Mood (how he or she sees world; says how he or she feels)

Active expression (describe emotional state)

Orientation:

Time (correctly identifies day, approximate date and time) ☐ Yes ☐ No

Place (athlete knows where he or she is) ☐ Yes ☐ No

Person (knows who interviewer is; others and their roles) ☐ Yes ☐ No

Thought process (preoccupations, major concerns, coherence)

Memory (concrete examples of immediate, recent, or remote memory problems)

Concentration (difficulty tracking own ideas)

Abstract thinking (understanding simple proverbs like "a rolling stone gathers no moss")

Judgment (understanding of the implications of the athlete's behavior)

Insight (awareness or understanding of problems (e.g. denial, blaming others, etc.)

Figure 9.2 Sample form for recording the results of the mental status examination.

Patient Education

Although some mental health professionals would not place patient education squarely within the conception of counseling, I believe patient education is one of the primary counseling roles of the sports medicine specialist. Although we frequently document the details of the athlete's history, physical exam, treatment, and progress, how often do average athletic trainers, physical therapists, or team physicians document their efforts at patient education? How often does the average sports medicine professional document the patient's understanding of this education? What about the athlete's reaction to the education? These are important elements of counseling documentation. They help document important aspects of the athlete's care. In a legal action, this documentation could play an important role in establishing not only that the athlete was provided with treatment, but that he or she understood his or her part in the treatment process.

Verbal Orders

Sports medicine is ideally practiced in a team environment, where athletic trainers, physical therapists, and other health care professionals work with physicians to care for injured athletes. Such collaboration is useful, but it does have drawbacks. One of the most common is that prescriptions for treatment or other forms of medical communication are transmitted orally. Such communications, especially when they involve the athlete's mental health, should be documented in the athlete's record. This helps ensure that the appropriate action is taken and followed up. It also helps the recipient of the communication to protect him- or herself legally.

Telephone Advice

Sports medicine professionals are frequently called on to give advice over the telephone. The range of advice certainly extends into areas defined as counseling in chapter 1. Telephone contacts are often interpreted as the initiation of a patient–practitioner relationship (Henry, 1994). Consequently, any time an athlete requests and receives advice by telephone, the sports medicine professional should be sure to document the call and its content in the athlete's record.

Suicidal or Violent Behavior

The first duty of any health care professional is to help prevent patients from injuring themselves or others. If a member of the sports medicine team encounters an athlete who threatens violence to him- or herself or another, there is a duty not only to act to protect the athlete, but to record the circumstances of the event in the medical record (Iyer and Camp, 1991; Soisson, VandeCreek, & Knapp, 1987). This is one of the few times when the confidentiality of the athlete–practitioner relationship should be violated (Keith-Spiegel & Koocher, 1985). Sports medicine professionals employed in school or university settings may be bound by institutional policies to inform the school's counselor or dean of students when such incidents occur.

Referrals

In addition to patient education and initial emotional counseling, one of the sports medicine professional's most frequent mental health activities is referring athletes to mental health professionals. It is difficult to overstate the importance of documenting such referrals in the athlete's medical record. Documentation of referral may be the only defense available to sports medicine professionals involved in litigation involving an athlete's mental health treatment (Soisson et al., 1987). Some athletes, unfortunately, refuse to accept a referral to a mental health professional. It is equally important that attempts to refer the athlete and any subsequent refusals are carefully documented in the medical record (Iyer & Camp, 1991).

WHAT NOT TO DOCUMENT

Although most of the details of counseling contacts between athletes and sports medicine professionals should be carefully and systematically documented in the medical record, good reasons exist to exclude some material from the record. Athletes, courts, and third-party payers can often find their way into the medical record if they want access. For this reason, Soisson and colleagues (1987) recommend that the following information be excluded from the athlete's counseling record:

- Emotional statements and personal opinions of the practitioner
- Information about illegal behavior
- Information about sexual practices
- Information not pertinent to the athlete's medical condition that is likely to embarrass or harm the athlete should the material be released

HOW TO DOCUMENT COUNSELING

The process of documenting counseling and other mental health information is not radically different from that used in the recording of physical complaints. A few differences exist, however. This section is intended to help you build on your present documentation skills so that you can include the counseling elements of your work in your patients' records. A basic understanding of medical record keeping is assumed.

Narrative Charting

narrative charting—Prose entries into an athlete's record; the most traditional form of record keeping for counseling and other mental health activities.

Narrative charting, which involves detailed prose entries into the athlete's record, is the most traditional form of record keeping for counseling and other mental health activities. Entries are usually made in either longhand script or are typed into the chart after being transcribed from dictation. Like any other record-keeping method, narrative charting has strengths and weaknesses. One of the most useful elements of the narrative-charting method is the facility with which direct quotations can be used to document an athlete's thoughts, feelings, and behaviors. Quotations are a particularly useful—and in many cases important—source of objective data to which both the sports medicine professional and the mental health professional can refer should follow-up be required. Quotations may be particularly important for documenting potentially violent, threatening, or suicidal thought processes (Fulero & Wilbert, 1988; Iyer & Camp, 1991).

The narrative-charting system has weaknesses as well. The most obvious drawback to this system is the amount of time it takes to write out detailed descriptions of counseling encounters. Although dictation can speed the process, it can still be laborious and time-consuming. The narrative process also requires the sports medicine professional to take detailed notes of very high quality—both in terms of description and legibility—during the counseling session. This is not always practical, especially when counseling involves a teaching emphasis in which the practitioner must demonstrate the technique to be mastered. Note taking, as previously mentioned, can also detract from the active listening process so important for counseling effectiveness. Finally, narrative charting is viewed by some as inefficient. It uses more words than may be necessary to convey the essence of the problem, the proposed solutions, and the athlete's response to the sports medicine professional's recommendations.

As previously mentioned, dictation of the narrative record can speed the process up significantly. Dictation is a difficult skill to master, however. If you choose to dictate your counseling records, the following tips will help improve the process (Ray, 1994):

- Organize the data from your notes before beginning dictation. Dictate a more comprehensive record from these notes.

- Always dictate mental health records in a private setting. Speak clearly and slowly into the dictation machine. This helps reduce noise on the tape and helps preserve the confidentiality of the information.

- Spell proper names and medical jargon. Provide your transcriber with a medical dictionary.

- Make sure your transcriber understands the importance of maintaining the confidentiality of mental health records. Transcription of mental health records should be done in an area where people cannot look at the records as they walk through the room or past the transcriber's desk.

- Review and initial all transcriptions before filing them in the medical record.

Problem-Oriented Medical Record

The **problem-oriented medical record** (POMR) was proposed by Dr. Lawrence Weed in the 1960s and is now widely used in both general medical practice and the mental health professions. The POMR is a record-keeping method that organizes the data around the patient's specific complaints (Berni & Readey, 1978). The POMR is constructed of four elements (Dayringer, 1978; see figure 9.3):

problem-oriented medical record (POMR)—A record-keeping method that organizes the data around a patient's specific complaints.

- The database. For sports medicine professionals this section includes sections on patient identification, primary complaint or problem, medical history, mental status, and a list of relevant social and family factors.

- The problem list. This is a numbered list enumerating the athlete's emotional-psychological problems. For many sports medicine professionals this list will be very short—perhaps limited to one or two entries—since sports medicine professionals are not trained to conduct a detailed psychological assessment. Only the most obvious problems are likely to be included here.

- The plan list. This is a list of the plans to be implemented to address each of the athlete's problems. It may—and probably should—include referral to a mental health professional for all but the most minor psychoemotional problems. It may include patient education plans to remediate gaps in the patient's understanding. Each plan should be cross-referenced to its appropriate problem.

- The follow-up list. This part of the POMR contains the patient's reactions to the various interventions based on the practitioner's follow-up of each problem. The **subjective–objective assessment plan** (SOAP) format is used to record this information. The subjective part of the record includes data that cannot be observed directly, but that the athlete reports to the sports medicine professional. Examples might include an athlete's comments that he or she "feels stressed" or "can't sleep." The objective part of the record includes things that the practitioner can directly observe. Mental health professionals will often use this part of the record to document the results of various mental status tests. The assessment is the practitioner's best judgment as to the nature of the athlete's problem. The plan should include any interventions undertaken to address the problem. In some cases follow-up may be limited to a notation that the athlete now understands and can perform his or her

subjective–objective assessment plan (SOAP)—A patient's reactions to the interventions based on the practitioner's follow-up of each problem.

exercises. In cases in which the athlete is referred to a mental health professional for a psychoemotional problem, follow-up may be more difficult. The mental health professional is not ethically permitted to correspond with the referring sports medicine professional in the absence of informed consent from the athlete. In cases in which the development of an effective therapeutic alliance would not be possible if the athlete's information was shared with others, such informed consent is not in the best interest of the athlete (Thompson & Sherman, 1993). In these cases, follow-up is limited to casual observations or follow-up conversations with the athlete, since no information will be forthcoming from the mental health professional. If it appears necessary or in the best interests of the athlete to communicate with the mental health professional, it is best to suggest to the athlete at the time of referral that, with his or her consent and support, the athlete can assist communications by asking the counselor for a release to sign at the first appointment.

Like narrative charting, the POMR has strengths and weaknesses for documenting counseling in sports medicine. Grant (1977) lists the following advantages:

- The POMR offers a clearly defined set of rules for recording counseling in sports medicine.
- The POMR encourages clarity and explicitness in counseling record keeping.
- The POMR enhances the sports medicine specialist's ability to retrieve counseling information from the record.

The POMR is not without its detractors, however. Hartman & Wickey (1978) assert that since the POMR was originally established for medical record keeping, it requires significant adaptation to fit a psychosocial model of care delivery. They also point out that the system takes time to master and implement, especially in large institutional settings. Reynolds's (1992) review of several studies revealed the POMR to have a low (.40) inter-rater reliability for some aspects of its content.

Documentation Pitfalls

All aspects of sports medicine practice are subject to mistakes and errors. Documentation of counseling is no different. Although documentation errors can always be costly, mistakes in the documentation of counseling can be particularly problematic because patients, including athletes, are very sensitive about references to their mental health.

Poor Handwriting

Illegible handwriting is the most commonly reported problem in mental health documentation, affecting 25 percent of the records in one study (Reynolds, 1992). If the patient records are written illegibly, the information becomes useless. Unfortunately, it is not unusual for practitioners to seek help from their secretaries in deciphering their own handwriting! If the practitioner's handwriting is not clear enough for everyone to read, dictation should be used to overcome the problem.

Premature Opinions and Judgments

Only facts should be entered as part of the counseling record (Fulero & Wilbert, 1988). This requirement contrasts with documentation techniques commonly employed for physical complaints. For instance, it would not be unusual for the sports medicine professional to enter the following statement into the record of a patient with a knee injury:

Based on the clinical signs and symptoms, the patient may have suffered a torn anterior cruciate ligament. He didn't feel a "pop" or "snap," but the swelling and sensation of laxity are suggestive of an ACL tear.

Data Base

Past medical Hx.

Family Hx.

Social Hx.

Habits

Tobacco:

Alcohol:

Drugs:

Seatbelts:

Exercise:

Nutrition:

Problems   **Dates**

1

2

3

4

Plans   **Dates**

1

2

3

4

Follow-up: See SOAP notes in record

Figure 9.3   Sample cover sheet for a problem-oriented medical record.

Consider the possible consequences, however, of similar speculation in a counseling setting:

> *Jenny seemed pretty "down." She was crying and had a hard time maintaining the conversation. Although I'm not exactly sure of the nature of her problem, I think she may be suffering from depression.*

There are at least two problems with this note. First, even though the sports medicine professional admits ignorance of the nature of the athlete's problem, an assessment is still provided, even though it is only a hypothesis. Since the practitioner lacks the training to make such a judgment, one wonders how valuable such an assessment can be. The second problem is integrally related to the first. If this record were to be released, either appropriately or inappropriately, the reader could be led to the conclusion that Jenny is clinically depressed, which may in fact be untrue. This could have damaging consequences for her future. If, on the other hand, the knee injury record was released, the impact is likely to be less consequential. The assessment in this case is more reasonable because it was made by someone with the expertise to render such an opinion. In addition, history of an ACL injury is likely to be met with far less prejudice in our culture (in most cases) than history of clinical depression. A good practice in writing counseling notes is always to consider the possible audiences for the records. If someone else were to read the note, how would it be interpreted? The following factual record of Jenny's counseling is more appropriate for inclusion in her file:

> *Jenny came to see me at 2:30 P.M. on Friday. She said she wanted to talk about her game the previous day. She said, "I played so bad. I'm afraid I'm going to lose my spot on the team." She cried for 5 minutes. She said, "This is the only thing I can think about. I can't get it out of my head. I can't concentrate in class." I suggested that Jenny visit with the counselor. She agreed. I walked her over to the Counseling Center and helped her make an appointment.*

---

10 Counseling Documentation Tips

Brown (1982) recommends that health care professionals adhere to the following 10 suggestions to help improve their counseling documentation, which have been modified for sports medicine professionals:

1. Record only observed behavior and factual information.
2. Use quotations to illustrate the athlete's feelings and thought processes.
3. Avoid recording hypotheses, hunches, or speculation.
4. Be brief.
5. Avoid making value judgments.
6. Describe behavior. Do not label the athlete or diagnose.
7. Inform the athlete that you will make a record of your counseling, the purposes of the record, and the confidential nature of the record.
8. Consider the athlete's rights and welfare in the construction and maintenance of records.
9. Keep counseling records up to date.
10. Follow the general guidelines for documentation of other health problems when documenting for counseling.

ACCESS TO COUNSELING RECORDS

Who should have access to an athlete's counseling records? Under what circumstances should such access be provided? These are important questions that sports medicine professionals should be prepared to answer before they take on a counseling role with the athletes under their care.

Confidentiality Versus Privilege

Two commonly misunderstood terms that have an important bearing on the disposition of the athlete's counseling records are confidentiality and privilege. **Confidentiality** is an ethical issue that requires the sports medicine professional to refuse to divulge any aspect of the athlete's medical or psychological history (Jacob & Hartshorne, 1991). It is an ethical agreement that frees the athlete to tell the professional whatever is necessary to enhance and improve the athlete's welfare. The confidential nature of an athlete's medical or psychological condition should be abrogated only if the athlete provides specific permission to do so (except in cases of suicidal or violent behavior as noted earlier).

Privilege, unlike confidentiality, is a legal term. It is the right of the athlete, established by law, to prevent the content of medical or psychological communications from being divulged (Keith-Spiegel & Koocher, 1985). Privilege is "owned" by the athlete and therefore may not be legally violated unless waived by the athlete, except in certain unusual circumstances. The question of whether an athlete's counseling record is privileged is complex. Privilege is established by statute and is therefore applied differently in different states. The physician–patient relationship for the purpose of maintaining the privacy of such records is fairly well established. Whether the athletic trainer–patient or physical therapist–patient relationship would be viewed by the courts in the same manner is not well known.

Informed Consent

Information related to the counseling provided by the sports medicine professional, as previously noted, should be held in confidence unless the athlete specifically agrees to allow the information to be released. This is often problematic, especially for athletic trainers and team physicians who are approached by coaches and administrators desiring access to such information. Unless the athlete has executed a properly written document of informed consent, it is inappropriate for the sports medicine professional to even acknowledge that the athlete is being treated or was referred for mental health services (Heil, 1993). Thompson and Sherman (1993) recommend that formal agreements specify the extent to which information will be shared with team personnel. In the absence of such agreements, all information should be held in confidence.

Keith-Spiegel and Koocher (1985) recommend that the following elements be included in the informed consent to release psychological information (see figure 9.4):

- Name of the person to receive the information
- The content of the records to be released
- The purposes for which the records will be used
- The date the form was signed and the information released
- Limitations or restrictions on the information to be released, including the dates for which the release is to remain in effect
- Name and signature of the person providing consent

confidentiality— An ethical position that requires the sports medicine professional to refuse to divulge any aspect of the athlete's *medical* or psychological history except under very rare circumstances.

privilege—An athlete's legal right, established by law, to prevent the content of medical or psychological communications from being divulged.

I,_____ , do hereby give consent for _____ ,or other medical or counseling personnel employed by_____ , to release such information regarding my medical history, counseling history, or results of medical or mental health tests as may be requested by _____ . I authorize release of this information in only the following forms (check any any for which authorization is granted):

☐ Complete written record
☐ Partial written record (specify authorized parts): _____
☐ Written summary
☐ Oral summary

I authorize the release of this information for only the following purposes (describe):

1._____   2._____

3._____   4._____

I understand that a record will be kept of all individuals requesting information and the date of the request. This information is normally confidential and except as provided in this Release will not be otherwise released by the custodian of the information. This Release remains valid until (check one):

☐ Revoked by me in writing   or   ☐ Until (enter date): _____

I have had an opportunity to ask questions regarding this Release and the process by which my medical information may be released. I understand that I can revoke this Release at any time. All of my questions have been answered to my satisfaction. Having read and understood the above, I freely sign this Release of Counseling Information Authorization.

_____   _____
Signature of athlete   Signature of witness

_____   _____
Date   Date

_____   _____
Signature of authorizing agent (if not athlete)   Relationship to athlete

Counseling Information Release Log

Date of release	Released to	Form of release	Content of release	Released by
1.				
2.				

Figure 9.4 Sample form authorizing release of counseling record information.

- The relationship of the authorizing agent to the athlete, if not the athlete him- or herself
- A statement advising the athlete that the consent can be canceled at any time should it become important to do so
- Name and signature of a witness

Access to Counseling Records by Family Members

Coaches and team personnel are not the only people who may desire access to confidential counseling information. It is not unusual for families to seek access to such records as well. If the athlete is under 18, the parents may have legal access to all their records. In many circumstances, the athlete's family has a personal relationship with the sports medicine professional. Athletic trainers and team physicians are frequently queried about the psychological state of athletes by the athletes' parents and other family members. These requests for information are often posed in informal or innocuous situations when the sports medicine professional's guard may be down.

The parents or legal guardians of minors generally have a legal right of access to medical and counseling records involving their children. Sports medicine professionals should exercise great caution, however, in informally divulging such information, even to parents of minor children. The trust required for an effective counseling relationship can be irreparably harmed if such confidences are broken. Clinicians should avoid divulging information in informal settings. The sideline of a high school football game is not the appropriate setting to bring Dad up to speed on Johnny's mental condition. Sports medicine professionals should generally insist that parental requests for information be provided in writing and that any release of information be thoroughly documented in the athlete's record.

When the athlete is an adult, requests for information from the family should always be denied unless the athlete gives permission (Keith-Spiegel & Koocher, 1985). Unless the athlete presents a danger to him- or herself or another, the same ethical requirements of confidentiality that apply in other cases also apply to the families of adult athletes.

RECORD HANDLING AND DISPOSAL

Although the protocols and requirements for counseling records management are similar to those for injury and illness documentation, there are a few differences and points of emphasis. Most of these differences arise out of the sensitive nature of the content of the mental health record. Surprisingly simple mistakes in records management can result in the loss of trust so important in the sports medicine professional–athlete counseling relationship.

File Management Tips

Bond (1993) recommends that health professionals involved in the generation of mental health records consider the following suggestions for managing counseling information.

Coded Entries

If the number of patients requiring counseling is small, as is likely for most sports medicine professionals, consider entering information using numbers, fictitious initials, or similar devices to help safeguard the confidentiality of the data.

Dual Records

Keep only the most pertinent and necessary information in the athlete's medical record. Highly personal, potentially embarrassing, or overtly speculative information should be kept in the sports medicine professional's personal files. This may be especially important in settings where many staff members have access to the athlete's records. In these settings formal agreements should be negotiated with both the institution and the athlete regarding the splitting of information between the athlete's and the practitioner's files. Even this may not be enough to safeguard the athlete's counseling records, however, since personal records of the sports medicine professional can be subpoenaed.

Computerized Records

Counseling records are theoretically safer when computerized. The chances of someone without a need to access the information simply stumbling across a file left open on a desk are reduced through computerization. Computers are not invulnerable to penetration, however. Sports medicine professionals should take reasonable care to safeguard mental health records using passwords, codes, and removable disk drives whenever possible.

Disposal of Records

The guidelines for disposal of mental health records are just that—guidelines. In the absence of state rules mandating a specific time period for retaining such records, there is little precedent to guide the practice of sports medicine professionals in this area. Keith-Spiegel and Koocher (1985) recommend that mental health records be retained for at least seven years from the last date of service, even if the state requires a shorter period. If the athlete is a minor, the records should be kept for seven years after the age of majority was obtained. Soisson et al. (1987) recommend full record retention for three years after the last date of service. They also recommend that either the full record or a summary be retained for another 12 years and that the record be destroyed no sooner than 15 years after the last contact with the athlete. In any case, when records are discarded, they should be shredded or burned, not simply thrown in the trash where someone could gain access to them.

CASE STUDY

Todd Blackwell, ATC, wasn't surprised when Bill came dragging into the training room on Friday morning for his daily knee rehabilitation. Bill was a wrestler at the university, but his season had been cut short by an ACL injury nine weeks ago. Since that time he had been working with Todd on a daily basis. Todd knew Bill pretty well before the injury—Bill was a senior who had been injured on many previous occasions—but since the knee injury they got to know each other a lot better. Todd knew that before the injury Bill had been a pretty typical college student—with typical alcohol consumption patterns. Since the injury, however, it seemed that Bill showed up for his morning rehabilitation hung over nearly half the time. Todd hadn't mentioned anything yet because he thought Bill was just a little depressed at not being able to wrestle in his senior year and that his increased drinking was simply a manifestation of this. Today, however, Bill looked worse than ever. Since it was a quiet morning in the training room, Todd decided to confront Bill on the issue of his drinking.

"Bill," Todd began, "I've been concerned about your drinking for some time now. Ever since the injury you seem to have really stepped it up." Todd was shocked when Bill began to cry. It was the last thing he ever expected Bill to do. "I did a really dumb thing last night, Todd," whispered Bill. "I was drunk, and I think I went too far with a girl I know in the same apartment building I live in. I don't

remember it all very well, but her roommate came looking for me this morning. She was screaming at me and asking how I could do something like this. I'll be honest, Todd, I'm scared to death."

Todd talked with Bill for a while and helped him compose himself. After the rehabilitation session ended, Todd dictated the following note:

> "I met with Bill for his rehabilitation today. He appeared hung over, as he has on many occasions since his injury. When I confronted him about his drinking he became upset, admitted the heavy drinking, and told me he may have sexually assaulted a fellow student last night. He seemed to feel remorse over the incident. I advised him to seek help from the counseling center for his heavy drinking and to find the woman and clarify the events of last night."

After the note was transcribed in the athletic office, Todd signed it and had it filed in Bill's medical record in the health center adjacent to the athletic training room.

QUESTIONS FOR ANALYSIS

1. What are the strengths and weaknesses of Todd's documentation of Bill's problems?

2. Would you have recorded the same information differently? What would you have done? How would you have documented the problems?

3. What potential complications is Todd likely to confront with his counseling documentation system? How could these problems be overcome?

4. Given Todd's record-keeping system, how likely is it that Bill's problems will remain confidential? Create a plausible scenario by which Todd's documentation of Bill's problems could be released inappropriately.

SUMMARY

The ability to document the counseling provided by the sports medicine professional is just as important as the ability to provide the counseling. Poorly documented counseling often reflects a lack of professionalism in the delivery of the counseling itself. Health care professionals, especially physicians, are poorly trained in this area and demonstrate a low level of skill in mental health documentation. Documentation of counseling can help the sports medicine professional avoid legal liability, enhance memory of events, adhere to professional standards, improve communications with mental health professionals, meet the requirements of third-party payers, and improve the quality of care for the athlete. Although counseling documentation can make the interpersonal process more cumbersome and could potentially lead to embarrassment of the athlete if released improperly, it is generally accepted as a standard for good professional care. Narrative charting and the problem-oriented record are the two most widely used systems for documenting mental health. The use of quotations to reflect the athlete's state of mind and thought process is important. Dictation can help improve the efficiency of the narrative system. The problem-oriented record uses codes and cross-references to document counseling in four parts: the database, problem list, plan list, and follow-up list. Poor handwriting and the inclusion of hunches or speculation are common documentation pitfalls. Sports medicine professionals should document the following as part of the counseling or mental health record: physical exam, mental status, patient education, verbal orders, telephone advice, suicidal or violent behavior, and referrals or refusal of referral. Highly personal or embarrassing information should be excluded from the counseling record. Sports medicine professionals have an ethical responsibility to hold their athletes' counseling records in confidence. Their records may or may not enjoy the legal protection of privilege. In any case, information should never be released without the informed consent of the athlete, although parents of minor children may have a legal right to the information even in the absence of consent. Sports medicine professionals should exercise diligence in protecting the privacy of the athletes they counsel by using coded mental health entries or maintaining dual records. The requirements for maintaining counseling records vary from state to state, but when records are discarded, they should be shredded or burned.

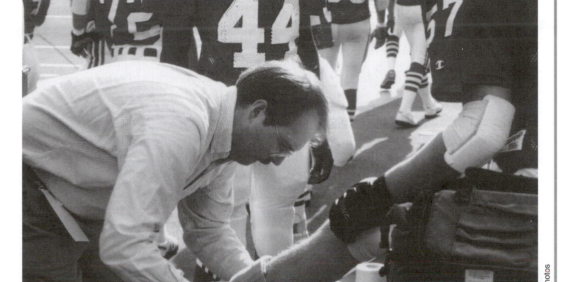
© Mike Morris, Unicorn Stock Photos

Ethical Perspectives in Counseling

Peter V. Loubert, PhD, PT, ATC, *Central Michigan University*

CHAPTER OBJECTIVES

Understand the definition and purpose of ethics relevant to the sports medicine professional

Identify resources that address standards for ethical behavior in your profession or in other professions for which counseling is a primary activity

Identify situations and circumstances in which counseling problems of an ethical nature most often occur

Avoid or deal appropriately with ethical problems that may arise when counseling athletes as a sports medicine professional *counselor—A person who provides personal advice or guidance to another. A professional counselor has formal educational training and professional credentials attesting to his or her competence for the role of counselor. Sports medicine professionals may serve in a nonprofessional counseling role by providing personal advice and guidance to athletes as part of their primary professional responsibilities.*

code of ethics—A systematic set of standards or principles that define ethical behavior appropriate for a profession. The standards and principles are determined by moral values.

competence— Adequate qualifications to conduct an activity. For counseling activities competence is most often determined by educational preparation.

As health care practitioners working with athletes, one of the most important roles we acquire is that of **counselor** to the athletes we treat. To be effective in this role requires that we have a clear understanding of the ethical principles applicable to the role. Without that understanding we risk harming the athletes we are committed to serve and potentially endangering our own livelihoods as sports medicine professionals. Appropriate understanding of ethics and application of ethical norms in our role as counselors will allow us to proceed with the understanding and wisdom of generations who have preceded us in dealing with the delicate and often sensitive matters inherent to the role of counselor.

A good place to begin studying ethics is the **code of ethics** of your profession. A common principle of these codes is that members should limit their practice to their specific areas of **competence**. Compliance with this principle requires that every sports medicine professional be acutely aware of their limitations in the role of counselor and that he or she recognize when there is need for referral to a **professional counselor**. We also must recognize counseling as a distinct professional discipline and be careful not to portray our activities in the role of counselor as professional counseling. Indeed, when we provide counseling support for an athlete, we do so as part of practice in our respective professions, not as professional counselors.

The purpose of this chapter is to introduce the topic of ethics as it applies to the role of counselor incumbent upon the sports medicine professional. We identify some of the most common situations in which ethical breaches can occur, and we consider recommendations for steps that the sports medicine professional can take to minimize the occurrence of ethical breaches.

WHAT IS ETHICS?

Ethics is the study of the rules, standards, and principles that dictate right conduct among members of a society. Such rules, standards, and principles are based on moral values, which serve as the basis for what is considered **right**. Moral values vary across time and among cultures and individuals according to acquired perspectives and experiences. Because of this, modern ethical principles are subject to continuous review and debate and represent the **consensus** within a society at any given time.

Ethics are derived from a long, rich history of philosophical debate. They are deeply embedded in our choices of how we govern and conduct ourselves as a civilized society and serve as the basis for many of our norms for social interaction. Ethics also reflect many of the tenets of a broad spectrum of religious beliefs and have been influenced by religious philosophies from around the world. All these influences and this history have led us to depend on the principles of ethics to form the moral backbone of the most important things that we do as contributors to a conscientious society. Among the professions, ethics provide a perspective from which to judge the goodness or badness of a professional's actions and are a reflection of the "conscience" of the profession (Appelbaum & Lawton, 1990).

WHY DO PROFESSIONS ESTABLISH ETHICAL STANDARDS?

Professions are defined by a commitment to certain characteristics that set them apart from nonprofessional groups within our society. One of the most important of these characteristics is a commitment to high standards of ethical behavior by the members of the profession. Among the professions that provide health care services to athletes, ethical standards are written in the form of a code of ethics by each of the respective professional organizations.

The purposes of these codes are to provide a guide for appropriate conduct by members, a reference by which to judge members when their conduct is brought into question, and assurance and protection to the public served by members of the profession. Furthermore, an important consequence of these purposes is protection of the individual members of the profession.

ETHICAL STANDARDS RELEVANT TO THE COUNSELING CARE OF ATHLETES

Sports medicine professionals should comply with the code of ethics of the national professional organization for their primary profession. For athletic trainers the appropriate code is the *NATA Code of Ethics* of the **National Athletic Trainers Association** (1995). Physical therapists are expected to adhere to the **American Physical Therapy Association**'s (1991) *Code of Ethics,* and physicians should comply with the *Principles of Medical Ethics* of the **American Medical Association** (1980). Contact information for each of these professional organizations is provided in table 10.1. The code-of-ethics documents provide guidelines for ethical conduct within the respective professions and are intended to apply to the entire range of practice patterns and settings applicable to the respective professions. Their standards are enforceable for the members of each organization but should also be considered applicable to nonmembers within the profession.

Codes of ethics from the disciplines in sports medicine provide little or no guidance specific to the counseling role. To develop a basic understanding of appropriate ethical conduct specific to the role of counselor, therefore, sports medicine professionals who spend time counseling athletes should go beyond their own profession's code of ethics. They should also consult the *Code of Ethics* of the **American Counseling Association** (1995) or the *Ethical Principles of Psychologists and Code of Conduct* of the **American Psychological Association** (1992). Contact information for these organizations is provided in table 10.2. The codes of ethics for both these associations provide minimal guidelines for standards of conduct that apply to the counseling role. These guidelines are more comprehensive and more applicable to

---

Table 10.1   Selected Organizations Involved in the Primary Care of Athletes

National Athletic Trainers Association
2952 Stemmons Freeway, Suite 200
Dallas, TX 75247
(800) 879-6282
http://www.nata.org

American Physical Therapy Association
1111 North Fairfax St.
Alexandria, VA 22314
(800) 999-2782
http://www.apta.org

American Medical Association
515 N. State St.
Chicago, IL 60610
(312) 464-5000
http://www.ama-assn.org

---

professional counselor—A person who has formal educational training and professional credentials attesting to his or her competence in the role of counselor.

ethics—The rules, standards, and principles that dictate right conduct among members of a society or profession. Ethics are based on moral values regarding what is considered right.

right—(noun) A moral or legal privilege inherent to membership in a community or society. (adj.) Fitting, proper, or conforming to legal or moral expectations.

consensus—The collective opinion of a group. A consensus usually does not represent the diversity of opinions within the group, nor does it necessarily well represent the preferred opinion of any individual within the group. It does, however, represent a position that all within the group are willing to abide by as members of the group.

National Athletic Trainers Association (NATA)—The primary professional organization for athletic trainers in the United States. The NATA provides national certification of qualified athletic training professionals.

American Physical Therapy Association (APTA)—The primary professional organization for physical therapists in the United States.

American Medical Association (AMA)—The primary professional organization for physicians in the United States.

American Counseling Association—A major national organization for professional counselors in the United States.

American Psychological Association (APA)—A major national organization for psychologists in the United States.

law—The rules and regulations governing the affairs of a community or society. Laws are enforced by administrative authority and an established judicial system of the community.

the counseling role than those of most other health care professions. These codes can be obtained through libraries or by contacting the associations directly.

THE RELATIONSHIP BETWEEN LEGAL AND ETHICAL CONSIDERATIONS

Ethical considerations often overlap, contradict, or otherwise interact with issues of **law**. It is convenient when a difficult ethical decision is consistent with the law; however, it is important to recognize that there are circumstances in which what is ethical may not be legal and what is legal may not be ethical. This is especially a problem in the context of counseling when there are issues of confidentiality and protection of individual rights to privacy. The right of an athlete to privacy may well conflict with the law when the law dictates that a specific type of information be reported. The multiple roles filled by sports medicine professionals make the issue even more difficult because of the many different types of information for which they are responsible. The most recent large-scale issue of this nature is the reporting of HIV status required by some health departments. Ideas regarding how the sports medicine professional can deal with such conflicts are included later in this chapter. What is clear is that professional codes of ethics almost always dictate that it is unethical to engage in any practice or activity that is illegal (Makarowski & Rickell, 1993).

THE SPORTS MEDICINE PROFESSIONAL AS A PRIMARY PARTY

The sports medicine professional may face ethical issues in many different forms. The most menacing forms are those where the sports medicine professional is a **primary party** to the ethical concern. To be a primary party means that the sports medicine professional is directly involved in the situation as a person who has behaved in an ethically questionable manner or who is the victim of an unethical act committed by another person. Of primary concern in this chapter is the former situation in which the sports medicine professional is the **perpetrator** of an unethical situation.

Table 10.2 Selected Organizations Involved in Professional Counseling as a Primary Responsibility

American Counseling Association
5999 Stevenson Ave.
Alexandria, VA 22304-3300
(800) 347-6647
http://www.counseling.org

American Psychological Association
750 First St., NE
Washington, DC 20002-4242
(202) 336-5500
http://www.apa.org

The following sections describe four types of situations in which the sports medicine professional could become entangled as a primary party in an ethical dilemma. These situations are also listed in table 10.3. Although this list is not exhaustive, these are the situations that occur most often or that have the greatest potential for harm to the individuals involved. It is apparent that the professional codes of ethics that address these situations are intended to protect the athlete from harmful actions on the part of a sports medicine professional who might be acting in a counseling role. It is fortunate that if the codes of ethics are adhered to, they also protect the professional.

primary party—A participant who is directly involved in an activity.

perpetrator—The person who is responsible for or has committed an act.

Table 10.3 Ways in Which a Sports Medicine Professional Can Become a Primary Party in an Unethical Situation

Breach of confidentiality

Conflict of interest

Exploitation

Dependency

Breach of Confidentiality

One of the most frequent ethical situations for the sports medicine professional is **breach of confidentiality**. This is an especially difficult situation for the sports health professional for several reasons. First, the sports medicine professional often assumes many roles in relation to an athlete. There is often a legitimate need for information to be shared with the team organization, with coaches, or with colleagues who are also responsible for some aspect of the athlete's care. Those needs, legitimate and illegitimate, sometimes conflict with what is in the best interest of the athlete and with the responsibilities that a sports medicine professional has in a counseling role. As an example, consider the professional basketball athletic trainer who has been told confidentially by an athlete that he is concerned that he may have a familial degenerative eye disease that could greatly affect his eyesight in the next three years. The athlete refuses to get tested for the disease and forbids the athletic trainer from sharing the information with anyone else because there is no proof that he has the disease.

breach of confidentiality—Violation of a commitment to privacy and to protection of information or communications.

In this example the athletic trainer is conflicted on the issue of confidentiality. On one hand he is bound to maintain the confidentiality of information provided in the counseling role, but on the other hand he is contractually obligated to act in the best interest of the basketball organization. Considering the upcoming contract negotiations for this athlete and the need for the team to carefully plan its roster, he clearly is pressured to commit a breach of confidentiality.

Confidential information obtained as part of the counseling relationship between a sports medicine professional and an athlete may be very personal, private, and sensitive. The sports medicine professional should handle such information very carefully to avoid ethical as well as legal breaches of confidentiality. In some situations the most appropriate ethical behavior may even jeopardize a sports medicine professional's job.

The second reason why maintaining confidentiality may be difficult for the sports medicine professional is because of the large number of people who are often involved in the care of an athlete. This is especially true where student and intern practitioners may not be fully cognizant of concerns for confidentiality. When sports medicine professionals are responsible for the supervision of students and interns, they will also be held responsible for student or intern actions. This makes the sports medicine professional a primary party in a breach of confidentiality even when he or she was not the immediate perpetrator of the breach.

The final concern regarding confidentiality is the high profile of athletes and the athletic industry in our society. Pressures from the press and from the public's desire to know everything possible about a high-profile athlete can be a significant threat to an athlete's right to privacy and the confidentiality of information to which the sports medicine professional is privy. To avoid breaches of confidentiality, sports medicine professionals should take proactive and diligent measures to protect information and communications. Several suggestions for such measures are listed in table 10.4.

There are three exceptions to the rule of confidentiality noted in the codes of ethics (see table 10.5). The sports medicine professional should recognize that no **reason** for a breach of confidentiality other than those in table 10.5 serves as an **excuse** for its occurrence. A professional should recognize the difference between a reason and an excuse, and accept a reason as an excuse only when it is both unavoidable and justifiable. The reasons in table 10.5 are considered excusable; any other reason would be inexcusable.

reason—*The basis or explanation for an action.*

excuse—*A reason that is considered justifiable.*

Conflict of Interest

conflict of interest—*Discordance or competition between the interests of one individual or group and those of another individual or group.*

The sports medicine professional serving in a counseling role is also susceptible to **conflicts of interest**. Again, the threat to ethical practice is a result of the multiple

Table 10.4 Measures to Protect the Confidentiality of Information and Communications

Establish and follow responsible procedures for documentation, and store records in a secure environment.

Only people with a legitimate role in providing health care to athletes should have access to athletes' records.

Information should be released only with written permission of the athlete involved.

A specific person should be designated to handle all requests for health-related information, and all people in the organization should be trained and reminded regularly to defer all inquiries to that person.

Sports medicine professionals should be trained never to discuss the health status of an athlete in public and never in private unless all people present have a legitimate need and authorization to have access to the information.

It may be necessary to keep documentation of interactions related to counseling functions separate from other health-related records for an athlete.

Table 10.5 Exceptions to the Rule of Confidentiality in a Counseling Relationship

When there is clear and imminent danger to the client

When there is clear and imminent danger to other persons

When legal requirements demand that confidential information be released roles that the sports medicine professional may fill. The responsibilities that sports medicine professionals have to a team organization, to the coaching staff, and to themselves often conflict with their responsibilities to the athlete. The temptation to act or to advise an athlete in a manner that serves the team or protects the job or other interests of the sports medicine professional may go unrecognized.

In the example of the athletic trainer holding confidential information about an athlete's possible eye disease, the threat to confidentiality of information comes about because the athletic trainer has a conflict of interest. The athletic trainer's personal concern for his job conflicts with the best interests of the athlete to keep the information confidential. These can be particularly difficult conflicts of interest to resolve because the coach and organization may have a legitimate need to know the information, and they may be able to invoke a threat of firing the athletic trainer.

Both the *Ethical Principles of Psychologists and Code of Conduct* of the American Psychological Association (1992) and the *Code of Ethics* of the American Counseling Association (1995) make it explicitly clear that the primary responsibility of the person serving in a counseling role is to his or her client. This standard must also apply to the counseling role of the sports medicine professional. The nature of the counseling role is a particularly sensitive one that involves a component of trust well beyond that of most other relationships. There is an implicit expectation of good will on the part of the person serving in the counseling role, and to act or to provide advice that in any way compromises the best interests of the athlete would be a violation of that trust. When sports medicine professionals serve in a counseling role for an athlete, they are obligated to resolve or set aside their own personal interests and those of any other allegiance they may have so that they can act in the best interest of the athlete.

The athlete's need for counseling is undeniably important and one that every sports medicine professional should do everything possible to accommodate. However, the threat of conflicts of interest often dictates that the counseling function be referred to someone outside the athletic organization. Referral is most important when the nature of the counseling is more serious, when the problem that needs attention is outside the scope of competence of the sports medicine professional, or when the threat of a conflict of interest is present. It is critical for the sports medicine professional to recognize that the appearance or perception of a conflict of interest can be very damaging, even when the intentions of the counselor are pure and when he or she believes his or her actions to be justified and appropriate. When the potential for a conflict of interest exists, the sports medicine professional should be very careful about taking on a serious counseling role with an athlete. In such situations the sports medicine professional would be well advised to refer the counseling to another qualified person for whom no conflict of interest is apparent.

Exploitation

Exploitation of an athlete by a sports medicine professional is a particularly manipulative and self-interested form of conflict of interest. It involves the intentional use of another person or group of persons to achieve some other selfish objective. When athletes confide in a sports medicine professional, as occurs in counseling, they become particularly vulnerable to exploitation because they may reveal things about themselves that would otherwise be unknown to the sports medicine professional. They may also become vulnerable because of the trust that is engendered as part of the counseling relationship. Under such circumstances athletes are vulnerable to exploitation for money, information, sex, self-endangerment, goods, or any number of other atrocities. For the sports medicine professional to perpetrate such a situation would be clearly unethical.

exploitation—Using another person for selfish purposes, particularly at the expense of that person or without that person's knowledge or full informed consent.

Dependency

dependency—Having a chronic, recurring need or perceived need. In a counseling relationship, dependency refers to a chronic need for the therapeutic relationship or a controlling relationship.

Dependency is another situation that can result from a counseling relationship. It typically occurs in an insidious and unintentional manner and is a product of the athlete's own psychological needs in the counseling relationship. Nevertheless, it remains contrary to the objectives of a healthy counseling relationship (American Counseling Association, 1995). The occurrence of a dependent relationship is not by itself an ethical concern, but rather it becomes one when the sports medicine professional fails to take appropriate action to deal with the dependency. Appropriate action may include referral, consultation, or other interventions to decrease the dependency without abandoning the athlete's other needs.

Dependency can also present as a subtle form of exploitation. In such cases it may be cultivated by the sports medicine professional (consciously or subconsciously) to meet his or her own psychological needs. Such a situation is clearly unethical and suggests that the sports medicine professional needs counseling of his or her own.

THE SPORTS MEDICINE PROFESSIONAL AS A THIRD PARTY

third party—A person who is affected by but not directly involved in a situation.

The sports medicine professional who fills a counseling role may also be involved in an ethical dilemma as a **third party**. To be a third party means that the sports medicine professional is not personally involved in the dilemma but has professional responsibilities because of his or her knowledge of the situation. The responsibility of the sports medicine professional is to intervene in the best interest of the client, but to also protect others from harm whenever there is apparent risk of harm occurring.

The sports medicine professional may be made a third party to an ethical situation as a result of knowledge that comes to their attention directly from the athlete they counsel or from other sources. Such knowledge can create very difficult circumstances because there are often conflicts between their responsibility to maintain confidentiality, their responsibility to protect the athlete from harm, their responsibility to protect others from harm, and their many other loyalties.

One of the primary differences between being involved as a third party and as a primary party is that as a third party the sports medicine professional can act more appropriately to manage a solution to the situation. When a sports medicine professional becomes involved in a situation as a primary participant, especially in the presence of a conflict of interest or exploitation, it is often necessary for the practitioner to remove him- or herself from the situation and request that someone else intervene to help resolve it. When the sports medicine professional is involved in an ethical concern as a third party, he or she is often in good position to orchestrate a solution to the situation. Often the solution involves providing information and perspectives to the athlete being counseled or managing other people and information to resolve the ethical dilemma.

Knowledge of Unethical Activity by Another Person

There are five categories of knowledge that are most likely to render a sports medicine professional a third party to an ethical dilemma (see table 10.6). The first of these is knowledge of the occurrence of a breach of confidentiality, conflict of interest, or exploitation involving the athlete being counseled. Just as when the sports medicine professional is directly involved, these situations can be very harmful to an athlete. Knowledge of such an occurrence requires the sports medicine professional to intervene on behalf of the athlete. Intervention usually does not mean that the sports medicine professional has responsibility for correcting the situation. It is usu-

> **Table 10.6**   Categories of Knowledge That Make a Sports Medicine Professional a Third Party to an Ethical Dilemma
>
> Knowledge of a breach of confidentiality, conflict of interest, or exploitation involving the athlete being counseled
>
> Forbidden knowledge
>
> Knowledge of high-risk behaviors
>
> Knowledge of illegal activities
>
> Knowledge of situations in which the welfare of the athlete conflicts with the welfare of another individual or group

ally sufficient to bring it to the athlete's attention so that the athlete is able to take responsibility for the situation him- or herself and can do so from a fully informed perspective. In the case of an athlete who is a **minor** or who might otherwise be unable to protect him- or herself in such a situation, the sports medicine professional should inform the parents or **guardians** of the athlete, refer the situation to the appropriate authorities (particularly when there are legal concerns), or intervene directly on behalf of the athlete.

Imagine, for example, that a college softball player goes to her athletic trainer for advice because she is frustrated about not getting enough playing time. She states that she feels the woman playing ahead of her is getting all the playing time, not because she is a better player, but because she sleeps with the coach. In this situation, if the allegations were true, as a third party having knowledge of this exploitation the athletic trainer would then be ethically bound to intervene on behalf of both athletes. Of course the first step in this intervention would be to investigate or otherwise verify that the story was true. The information should not be considered "knowledge" on the basis of the story of the first athlete alone, who probably has a conflict of interest and may be misinformed or may be trying to manipulate the athletic trainer. If it turns out that there is reason to believe that the story is true, what would be an appropriate next step for the athletic trainer? Confront the teammate? Confront the coach? Report it to the athletic director? Other action?

Forbidden Knowledge

Forbidden knowledge is information about a situation that you are forbidden to act on. Such information can involve the athlete being counseled or others and can come to a sports medicine professional from the athlete or from another person. Typically the sharing of such information is preceded with a phrase such as, "If I tell you this, you must promise not to share it with anyone" (Makarowski and Rickell, 1993).

As an example, consider how you would react if an athlete came to you for advice in the following manner during the off-season: "I need to talk to you about a health-related problem, but I don't want the coaches or my parents to know about it. It's kind of serious, but private." It is clearly appropriate for an athlete to approach a sports medicine professional about a health concern, but the restriction on use of the information has considerable potential for requiring an inappropriate compromise by the clinician. Under circumstances such as this it may be necessary to interrupt the exchange before the disclosure progresses any further. As soon as athletes share privileged information, they are likely to expect compliance with their wishes. The athlete of our example could be planning to disclose information about any number of issues, some quite serious, such as steroid use, pregnancy, or an acquired disease that may affect his or her ability to participate in athletics.

minor—A person under legal age for adult responsibilities and decisions.

guardian—A person who has legal responsibility for the care and decisions of someone who is incompetent to do so for him- or herself or who is a minor.

forbidden knowledge—Information about a situation upon which a person in a counseling role is forbidden to act.

The sports medicine professional taking on a counseling role should be wary of anyone wanting to share information but refusing to allow it to be acted on. To agree to such terms might preclude the sports medicine professional from taking necessary actions that would otherwise supersede the promise, including the reasons cited in table 10.5. If an athlete offers forbidden information, the sports medicine professional would be well advised to insist that the athlete trust him or her to act on the information in the athlete's best interest. The sports medicine professional should assure the athlete that he or she will maintain the confidentiality of information as long as there is no threat of harm to the athlete or to other persons affected by the information and as long as the release of the information is not legally required. If an athlete is unable to agree to those terms, he or she should be offered a referral to someone with whom he or she can trust the information and they should be strongly encouraged to follow through with the referral. An appropriate response for the example mentioned previously might be "Before you tell me anything more, you need to understand that my first and foremost concern is the health of the individuals on this team. I will not be able to keep the information private if I feel that it is necessary to disclose the information to protect your health or the health of other members of the team. In addition, if you are involved in any illegal activities or in violation of team rules I may have to take other actions. I will do my best to keep your confidence, but I will not have my hands tied if it is not appropriate for me to do so. If you can live with these conditions, let's sit down and talk, otherwise I will help you find someone else to talk to."

When someone other than the athlete being counseled offers forbidden information, it is also essential that you make it clear that you are obligated to act in the best interest of the athletes under your care. It may be appropriate to offer to use the information in an anonymous fashion, if possible, but you must not forfeit the right to use it when necessary.

A word of caution regarding the use of knowledge in a counseling role is in order, particularly in the context of forbidden knowledge. To take action on knowledge that is inaccurate or untrue can be very harmful to you, to the athletes for whom you are responsible, or to others. The offer of forbidden knowledge by an athlete or by others is a common avenue by which a person in a counseling role is at risk for being manipulated, particularly when the information is about another person. The sports medicine professional should use any such information cautiously, particularly when the accuracy of the information is in doubt. In some circumstances it may be appropriate to delay action on a piece of information until it can be verified.

Knowledge of High-Risk Behaviors

high-risk behaviors— *Behaviors that expose a person to an unnecessarily high degree of physical or psychological jeopardy.*

Knowledge of **high-risk behaviors** is another area of potential ethical concern for the sports medicine professional. Knowledge of high-risk behaviors may come to your attention by your own observation, by report from the athlete being counseled, or by others. This particular concern extends to situations in which the athlete being counseled is at risk of harm as a result of his or her own high-risk behaviors or the high-risk behaviors of others. It also includes situations in which the athlete's high-risk behaviors may put others at risk.

Examples of high-risk behaviors include such things as engaging in unprotected sex, being involved with multiple sex partners, use of drugs, owning or carrying handguns, drinking and driving, cigarette smoking, dangerous weight control or eating habits, and disregard for normal safety practices such as use of protective equipment or obeying traffic signals while driving. Of course there are many other possible examples, some carrying a more serious or more immediate threat than others. The need for intervention can vary according to the seriousness or immediacy of the threat.

When the sports medicine professional has knowledge of potentially harmful high-risk behaviors, the ethical responsibility is not so much to prevent the behaviors as it is to be sure that the individuals involved are aware of the behaviors and of the associated risks. The sports medicine professional may also be required to assist the people involved in finding alternatives to the high-risk behaviors. The sports medicine professional's responsibilities therefore are to provide information, education, or counseling to the parties involved so that they can make an informed choice regarding their participation in the behaviors.

When the high-risk behavior of an athlete puts others at risk, it is the responsibility of the sports medicine professional to intervene, if only to be sure that the other individuals being put at risk are aware of the risk so that they can protect themselves.

Knowledge of Illegal Activities

Knowledge of illegal activities involving an athlete can also create a difficult ethical situation. An athlete may admit to illegal activities as part of an advising session, or the knowledge may come to the attention of the sports medicine professional from an outside source. One of the difficulties occurs when legal authorities are aware of the illegal activities and seek information from the sports medicine professional. Another difficulty occurs when legal authorities are unaware of the illegal activity. Both of these circumstances demand that the sports medicine professional be familiar with his or her legal obligations as a professional, and they also demand very careful consideration of the specific situation encountered. Legal concerns become entangled with issues of confidentiality, responsibility to the client, privileged communication status, legal reporting requirements, and many other issues. Legal counsel may be required for the sports medicine professional to protect his or her own status as well as that of the athlete.

It would be impossible to provide a comprehensive list of illegal activities of which sports medicine professionals might become aware among the athletes they serve. However, the following single example can illustrate many of the difficulties that one might encounter.

> *A college hockey player confided in a team physician that he had injured his knee in a car accident the prior evening. When asked if anyone else had been hurt, the player replied that he didn't think so, but he didn't stop to find out. Earlier in the day the physician had read a newspaper article about a hit-and-run accident that same evening in which a victim had been severely injured and drunk driving was suspected. A police investigation was underway. When confronted about the situation, the athlete denied having anything to do with the accident in the paper and refused to talk about it any further.*

In this case the physician has confirmation of an illegal activity (the athlete admitted failing to stop at the scene of an accident) but only suspects anything further. The ethical responsibilities of the physician in this scenario may be very difficult to sort out, and there are likely to be significant legal ramifications to carrying out those responsibilities. Legal consultation would clearly be appropriate to clarify what options for action or inaction would be legal. To report that this athlete had fled the scene of an accident would clearly be a violation of the athlete's confidence. In many cases it might be illegal to make such a report. However, in some cases it might be illegal *not* to report this knowledge.

If there were no legal ramifications to be concerned about, what would be the right (ethical) thing to do? Each of us would have to consult our own conscience and perhaps other professional colleagues, friends, clergy, counselors, or the relevant code of ethics to determine our ethical responsibility. It may well be that the determination of ethical responsibility would be different for different people. There may also be conflicts between what is ethical and what is legal. If there were a conflict between what was right to do and what was legal to do, what would you do?

Knowledge of Situations in Which the Welfare of the Athlete Conflicts With the Welfare of Others

self-determination—
Free will to judge for oneself, to determine one's own course of action, and to manage one's own affairs.

A central concept in ethics is that individuals have a right to **self-determination** (Appelbaum & Lawton, 1990). This right, however, can come into conflict with the rights and welfare of other individuals or groups in society. An example of this is when an athletic trainer has knowledge of a wrestler with a contagious skin disease that may be difficult to see. In this example the right of a capable and otherwise healthy athlete to compete conflicts with the right of other athletes not to be exposed unnecessarily to the skin disease.

Knowledge of situations in which the welfare of the individual athlete conflicts with the welfare of another individual or group can present challenging ethical questions for the sports medicine professional. The action to take in many such situations is directed by social conventions or by law. However, there are also many areas that are not so clearly defined. The sports medicine professional serving in a counseling role may have the opportunity to remediate some of these difficult ethical situations. Many of them can be resolved by seeking permission to take action or disclose information or by bringing the involved parties together to develop a mutually acceptable solution to the problem. Indeed, most situations that present a conflict between the rights and welfare of individuals can be resolved by providing an opportunity for the affected parties to become familiar with the perspectives of the other party. Most people are reasonable and willing to compromise when they are faced with the concerns of others who may be affected by their actions.

ETHICAL COUNSELING IN SPORTS MEDICINE: SPECIFIC RECOMMENDATIONS

Most sports medicine professionals are committed to ethical practice; however, they are not interested in becoming ethicists in order to do so. Fortunately, ethical practice doesn't require becoming an ethicist, but it does require understanding of the meaning and intent of the relevant codes of ethics, reflection on the situations and actions that occur in practice, and development of professional habits and awareness that are consistent with ethical practice. The following list of recommendations is intended to serve as a functional guide to ethical practice that will assist the sports medicine professional who serves athletes in a counseling role. It is hoped that the guidelines provided in this list will minimize the occurrence of ethical conflicts and facilitate the resolution of those that do occur.

• *Study the relevant professional codes of ethics.* Begin first with the code of ethics of your own profession, then review the code of ethics of a counseling profession such as the American Counseling Association or the American Psychological Association.

• *Learn to recognize situations where ethical concerns may be present or appear to be present.* This requires careful consideration of all your personal and professional relationships and how they affect the athletes that you treat.

• *Increase your sensitivity to situations where ethical concerns are present.* Sensitivity requires that you be able to appreciate a situation from the point of view of others who are affected, particularly the athletes under your care. It is important to treat every ethical concern seriously, or you will be perceived to be insensitive and uncaring—and there is no better formula for professional trouble than that.

• *Consult whenever there are ethical questions, especially when the answers are not clear or not clearly defensible.* Good consultation serves to protect the sports medicine professional as well as the athlete because it provides an outside, objective perspective on the situation of concern. In addition, there is often more wisdom in the careful consideration of a small group than there is within any individual.

• *Refer when the ethical or counseling concern is beyond your legal scope of practice or your competence.* Professional counselors have education and counseling skills well beyond those of most sports medicine professionals. It is in the best interest of everyone involved to make prudent use of referrals in critical, complicated, and difficult counseling cases. To do this, however, you must use the screening tools provided elsewhere in this text and be acutely aware of your own limitations as a sports medicine professional serving in a counseling role.

• *Refer when you become a primary party in an ethical dilemma or when you might be perceived by the athlete or outside observers to be a primary party.* When a sports medicine professional becomes a primary party in a situation of ethical concern, both the professional and the athlete are at risk, and the situation can become worse. In addition, you should consider that even the perception of such a situation could be destructive. Referral to an unconflicted counselor is generally considered necessary and prudent in such situations.

• *Document carefully and often.* As in most other areas of practice, careful and accurate documentation is essential in any counseling role.

• *Follow your conscience.* Good conscience requires knowledge and awareness. For the sports medicine professional serving in a counseling role, it requires knowledge of the moral and ethical standards applicable to counseling and awareness of the individual circumstances each athlete faces. Where we most often fail to be conscientious is not so much in knowledge as it is in awareness. To be aware we must be reflective and considerate, both of which take time and effort. As sports medicine professionals we must guard against becoming too busy or too entrenched in routine to allow ourselves the time and energy to be reflective and considerate. Otherwise we will fail to follow our conscience.

• *Fully disclose to athletes all of your roles that might involve them directly or indirectly.* More than anything else, disclosure is an ethically critical component for informed consent in a sports medicine professional's relationship with an athlete. Avoid circumstances that cause you conflicting interests regarding the athlete, and be sure to fully disclose your roles to the athlete. Furthermore, be sure to make the athlete aware of the risks of using you as a counselor or otherwise confiding in you. This allows the athlete to make an informed choice to trust you or not to trust you. Some examples of situations that warrant disclosure include, but are not limited to, the following:

1. Athletes should be made to understand that you also have responsibility for other athletes on a team. Because of this you may be obligated to disclose or act on information that affects the health or safety of other athletes.

2. Sports medicine professionals are often employed by the same organization for which the athlete plays. This is a potential conflict of interest that the athlete needs to understand because the practitioner may be required or have strong incentives to act in the best interest of the organization rather than of the athlete.

3. Sports medicine professionals often make available services, referrals, or goods in which they have a financial interest. This is a conflict of interest that should be disclosed to the athlete and to which alternatives should be provided.

4. Athletes should be informed that the sports medicine professional also has social and legal obligations that may require him or her to divulge information that could be in conflict with the athlete's own best interest. If the athlete tells a practitioner about certain illegal activities, the practitioner may be required by law to report that information. Furthermore, the athlete should be informed that information may be divulged when it indicates that the athlete or others may be in imminent danger.

• *In dealing with an ethical dilemma consider possible courses of action carefully.* When confronting an ethical dilemma, (1) identify the greatest variety of choices possible, including those that may seem extreme; (2) investigate each of the possible choices identified; and (3) judge your choices from an other-centered perspective rather than from a self-centered or egocentric perspective.

• *Whenever possible have the athlete make his or her own fully informed choices in a counseling relationship rather than imposing a solution on the athlete.* An informed perspective requires exploration of the positive and negative implications of every conceivable choice. It empowers the athlete to best judge what course of action is in his or her best interest and is a necessary prerequisite to self-determination. Having athletes make their own choices helps them take responsibility for their destiny.

These actions, when combined, dramatically reduce the occurrence of ethical conundrums.

CASE STUDY

Gerry Cramer is an athletic trainer at a large university with a very successful athletic program. One morning Gerry made a routine trip to the student health service to pick up lab reports and X rays, and a secretary asked Gerry whether Sean O'Connor (a star basketball player) had been dating a student named Sandra Johnson (a nonathlete student on campus). When Gerry responded that Sean had been dating Sandra a few months ago, the secretary expressed how unfortunate it was that Sandra had recently tested positive for HIV. Gerry was startled to hear this news. Sandra wasn't an athlete under care of the athletic training room, nor did Gerry really even know Sandra. Gerry was concerned, however, about how this might affect Sean O'Connor, who was under the care of the athletic training room.

Questions for Analysis

1. What are the major ethical issues Gerry should be concerned about following this exchange? Should Gerry pursue additional details and information from the secretary? If so, what?

2. To whom is Gerry primarily responsible in this situation? What responsibilities does Gerry have toward Sean, and what responsibilities does Gerry have toward Sandra? What other persons may be involved and warrant consideration?

3. What should Gerry do with the information about Sandra's HIV status? Should Gerry use the information as a basis for counseling advice to Sean? Under what conditions should Gerry use the information? What alternatives should Gerry be investigating?

4. What is the worst mistake that Gerry could make in trying to fulfill the responsibilities of an athletic trainer to an athlete in this situation? What would be the ideal resolution to this ethical situation? What alternatives fall in between the two extremes? How should Gerry proceed?

5. If it is determined at some time that Sean O'Connor is HIV positive, how should this be handled in the athletic training room? Who needs to know? What permission is necessary for the information to be relayed? Who is responsible for the safety of other athletes, coaches, the training staff, and officials with regard to their risk of exposure?

6. What risks does Gerry face as a result of having this information? What steps should Gerry take to avoid becoming another victim in this ethical dilemma?

SUMMARY

Sports medicine professionals are often called to serve in a counseling role while working with athletes. To carry out this role well it is essential that they be familiar with the ethical standards that are customarily applied to the role. Sports medicine professionals are encouraged to review the code of ethics of their primary profession from the perspective of their counseling role and to study the code of ethics of the American Counseling Association or the American Psychological Association for interpretations and standards specific to counseling.

The most common types of ethical problems that directly involve the sports medicine professional are breach of confidentiality, conflict of interest, exploitation, and dependency. Sports medicine professionals may also have ethical responsibilities when they have knowledge of the occurrence of ethical breaches by others, when they are privy to forbidden knowledge, or when they have knowledge of high-risk behaviors, illegal activities, and conflicts between the welfare of different parties involved in a situation.

Sports medicine professionals may reduce the occurrence of ethical dilemmas by studying the appropriate codes of ethics and learning to recognize and be sensitive to situations that present ethical concerns. It is considered prudent practice to consult with an uninvolved professional whenever there are questions about an ethical situation and to refer the athlete for counseling by a professional counselor when the counseling need is beyond the legal scope of practice or competence of the sports medicine professional. The sports medicine professional should present an athlete seeking counseling with the conditions of counseling, including disclosure of potential conflicts between roles and the circumstances that affect the confidentiality of information transmitted in the counseling relationship. Counseling activities should be documented prudently, and referral is recommended whenever a professional becomes involved as a primary party in an ethical dilemma. Whenever possible athletes should be encouraged to make their own fully informed choices in a counseling relationship.

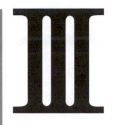

Specific Counseling Issues in Athletic Health Care

The chapters in this part of the text will help readers develop specific strategies for counseling patients in the most common situations found in sports medicine settings. Although athletes can experience all of the psychoemotional problems that other people do, sports medicine professionals are most concerned with a few issues that seem to be especially problematic for athletes. Eating disorders, nutritional concerns, rehabilitation adherence, and substance abuse are all addressed in this part of the book. In addition, information on how to counsel athletes who suffer from stress and anxiety and those who have experienced catastrophic injury is provided in this part.

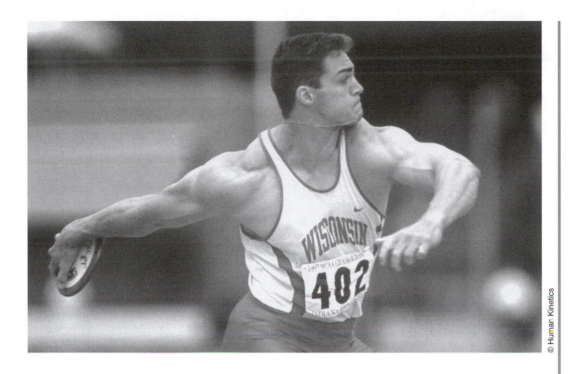

© Human Kinetics

Counseling for Substance Abuse Problems[1]

Kirk J. Brower, MD, *University of Michigan, Ann Arbor*
Jonathan H. Rootenberg, FRCPC, MD, *University of Toronto*

CHAPTER OBJECTIVES

Understand how to screen and assess athletes for the signs, symptoms, and indicators of hazardous use, substance abuse, and substance dependence

Learn to use the assessment to determine the severity of problems and the athlete's motivation for change

Learn to set goals for counseling based on the assessment, such as the need for abstinence or the need for referral for specialized treatment

Understand how to differentiate between enabling and helping the athlete

Practice techniques for motivating athletes to change and for managing their resistance to change

Learn how to use the FRAMES mnemonic to optimize brief interventions for athletes with substance problems

[1]Portions of this chapter were modified from K.J. Brower & J.D. Severin (1997). Alcohol and other drug-related problems. In D.J. Knesper, M.B. Riba, & T.L. Schwenk (Eds.), *Primary care psychiatry* (pp. 309-342). Philadelphia: Saunders.

The use of alcohol and other drugs is highly associated with injuries, and approximately 30 percent of patients hospitalized on orthopedic units suffer from alcoholism (Beresford, Low, Adduci, & Goggans, 1982; Moore et al., 1989). Athletes appear as likely as, or perhaps less likely than, the general population to use substances. Nevertheless, athletes may be more vulnerable than nonathletes to abuse ergogenic drugs in order to enhance performance in sport (see table 11.1). Because of the relationship between substance use and injuries and because athletes may experience unique pressures to use potentially harmful substances, athletic trainers, physical therapists, and sports physicians will encounter high-risk athletes who could benefit from early recognition and counseling.

The purpose of this chapter is to provide you with some techniques for recognizing, assessing, and counseling athletes who need to reduce or eliminate their use of substances. Although patients with alcohol and drug problems commonly remain undiagnosed and untreated because of the shame and stigma attached to these problems, most patients who do receive treatment have favorable outcomes. Moreover, the earlier a problem is detected and treated, the better the expected outcome. The skills for early recognition and initial counseling are readily learned and easily applied, and they constitute the major content of this chapter. It is beyond the scope of this chapter to review the epidemiology and pharmacology of each of the major classes of abused substances, so you are referred to several good medical reviews of these subjects (Fleming & Barry, 1992; Schuckit, 1995; Wadler & Hainline, 1989; Yesalis, 1993).

SIGNS AND SYMPTOMS OF SUBSTANCE USE PROBLEMS

substance abuse—The persistent use of a substance despite problems or adverse consequences, in the absence of impaired control, tolerance, or withdrawal.

substance dependence—A compulsion to take a substance for its psychological effects despite recurrent, adverse consequences, accompanied by impaired control over use, with or without tolerance and withdrawal.

It is helpful for all health care professionals, including athletic trainers, physical therapists, and sports physicians, to have the knowledge and skills to identify substance use problems in their patients. In recognizing and diagnosing substance problems, it is important first to know the signs and symptoms of substance use disorders and then to know how to elicit them in the clinical interview. The diagnoses of **substance abuse** and **substance dependence** are made on the basis of specific

Table 11.1 Reasons Athletes Take Ergogenic Drugs
Increase in strength and power
Increase in endurance
Increase in aggressiveness
Increase in speed and acceleration
Enhancement of competitive attitude
Enhancement of concentration
Enhancement of fine motor coordination
Enhancement of eye–hand coordination
Diminishment of pain perception
Diminishment of anxiety
Diminishment of tremor
Delay in onset of fatigue
Weight control

signs and symptoms (American Psychiatric Association, 1994), which are grouped into the following three categories.

Continued Use Despite Recurrent Problems

When using a substance causes problems and the individual continues to use it anyway, the individual is abusing the substance. This defining symptom of substance abuse is easily remembered by the UCR mnemonic: *Use,* followed by adverse *consequences,* followed by *repetition* of use and consequences (Fleming & Barry, 1992). The adverse consequences may occur in the areas of physical health, emotional health, or social functioning.

Impaired Control

People with impaired control take more substance than they intend, try to make rules about their use that they are unable to keep, or are unable to cut down their use despite wanting or trying to. For example, when a person intends to have only two drinks in an evening and then has six drinks, impaired control over drinking can be inferred. Although the athlete may argue that there were other times when the amount was predicted ("I said I'd have two, and I did have two"), it is the inability to predict consistently from one drinking occasion to another that is characteristic of impaired control.

Tolerance and Withdrawal

Tolerance and **withdrawal** indicate that a physiological adaptation has occurred. As a result of taking a substance chronically over time, the body changes in such a way that it takes more of the substance to get the same effect that smaller doses once produced (tolerance) or that a person feels physically ill when he or she stops or cuts down use of the substance (withdrawal). Athletes with withdrawal syndromes, by definition, have **physical dependence**. For diagnostic and treatment purposes, it is important to distinguish physical dependence from the full syndrome of substance dependence and from substance abuse (discussed later). In this chapter the term *dependence* (when used without a qualifier) refers to the full syndrome of substance dependence, whereas *physical dependence* is always qualified as such.

PATTERNS OF USE, DIAGNOSES, AND STAGE OF PROBLEM DEVELOPMENT

The type of treatment and counseling that an athlete needs depends on the particular diagnosis and stage of problem development (see figure 11.1). Athletes who need counseling generally fall into one of three patterns of use: at-risk use, problem use, and dependent use. The three categories lie along a continuum: At-risk use represents an earlier stage that precedes problems, and dependent use represents a later and severe stage of problem development. Problem use and dependent use are also referred to by the diagnostic terms *substance abuse* and *substance dependence,* respectively. At-risk use, also called **hazardous use**, is a prediagnostic term, meaning that the athlete's pattern of use places him or her at risk to develop a diagnosis of substance abuse or dependence.

Hazardous Use (At-Risk Use)

Hazardous use refers to a pattern of use that places the athlete at risk of developing problems. At this stage, the athlete has not developed problems that would qualify

tolerance—The need for greatly increased amounts of a substance to achieve a desired effect, or a markedly diminished effect with continued use of the same amount of the substance.

withdrawal—A syndrome of physical and emotional distress that occurs when an individual reduces or stops heavy or prolonged use of a substance.

physical dependence—The occurrence of withdrawal symptoms after stopping or reducing substance use. Also called physiological or pharmacological dependence.

hazardous use—A pattern of substance use that puts a person at high risk to develop problems or dependence. Also called at-risk use.

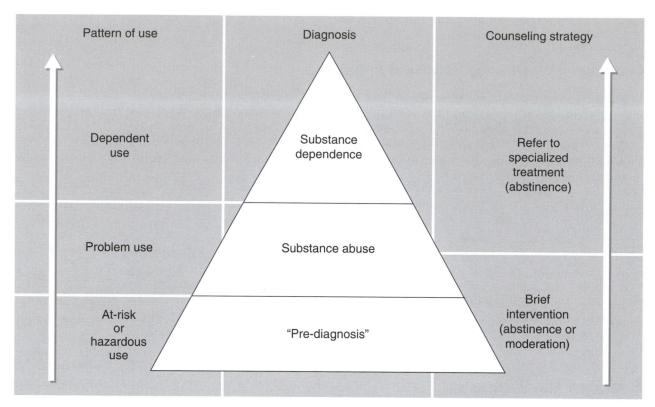

Figure 11.1 The relationship between pattern of use, diagnosis, and counseling strategy. Increasing intensity and severity of the problem are indicated by the arrows. The assessment establishes the pattern of use and diagnosis. Sports medicine professionals can attempt brief interventions for athletes with hazardous use and mild to moderate substance abuse problems. Abstinence or moderation can be negotiated as appropriate. For athletes with severe substance abuse problems, substance dependence, significant psychosocial comorbidity, or problems resistant to brief interventions, refer the athlete to specialized treatment for abstinence.

for a diagnosis of abuse or dependence. Counseling the at-risk athlete is best done by a knowledgeable professional whom the athlete trusts. As such, the athletic trainer, physical therapist, and sports physician are ideally suited for counseling this type of patient.

There are various definitions as to what constitutes hazardous drinking of alcohol. The National Institute on Alcohol Abuse and Alcoholism (1995) defines moderate drinking as no more than 3 drinks a day for women, 4 drinks a day for men, 7 drinks a week for women, and 14 drinks a week for men (3-4-7-14 rule). Of course, athletes who are alcoholic, pregnant, underage, taking medications that interact adversely with alcohol, or have medical illnesses such as liver disease should not drink at all. Therefore, the rule should be expanded to include abstinence (0-3-4-7-14). Hazardous consumption of prescription drugs can be defined as using more than prescribed or using the medication for reasons other than prescribed (e.g., to get high). For illicit drugs, any use is considered hazardous, due to legal risk and the unknown composition of illicitly sold substances.

Substance Abuse (Problem Use)

Substance abuse is defined as the continued use of a substance despite harmful problems or adverse consequences resulting from its use. The definition of substance abuse is the same for alcohol, prescription drugs, and illicit drugs. Substance abuse can be thought of as generating adverse consequences in the absence of impaired control or physical dependence. Substance abuse usually precedes and may develop into substance dependence. The adverse consequences may be medical, psychological, social, or legal. When the adverse consequence takes the form of an injury or when continued substance use interferes with recovery from an injury, the sports medicine professional has a definite role in counseling the athlete about substance abuse.

Substance Dependence (Dependent Use)

Substance dependence is the most severe form of substance problems and is characterized by impaired control over use, adverse consequences, and sometimes tolerance and withdrawal. The definition of substance dependence is the same for alcohol, prescription drugs, and illicit drugs. For purposes of this chapter, alcoholism is considered to be a severe form of alcohol dependence. The role of the sports medicine professional for dependent athletes is to facilitate referral to and continued participation in specialized addiction treatment.

The full syndrome of substance dependence must be distinguished from the limited syndrome of physical dependence. The distinction is important for treatment and counseling. Physical dependence simply denotes the occurrence of withdrawal symptoms when the athlete stops or cuts down use. Substances that are most commonly associated with withdrawal symptoms are alcohol, amphetamines, cocaine, nicotine, opioids, and sedative-hypnotics. Marijuana and **anabolic steroids** have also been associated with withdrawal symptoms, although these have been less well established and studied than for other drugs. Physical dependence may occur as part of the full syndrome of substance dependence, but it may also occur on its own. When physical dependence occurs by itself, then treatment is a relatively simple procedure, and the physician gradually tapers the athlete off the substance. However, if the athlete also suffers from the full syndrome of substance dependence, then simple tapering is insufficient treatment because the athlete will likely relapse to using substances. Athletes with the full syndrome of substance dependence are likely to use more medication than prescribed, to use the medication for purposes other than the prescribed reason (such as to get high or to numb their emotions), to obtain prescriptions from more than one doctor, to mix the prescribed medication with alcohol or with street drugs, and to evidence impaired functioning due to **intoxication**. When one or more of these manifestations of impaired control and use despite adverse consequences are present, referral to specialized addiction treatment is recommended because controlled use or attempts to taper the medication in a nonspecialized setting are likely to fail and to frustrate both the athlete and staff.

> *anabolic steroids—Synthetic derivatives of testosterone that have both anabolic (tissue-building) and androgenic (masculinizing) effects.*

> *intoxication—Clinically significant and potentially harmful physical or psychological changes that are due to the acute effect of a substance.*

SCREENING

Once the clinician has a solid understanding of the three patterns of substance use for which counseling is helpful and of the signs and symptoms of substance abuse and dependence, the clinician needs to know how best to screen for these patterns in the clinical setting. Screening refers to the detection of a potential problem and can be done by the sports medicine professional. Interviewing and questionnaires are by far the best approach to screening for substance problems because of their higher sensitivity and specificity compared with physical and laboratory exams. Screening questions can be introduced during a discussion of other personal health habits, such as wearing seat belts or diet.

Alcohol Screening

The following sections describe the recommended approach for alcohol screening.

Frequency–Quantity (F-Q-Max) Questions

First, screen for at-risk or hazardous drinking using three simple questions for frequency (F), quantity (Q), and maximum quantity (Max; see table 11.2).

- How many days in a week do you typically have something to drink? (F)
- On days that you drink, how many drinks do you typically have? (Q)
- What is the most you had to drink in any one day during the past month? (Max)

Use the 3-4-7-14 rule previously described for determining at-risk drinking: If the maximum is greater than 3 for women or 4 for men or if frequency times quantity is more than 7 for women or 14 for men, then the athlete is at risk to develop alcohol problems and should be counseled and referred accordingly.

Avoid asking "How much do you drink?" as the first screening question, or else be prepared for vague answers such as "not that much." Rather, specific questions that focus on frequency, then quantity, and finally on heavy consumption are more likely to evoke meaningful responses. In asking about quantity the interviewer should define what is meant by a drink (a can of beer = a glass of table wine = a shot of 80 proof liquor = about 0.5 oz or 12 g of absolute ethanol). General equivalencies of alcoholic beverages are listed in table 11.3.

CAGE Questions

Next, ask the four CAGE questions (table 11.2), which are probably the briefest and simplest screen for alcohol abuse and dependence (Ewing, 1984). If an individual answers "yes" to a CAGE question, then he or she should be prompted to elaborate:

Table 11.2 Screening for Alcohol Problems

Ask about level of consumption (F-Q-Max questions):

1. How many days in a week do you typically have something to drink? (Frequency)
2. On days that you drink, how many drinks do you typically have? (Quantity)
3. What is the most you had to drink in any one day during the past month? (Maximum)

If Frequency × Quantity > 7 drinks per week for women and > 14 drinks for men, or if maximum is > 3 for women and > 4 for men, then patient exceeds low-risk drinking.

Ask the CAGE questions:

1. Have you ever felt you should *cut down* on your drinking?
2. Have people *annoyed* you by criticizing your drinking?
3. Have you ever felt bad or *guilty* about your drinking?
4. Have you ever had a drink first thing in the morning to steady your nerves or to get rid of a hangover (*eye-opener*)?

Scoring: One or more "yes" answers screens for hazardous drinking. Two or more "yes" answers is a positive screen for an alcohol disorder.

If consumption or CAGE questions are positive, then assess for consequences, dependency symptoms, and severity.

Table 11.3 General Equivalencies of Alcoholic Beverages

Hard liquor (~40% alcohol or 80 proof)

1 shot or highball (1.5 oz, 44.4 ml)	= 1 drink
1/2 pint (237 ml)	= 6 drinks
1 pint (473 ml)	= 12 drinks
1 fifth (757 ml)	= 20 drinks
1 quart (946 ml)	= 24 drinks

Beer (4-5% alcohol)

One 12-oz (355-ml) bottle or can	= 1 drink
One "40-ouncer" (1.2 L)	= 3.3 drinks
One 6-pack (2.1 L)	= 6 drinks
1 case (8.5 L)	= 24 drinks

Wine (11-12% alcohol)

1 glass (5 oz, 148 ml)	= 1 drink
1 bottle (750 ml)	= 6 drinks
1 gallon (3.8 L)	= 30 drinks

Wine coolers (5% alcohol)

One 12-oz (355-ml) bottle	= 1 drink

Note. One drink contains approximately 0.5 oz or 12 g of absolute ethanol.

"Tell me more about that." When asking any questions about substance abuse, the interviewer should pay attention to both the content of the answers and the manner in which the person responds. If defensiveness or anger is manifested, then the CAGE question about feeling annoyed is already answered. Maintaining rapport and a nonjudgmental attitude are critical to the screening process. Two or more "yes" responses indicate a positive screen for alcohol dependence; however, even one "yes" may indicate problem drinking.

The Alcohol Use Disorders Identification Test (AUDIT)

The AUDIT (Saunders, Aasland, Babor, de la Fuente, & Grant, 1993) is a self-administered, 10-item screening instrument that assesses both the level of alcohol consumption and related problems, including symptoms of dependence (see table 11.4). It can be used as an alternative to the CAGE and F-Q-Max questions. The score ranges from 0 to 40, and a score of 8 or above indicates hazardous or problem drinking and the need for further assessment. The wide scoring range on the AUDIT also allows the screener to determine the severity of drinking problems, with higher scores indicating greater severity. Feedback about the score can be given in a manner similar to informing athletes about their laboratory values.

Drug Screening

There are two methods recommended for drug screening: the CAGEAID questions and the drug abuse screening test (DAST-10).

The CAGEAID Questions

The CAGEAID questions are the CAGE questions (table 11.2) that have been adapted to include drugs (Fleming & Barry, 1992):

- Have you felt you ought to *cut down* on your drug use?
- Have people *annoyed* you by criticizing your drug use?
- Have you felt bad or *guilty* about your drug use?

Table 11.4 Alcohol Use Disorders Identification Test (AUDIT)

Please circle the answer that is correct for you.

1. How often do you have a drink containing alcohol?

Never	Monthly or less	Two to four times a month	Two to three times a week	Four or more times a week

2. How many drinks containing alcohol do you have on a typical day when you are drinking?

1 or 2	3 or 4	5 or 6	7 to 9	10 or more

3. How often do you have six or more drinks on one occasion?

Never	Less than monthly	Monthly	Weekly	Daily or almost daily

4. How often during the last year have you found that you were not able to stop drinking once you had started?

Never	Less than monthly	Monthly	Weekly	Daily or almost daily

5. How often during the last year have you failed to do what was normally expected from you because of drinking?

Never	Less than monthly	Monthly	Weekly	Daily or almost daily

6. How often during the last year have you needed a first drink in the morning to get yourself going after a heavy drinking session?

Never	Less than monthly	Monthly	Weekly	Daily or almost daily

7. How often during the last year have you had a feeling of guilt or remorse after drinking?

Never	Less than monthly	Monthly	Weekly	Daily or almost daily

8. How often during the last year have you been unable to remember what happened the night before because you had been drinking?

Never	Less than monthly	Monthly	Weekly	Daily or almost daily

9. Have you or someone else been injured as a result of your drinking?

No	Yes, but not in the last year	Yes, during the last year

10. Has a relative or friend or a doctor or other health worker been concerned about your drinking or suggested you cut down?

No	Yes, but not in the last year	Yes, during the last year

(continued)

Table 11.4   *(continued)*

Procedure for Scoring AUDIT

Questions 1-8 are scored 0, 1, 2, 3, or 4. Questions 9 and 10 are scored 0, 2, or 4 only. The response coding is as follows:

	0	1	2	3	4
Question 1	Never	Monthly or less	Two to four times per month	Two to three times per week	Four or more times per week
Question 2	1 or 2	3 or 4	5 or 6	7 to 9	10 or more
Questions 3-8	Never	Less than monthly	Monthly	Weekly	Daily or almost daily
Questions 9-10	No		Yes, but not in the last year		Yes, during the last year

The minimum score (for nondrinkers) is 0, and the maximum possible score is 40.

A score of 8 or more indicates a strong likelihood of hazardous or harmful alcohol consumption.

- Have you ever used drugs the first thing in the morning to steady your nerves or to get the day started (*eye-opener*)?

Scoring is the same as for the CAGE questions.

The Drug Abuse Screening Test (DAST-10)

The Drug Abuse Screening Test (DAST-10) is a 10-item, yes/no, self-administered questionnaire (table 11.5). It is a shortened version of the original 28-item DAST (Skinner, 1982). Scoring ranges from 0 to 10. A score of 1 to 2 indicates a low level of problems, 3 to 5 indicates a moderate level of problems, 6 to 8 reflects a substantial level of problems, and 9 to 10 represents severe difficulties.

ASSESSMENT

A positive screen for substance abuse or dependence is followed by an assessment. Whereas the purpose of screening is to identify a possible problem, the purpose of an assessment is to confirm the problem and determine its extent, which will guide treatment planning. The sports medicine professional may prefer to refer athletes who screen positive to an addiction specialist for an assessment. In this case the goal of counseling is to facilitate a referral. Alternatively, the sports medicine professional may wish to assess further, particularly with athletes who initially seem resistant to a referral but who otherwise trust the clinical team. The assessment establishes the diagnosis, the severity of problems, and the athlete's **motivation** to change.

motivation—A state of readiness or eagerness to pursue an action or to change, which can be influenced by the counseling process.

Assessing Signs and Symptoms of Substance Abuse and Dependence

Sports medicine professionals should be aware of the following interview techniques. They can help identify a substance abuse problem.

Table 11.5 Drug Use Questionnaire (DAST-10)

The following questions concern information about your possible involvement with drugs *not including alcoholic beverages* during the past 12 months. Carefully read each statement and decide if your answer is "Yes" or "No." Then circle the appropriate response beside the question.

In the statements "drug abuse" refers to (1) the use of prescribed or over-the-counter drugs in excess of the directions and (2) any nonmedical use of drugs. The various classes of drugs may include cannabis (marijuana, hashish), solvents, tranquilizers (e.g., Valium), barbiturates, cocaine, stimulants (e.g., speed), hallucinogens (e.g., LSD), or narcotics (e.g., heroin). Remember that the questions do not include alcoholic beverages.

Please answer every question. If you have difficulty with a statement, then choose the response that is mostly right.

These questions refer to the past 12 months.

		Circle Your Response	
1.	Have you used drugs other than those required for medical reasons?	Yes	No
2.	Do you abuse more than one drug at a time?	Yes	No
3.	Are you always able to stop using drugs when you want to?	Yes	No
4.	Have you had "blackouts" or "flashbacks" as a result of drug use?	Yes	No
5.	Do you ever feel bad or guilty about your drug use?	Yes	No
6.	Does your spouse (or parents) ever complain about your involvement with drugs?	Yes	No
7.	Have you neglected your family because of your use of drugs?	Yes	No
8.	Have you engaged in illegal activities in order to obtain drugs?	Yes	No
9.	Have you ever experienced withdrawal symptoms (felt sick) when you stopped taking drugs?	Yes	No
10.	Have you had medical problems as a result of your drug use (e.g., memory loss, hepatitis, convulsions, bleeding, etc.)?	Yes	No

©1982 by the Addiction Research Foundation. Author: Harvey A. Skinner, PhD.

For information on the DAST, contact Dr. Harvey Skinner at the University of Toronto, Department of Public Health Sciences, McMurrich Building, Toronto, ON, Canada M5S 1A8.

Adverse Consequences

The following areas should be assessed: medical, psychiatric, and social (job, school, family, other relationships, financial, legal). Medical problems are determined by the athlete's medical history and physical exam (discussed later in this chapter). For eliciting other consequences, there are two approaches. One is by direct questioning: *Have substances caused any problems for you or your family? For you emotionally? At your job or school? For your social life? For your finances? Do you have any legal problems?* This approach is effective for athletes who admit they have a problem and want help. However, the questions may evoke **resistance** in other athletes and are easy to deny. The other approach is to assess problem areas first, then link adverse consequences in these areas to substances. A psychosocial history is obtained that is empathically related back to substances. For example, "How are things on the job? At home? With your family? . . . It sounds like things are pretty difficult right now, and you are feeling frustrated. I want to help in whatever way I can. How does your use of substances fit in with this?"

resistance—An athlete's opposition to a counselor's approach. Also, a reluctance to consider change; the opposite of motivation.

Impaired Control

Impaired control is displayed, for example, when the athlete decides to drink only four beers in the evenings on weekends but eventually drinks hard liquor throughout the week. To elicit information about impaired control, ask questions such as "Do you use more than you intend to? Have you tried or wanted to cut down? What happened? Do you ever make rules for your drinking or drug use? Do you always keep them?"

Tolerance

To elicit information about the athlete's substance tolerance, ask questions such as "Do you need more to get the same effect? Do you get less of an effect with the same amount?" Determine what the athlete's desired effect is: getting high, reducing anxiety, getting to sleep, or pain reduction.

Withdrawal

To determine whether the athlete experiences withdrawal, ask "Do you ever feel sick when you try to stop or cut down your use? What symptoms do you have?"

Assessing Problem Severity

Some of the screening questionnaires previously discussed can also be used to assess problem severity because they have a wide scoring range above the cut-off score for a positive screen. The higher the score, the more severe the problem. The AUDIT for alcohol problems (see table 11.4) and the DAST-10 (see table 11.5) are recommended.

Assessing Motivation

The clinician may be convinced on the basis of screening and further assessment that the athlete has a problem, but the athlete may not think so. Before counseling an athlete to change, it is wise to assess the athlete's perception of the problem and his or her motivation for change with questions such as these: "How do you feel about your substance use? Do you have any concerns we have not talked about? Are you interested in changing?"

PHYSICAL EXAM

The physical exam is usually performed by the sports physician; however, the other members of the sports medicine team may detect signs of drug use during the course of their work with an athlete. The physical exam may provide clues to intoxication, withdrawal, or chronic substance use. Although the physical exam is not sensitive as a screening test for substance use, positive findings need treatment. Equally important, when counseling the athlete, objective findings should be linked to the substances used as the practitioner expresses concern for the athlete's health. Nevertheless, an absence of findings on the physical exam does not imply an absence of a substance problem because most of the early manifestations of substance abuse are psychosocial in nature.

General Appearance

Weight loss and an emaciated appearance can be seen in chronic alcoholics due to poor nutrition and in chronic cocaine and stimulant users due to anorexic effects. Chronic users of other substances may neglect their health and appear poorly nourished. By contrast, anabolic steroid users show evidence of muscular hypertrophy and an athletic appearance. Shivering and huddling for warmth may be seen during opioid withdrawal.

Vital Signs

In general, one or more vital signs will be elevated during intoxication with cocaine, stimulants, hallucinogens, phencyclidine (PCP), and marijuana and during withdrawal from alcohol, sedatives, and opioids. Marijuana intoxication typically increases heart rate without affecting other vital signs. Respiration may be depressed with opioid intoxication. Mild increases in blood pressure may be seen with anabolic steroid use. Although nitrite inhalants can lower blood pressure and increase heart rate acutely, these effects last only for five minutes and so are unlikely to be observed during an office physical exam.

Skin

Several signs and symptoms of substance abuse are manifested as changes in the skin. Needle tracks may be the most easily recognized of these signs, but there are others to look out for as well.

Signs Associated With Injectable Drug Use

Needle tracks along the forearm and other veins (such as in the hands, feet, and groin) are visible with intravenous drug use (most often heroin or cocaine). Thrombosed or hardened veins may be palpable beneath the skin in intravenous users, and it may be difficult to find viable veins from which to draw blood. Subcutaneous injections ("skin popping") may leave circumscribed, pocklike depressions in the skin. Anabolic steroid users typically inject into large muscle groups such as the deltoids or gluteals, with a preference for the gluteals so that marks will be hidden during bodybuilding competitions. Abscesses, cellulitis, and other infections are possible with injectable drug use.

Other Cutaneous Signs

Diaphoresis (sweatiness) accompanies intoxication with stimulants, cocaine, or hallucinogens and withdrawal from alcohol, marijuana, sedatives, or opioids. Piloerection (goose bumps) is seen during opioid withdrawal. Self-induced excoriations may result from cocaine- or stimulant-induced formication (the sensation of bugs crawling under the skin). Abnormal vascularization of the facial skin is seen in chronic alcoholics. Jaundice may result from alcohol-related liver disease, steroid-related liver disease, or viral hepatitis transmitted from contaminated needles. Acne can be seen with anabolic steroid use. Hirsutism (excessive hair growth) in females and male pattern baldness in males may be associated with anabolic steroid use. Burns, especially on the fingers, may be associated with smoking drugs. Traumatic bruises may result from falls, accidents, or fights while intoxicated. Flushing can be seen with alcohol, hallucinogens, and opioid intoxication.

Eyes

Dilated pupils are seen during intoxication with cocaine, stimulants, or hallucinogens and during opioid withdrawal. Pinpoint pupils are seen with opioid intoxication. Lacrimation (watery or tearful eyes) is seen during opioid withdrawal. Conjunctival erythema (reddened eyes) is seen with marijuana or inhalant intoxication and in chronic alcoholics. Nystagmus (abnormal jerking of the muscles controlling eye movements) is seen during intoxication with alcohol and other sedatives, phencyclidine, and some inhalants. Nystagmus is also seen as part of Wernicke's encephalopathy in thiamine-deficient alcoholics. Jaundice may be apparent in the eyes as well as in the skin, as previously described.

Nose, Mouth, and Throat

Rhinorrhea (runny nose) is seen during opioid withdrawal. An infected, ulcerated, or perforated nasal septum may be seen with intranasal cocaine use. Glue sniffer's rash may occur around nose and mouth. Dry mouth may occur with marijuana intoxication. Pharyngeal erythema (inflamed, reddened throat) may occur with smoking drugs (tobacco, marijuana, cocaine, PCP). Oral cancers may occur with heavy alcohol and tobacco use. Coated tongue may be seen in chronic alcoholics. Poor dentition may be seen in chronic substance users who neglect their health. Deepened voice is heard in female anabolic steroid users. Yawning is observed during opioid withdrawal but may also occur during cocaine or stimulant withdrawal due to sleep deprivation after a multiple-day binge.

Chest

Rhonchi, sounds heard over the chest with a stethoscope during respiration, are produced by the flow of air through narrowed breathing passages. Rhonchi are associated with upper-airways irritation and coughing and may occur in chronic smokers of marijuana or cocaine. Gynecomastia (enlargement of male breast tissue) with painful lumps is seen with anabolic steroid use.

Abdomen

Hepatomegaly (enlargement of the liver) and right upper-quadrant tenderness may occur in alcohol-related liver disease and with anabolic steroid use. Diffuse abdominal tenderness accompanied by nausea, vomiting, and diarrhea may occur during withdrawal from opioids, alcohol, and sedatives.

Genitourinary System

Testicular atrophy may be seen with chronic, heavy alcohol or anabolic steroid use. Clitoral hypertrophy and prostatic hypertrophy occur in female and male anabolic steroid users, respectively.

Neurological Exam

Slurred speech, ataxic (wide-based, staggering) gait, and incoordination occur during intoxication with alcohol, sedatives, marijuana, opioids, hallucinogens, PCP, and inhalants. Persistent ataxia and incoordination may occur with alcohol- or inhalant-related cerebellar degeneration. Tremor occurs during intoxication with cocaine, stimulants, hallucinogens, and inhalants and during withdrawal from alcohol, sedatives, and opioids. Hyperreflexia (an increase in deep-tendon reflexes) occurs during intoxication with cocaine, stimulants, PCP, and hallucinogens and during withdrawal from alcohol and sedatives. In some instances hyperreflexia precedes seizures. Depressed reflexes are seen during inhalant intoxication. Diminished response to pain and numbness is seen especially with PCP intoxication due to its anesthetic properties but may also be seen with alcohol, sedative, and opioid intoxication. Peripheral neuropathy (disease of the peripheral nerves resulting in muscle weakness, sensory loss, and abnormal sensations in the limbs) is seen with chronic alcohol and inhalant use.

LABORATORY EXAM

Several laboratory tests can serve as useful adjuncts in the assessment process. Laboratory tests should ordered and interpreted by the sports physician.

Urine Drug Screening

How long a substance can be detected in urine depends on the amount, frequency, and duration of use; the individual's metabolism; the pharmacokinetics of the particular substance; and the sensitivity of the assay (American Psychiatric Association, 1994; Hawks & Chiang, 1986; Vereby, 1991). General guidelines appear in table 11.6.

Table 11.6   Urine Drug Screening

Substance	Duration in urine (days)[a]
Alcohol	1
Amphetamines	1-3
Barbiturates	
Short-acting	3-5
Long-acting	10-14
Chronic phenobarbital	Several weeks
Benzodiazepines	
Long-acting, chronic use	Several weeks
Cannabinoids (marijuana; THC)	
Acute use	2-8
Chronic daily use	14-42
Cocaine (benzoylecgonine)	
Single dose	1-3
Repeated high doses (possibly)	7-12
Lysergic acid diethylamide (LSD)[b]	2-4
Methylenedioxymethamphetamine (MDMA)[b]	2-4
Methaqualone	7-14
Opioids (except methadone)	1-2
Phencyclidine (PCP)	
Single dose	2-8
Prolonged or high doses	Several weeks

[a]Duration depends on an individual's level of consumption and metabolism, pharmacokinetics, and the sensitivity of the assay. The values in the table are estimates from the American Psychiatric Association (1994), Hawks and Chiang (1986), and Vereby (1991).

[b]Must be specially ordered; not included in most routine drug screens.

Modified with permission from Brower & Severin (1997). Alcohol and other drug-related problems. In D.J. Knesper, M.B. Riba, & T.L. Schwenk (Eds.), *Primary care psychiatry* (pp. 309-342). Philadelphia: Saunders.

Blood Alcohol Levels

Blood alcohol levels (BALs) are especially indicated when an injury is associated with acute intoxication. The lab value can be used at a later time to provide feedback to the athlete about hazardous drinking. Tables are available that allow the clinician to calculate how much alcohol was consumed when the athlete's BAL, weight, and sex are known (Kishline, 1994). This allows the athlete and counselor to be more exact when, for example, an athlete insists, "I only had a couple of beers." Kishline (1994) recommends that a moderate drinker should not exceed a BAL of 55 mg%, the so-called 55 limit, while also recognizing that the only safe BAL prior to some activities, such as driving, is zero. (Note: 100 mg% = 100 mg/100 ml = 0.1 g/dl, which is the legal limit for intoxication or drunk driving in many states.)

Other Laboratory Tests

Several other laboratory tests provide useful information regarding an athlete's alcohol and drug use, including the following:

- Gamma-glutamyl-transferase (GGT), also called gamma-glutamyl-transpeptidase (GGTP)—Elevated with chronic, heavy drinking
- Aspartate aminotransferase (AST or SGOT) and alanine aminotransferase (ALT or SGPT)—Elevated in alcoholic liver disease and in anabolic steroid users because of intramuscular injections and intensive weight training
- Mean corpuscular volume (MCV)—Increased with heavy drinking
- Tuberculosis (TB) skin test—Recommended for confirmed cases of substance problems because of the association between tuberculosis and substance abuse
- HIV and hepatitis B and C—Indicated for athletes who share needles or engage in high-risk sexual practices

SUMMARY OF SCREENING AND ASSESSMENT

After conducting the various assessments and examinations previously described, the sports medicine professional will know whether a problem with substances exists, the extent of the problem, and the athlete's motivation to change the problem. The results of the assessment guide the goals and nature of the counseling to follow. Athletes who use illicit or banned substances or whose problems with alcohol are assessed as severe should be counseled toward abstinence. Athletes who have severe problems with any substance are counseled to accept referral for specialized treatment, whereas athletes with mild problems can be counseled with brief interventions as described later. Regardless of problem severity, athletes who resist change should be counseled using motivational techniques. In all cases, the results of the assessment are shared with the athlete in a nonjudgmental manner using the feedback technique described later.

COUNSELING SKILLS IN SUBSTANCE ABUSE CONTEXTS

In this section the goals of counseling people with substance use problems are discussed, followed by special considerations for counseling athletes with substance use problems. Next, the concept of enabling is introduced. Our attention then shifts to motivating athletes who either do not think they have a problem or do not feel ready to change their substance-using behavior. The section concludes with a discussion of brief interventions and referrals to specialized treatment.

Which member of the sports medicine team should provide counseling? The answer depends in large part on the inclination and interest of the sports medicine professional and on the quality of the therapeutic relationship. The principles and techniques elaborated in this section can be employed by a wide range of professionals oriented to helping people change their behavior. Athletic trainers, physical therapists, and sports physicians are all involved in motivating patients to do what is needed for recovery from injury. In this sense, counseling the athlete to do what is needed for recovery from substance-related problems is analogous. On the other hand, substance abuse counseling is not so simple that it can be mastered by reading one chapter. Interested professionals, regardless of previous experience or professional degree, will benefit from additional training and supervision. Moreover, treatment success is optimized when all members of the treatment team agree on a plan and support each other's efforts.

Goals

Two sets of goals are negotiated with athletes after an assessment determines the stage of problem development. The first goal may be to refer the athlete to an addiction specialist. For at-risk and early-problem athletes, counseling by the sports medicine team is sufficient in many cases. For athletes with severe problems or dependence, referral to a specialist will be the goal of counseling (refer back to figure 11.1). The second set of goals is whether to advise abstinence or moderation. For at-risk drinkers, prescription drug users who do not meet criteria for substance abuse or dependence, and some problem drinkers, moderation is an option. Abstinence is clearly recommended for athletes with severe problems or dependence and for any use of illicit substances. Abstinence is also the treatment goal of choice for athletes who use anabolic steroids to enhance athletic performance or physical appearance. Finally, abstinence is generally recommended for athletes who abuse prescription drugs such as opioids and sedative-hypnotics. Before initiating abstinence, the athlete should consult a physician to determine whether life-threatening or severe withdrawal symptoms are likely and whether medical detoxification is needed.

Research to date supports moderation for those with hazardous drinking patterns or mild to moderate drinking problems. In addition, outcomes are improved when athletes are made partners in the selection of treatment goals. Therefore, the wise counselor will negotiate the treatment goal with the athlete when this does not jeopardize health rather than prescribe a rigid goal that the athlete rejects. Athletes who fail moderation trials may then be inclined and advised to set an abstinence goal.

Individuals who are able to abstain from alcohol entirely for a two-week period at the beginning of treatment are more likely to attain their ultimate goal, whether abstinence or moderate drinking. Moreover, this initial period of abstinence allows the sports medicine professional and athlete to assess further the effect of alcohol on the athlete's well-being as the alcohol is eliminated. Situations that trigger urges to use also become more apparent during abstinence and can be targeted for treatment purposes.

Important Treatment Considerations for Athletes

Several suggestions should be considered when working with athletes with substance use problems. Those discussed in the following sections are

- Understand the pressures associated with athletic excellence
- Consider yourself a team member

- Recognize competitive themes in counseling relationships
- Beware of providing "special treatment"

Understand the Pressures Associated With Athletic Excellence

When counseling athletes, it is extremely important to understand the purpose, intent, and pressures for the drug taking. When you understand the motivation for use, counseling can address those pressures. In general, athletes use drugs for all the same reasons as other people, but they also experience somewhat unique pressures to use. They may use drugs to enhance performance, to mask pain, to alleviate the emotional pressure of competition, and to socialize with team members. Athletes may be more likely than nonathletes to use **ergogenic** and **restorative drugs** (Nuzzo & Waller, 1988). Ergogenic, or performance-enhancing, aids refer to drugs (e.g., amphetamines, anabolic steroids) or methods (e.g., blood doping) that are used to gain athletic advantage.

Restorative drugs are taken in an attempt to return (or restore) function to "normal." The athlete takes restorative drugs to perform despite an underlying illness or injury. The current literature does not indicate that otherwise healthy athletes use analgesics to gain a competitive advantage. The real hazard lies with the injured athlete who requires analgesia to compete fully with minimal pain. Pain reduction may allow the athlete to continue performing while masking warning pain and causing increased (and possibly irreversible) tissue damage. Considerable effort might have to be expended to protect the athlete from either external or internal pressure to compete.

Sports are very competitive and goal oriented, which in our society often manifests as a "winner take all" philosophy. Professional athletes have their livelihoods to protect, and college-bound athletes have scholarships at stake and a desire to uphold the honor and tradition of the school and team that they represent. In the mind of an athlete seeking a competitive edge, the benefits of drug use may outweigh the perceived risks.

ergogenic drugs—Substances (e.g., amphetamines, anabolic steroids) that are taken for the purpose of enhancing athletic performance.

restorative drugs—Substances that are taken in an attempt to restore function and performance to "normal," despite underlying illness or injuries.

Consider Yourself a Team Member

The principle here is to keep the twin goals of health enhancement and performance enhancement in alignment rather than in conflict. Accordingly, the counselor takes the position that an athlete performs best when optimally healthy. However, this position is challenged by the alternative notion that drugs that are potentially dangerous to health may improve athletic performance. The athlete and other members of the team may focus primarily on performance. Therefore, the responsibility for helping the athlete maintain an alignment between health and performance goals falls more on the clinical member of the athlete's team than on anyone else.

Recognize Competitive Themes in Counseling Relationships

Athletes tend to view themselves as being "young, tough, and almost indestructible," and they may discount the hazards and toxicity of alcohol and other drugs (Brown & Benner, 1984). Some athletes take pride in being able to drink others "under the table" or in performing well while intoxicated or hung over. These competitive themes may carry over into the counseling session as well. For example, some anabolic steroid users initially exhibit a competitive stance with the counselor (Brower, 1992). As in athletic competition, the counselor may be perceived as an opponent or even "sized up" in terms of both body build and knowledge about anabolic steroids. If the counselor is an athlete or a past anabolic steroid user, this can be used to therapeutic advantage, similar to the work of a recovering counselor with other substance-dependent patients. What is most important, however, is that the athlete feels understood by the counselor. When the counselor is perceived as being on the athlete's side or team, competitiveness should diminish.

Beware of Providing "Special Treatment"

The counselor must always remain cognizant of therapeutic roles and boundaries to avoid being placed in an untenable therapeutic position. A common problem of this type is seen when a counselor becomes overly invested in his or her patient's athletic performance and derives vicarious gratification from the athlete's exploits. In this manner **countertransference** issues may be influenced by the athletic context. Although performance outcomes are of interest and are related to treatment, overall health and symptom management should be the primary goals.

countertransfer-ence—The conscious and unconscious emotional responses of the counselor to the athlete.

Know Which Drugs Are Banned

Drug-testing policies constantly change, as do the lists of drugs that are banned. These are influenced by legal challenges, ethical issues, public opinion, and collective bargaining. Both the United States Olympic Committee [(800) 233-0393] and the National Collegiate Athletic Association [(800) 546-0441] maintain confidential, toll-free hot lines for accurate, updated information on which substances are banned.

Helping Versus Enabling

enabling—The actions of people close to the athlete that make it easier for the athlete to continue using substances by protecting the athlete from the negative conse-quences of using.

The term **enabling** describes the behaviors of others that may be intended to help the athlete but unwittingly protect the athlete from the negative consequences of substance use. Consequently, enabling makes it easier for the athlete to continue using substances. For example, family members or teammates may "cover" the athlete's responsibilities so that the athlete's dysfunction from substance abuse goes unnoticed by employers, coaches, or health care professionals. Sports medicine professionals can also unwittingly become enablers, for example, by failing to intervene with athletes who abuse substances, prescribing addictive drugs for athletes with substance abuse or dependence, or clearing athletes for competition who need substance abuse treatment. The sports medicine professional avoids the enabler role by asking himself or herself honestly, "Do my actions with this athlete make it easier or harder for the athlete to continue using harmful substances?"

People who enable patients with substance problems are sometimes called *codependent*. Codependency refers to a style of relating to the addicted person, not to a partner who also is substance dependent. Codependents often benefit from counseling to cope better with the stresses of living or working with an active alcoholic or addict. Referral to Al-Anon or Nar-Anon (addresses given later in this chapter) may be especially helpful. These are 12-step groups that help people understand that they did not cause the problem, they cannot control the problem, they cannot cure it, and the alcoholic or addict is responsible for his or her own recovery. When sports medicine professionals have the athlete's consent to talk with people who may be enabling the athlete's drug use, they can educate those people about the enabling process and how to avoid it.

Motivational Counseling

Motivational counseling is used when an athlete with substance abuse or dependence either does not believe there is a problem or lacks a commitment to change. These attitudes are readily identified during the assessment process by asking athletes whether they have any concerns about their use of substances and whether they are interested in changing.

Motivation is defined as a state of readiness to change, which can be influenced by the counseling process (Miller & Rollnick, 1991). Although some counselors tend to view their patients as either motivated or unmotivated to change, motivation is not a fixed personality trait that the patient either has or does not have. Rather, motivation is a changeable state of mind that can be influenced by what the counselor says and does.

Motivational counseling is based on a model of how people change, called the stages-of-change model. Prochaska and DiClemente (see Miller & Rollnick, 1991) developed the model by studying how change occurs naturally, outside of treatment—for example, people who stop smoking on their own without formal outside help. When comparing self-change to change that occurs in counseling, they noticed many similarities; this led them to describe change as occurring in steps, or stages. They described five **stages of change**: precontemplation, contemplation, preparation, action, and maintenance.

Precontemplation

Athletes at the **precontemplation** stage have not yet begun to think they have a problem. Thus it does not occur to them to change their behavior. If asked to change, they typically deny having a problem. Rather than oppose the denial, the counselor aims only to help move the athlete to the next stage of contemplation.

Contemplation

In the **contemplation** stage, athletes begin to consider that they may have a problem but don't think that they really do. Ambivalence is the hallmark of this stage as athletes struggle to understand their problems with substances. A common mistake of counselors is to tell the athlete all the problems that a substance is causing, which forces the athlete to take the other side of the ambivalence and tell the counselor all the reasons it really isn't such a problem. Instead, the sports medicine professional should help athletes to explore their own concerns about their substance use. The counselor should summarize both sides of the ambivalence while particularly affirming the athlete's concerns soon after they are stated.

Preparation

At the preparation stage, athletes need help sorting out the alternative change strategies that are available and choosing the one most likely to be effective for them. People will commit to action only when they find the change strategy acceptable and when they believe their efforts to change will be successful.

Action

Action refers to the stage in which people overtly modify their behavior and their surroundings. In short, they make the move for which they have been preparing. The action phase is what most people think of as formal substance abuse treatment.

Maintenance

There is an old joke about an alcoholic who quit drinking a thousand times but started drinking again each day after quitting. Athletes may find it easier to stop using substances than to remain stopped. In the maintenance stage, the athlete learns to prevent relapses by identifying triggers to using substances and developing alternative coping responses. Maintenance is a critically important stage that can last from six months to a lifetime. When athletes relapse, the challenge is to recover from the relapse as quickly as possible and to resume the change process. Recovery from relapses may involve cycling again through some of the earlier stages of change.

Athletes need different kinds of counseling, depending on where they are in the cycle of change. Problems arise when counselors want athletes to move too fast or to skip stages. For athletes to move through the stages successfully, the counseling

stages of change—A series of phases that people move through during the process of changing a behavior. Movement from one stage to the next requires motivation, time, and completing specific tasks.

precontemplation—The first or earliest stage of change in which athletes usually have no intention of changing their behavior and typically deny having a problem.

contemplation—Stage of change in which the athlete begins to think a problem exists but is ambivalent about changing it.

approach should target the stage that the athlete is in. A mismatch between the counselor's approach and the athlete's stage of change will evoke resistance and denial from the athlete. For example, advising an athlete in the precontemplation stage to attend meetings of Alcoholics Anonymous will likely fail, whereas it can be appropriate advice for an athlete in the action stage. Usually the most challenging athletes for counselors are those in the precontemplation and contemplation stages. The purpose of motivational interviewing is to help people move from precontemplation and contemplation to preparation and action.

Helping Precontemplators or Contemplators Strengthen Their Motivation for Change

Miller and Rollnick (1991) described five general principles underlying motivational interviewing. It should be noted that these techniques require skill developed by experience and practice. Wise sports medicine professionals should recognize that only through practice and experience will they become expert in their use of these skills.

Express Empathy

Empathy and the therapeutic alliance are essential for effective treatment. Athletes must feel that the sports medicine professional is on their side rather than feeling pressured to change. Empathy makes the athlete feel understood. The sports medicine professional conveys empathy by reflecting back the athlete's point of view. For example, "You're not sure you have a problem" is more empathic than "You have a problem whether you see it or not!" Empathy starts where the athlete initially presents, not where the sports medicine professional wants the athlete to be. Paradoxically, by communicating understanding of athletes as they are, they are freed to change.

Develop Discrepancy

Help individuals to see and feel how their current behavior threatens personal goals or is inconsistent with more central personal values. For example, a recent high school graduate may value his independence from his parents yet be tied to living at home because drugs "rob" him of most of his earnings. The same athlete may not be very concerned that cocaine can cause heart attacks and may tune out the sports medicine professional who provides that information. The key is to "let in" the awareness of adverse consequences that are personally meaningful, in a safe environment in which the pros and cons can be explored openly without criticism or coercion.

Avoid Argument

It is counterproductive for the sports medicine professional to argue with an ambivalent athlete. Arguing just breeds resistance.

Roll With Resistance

Resistance is commonly thought of as the opposite of motivation. If motivation is a readiness to change, then resistance is a reluctance to change. Resistance is mistakenly thought of as something inside the athlete that the counselor needs to help overcome or get rid of. Instead, resistance reveals the interpersonal process between the sports medicine professional and the athlete. In other words, the athlete is resisting something that the sports medicine professional is doing in the interview. Resistance therefore can be influenced by the practitioner's manner and approach. The overt behaviors of resistance are easy to detect in the interview as denying, minimizing, changing subjects, blaming, arguing, or complying superficially. Resistant behaviors occur because of underlying feelings of shame, guilt, anxiety, or pessimism about change. These behaviors indicate that the sports medicine professional has "lost" the athlete and gotten too far ahead of the athlete in the stages of change. Thus the sports medicine professional needs to shift strategies and return to where the athlete is.

Miller and Rollnick (1991) compare the counselor's management of resistance to a judo master's response to an opponent's line of force. The master does not oppose the force directly, but rather "rolls" with its momentum and turns it to good advantage. Likewise, the counselor does not oppose an athlete's denial directly. Rather, the counselor employs a number of techniques that help the athlete and counselor move together in the same direction. In managing resistance, the sports medicine professional should acknowledge the athlete's point of view and emphasize the athlete's personal choice and responsibility. The specific techniques of reflection, double-sided reflection, shifting focus, and reframing are exemplified next.

One way to let the athlete know that you have "returned" is to reflect what the athlete is saying. Reflection restates the meaning of the athlete's words and lets the athlete know that you hear and understand what he or she is saying. For example:

Athlete: I'm not an alcoholic. My wife's the alcoholic.

Sports medicine professional: It seems to you that your wife has more of a drinking problem.

Double-sided reflection helps move athletes to contemplation by helping them own both sides of their ambivalence:

Athlete: I don't think I have a problem with drinking. I just don't like my wife's criticism of it.

Sports medicine professional: On the one hand, it's hard for you to see what all her fuss is about. On the other hand, you would like things to be different with your wife, and you know that has something to do with your drinking.

Shifting focus can be used to avoid arguing with an athlete who is confronting the sports medicine professional.

Athlete: You think I'm an alcoholic, but I'm not!

Sports medicine professional: I'm not really concerned with labels. I'm concerned about how things are going for you, and how alcohol fits in. Tell me more about what happened with your coach last week.

Reframing is a technique for helping people achieve a new perspective on an old point of view. In the following example, the athlete is encouraged to see the hidden danger in a perceived strength.

Athlete: I don't have a problem with alcohol. In fact, I can drink more than most people and not even feel it.

Sports medicine professional: We call that tolerance. Most people will stop drinking before you do. But with tolerance, you can damage yourself and not even know it because you can't feel it. That can be a problem.

Support Self-Efficacy

Self-efficacy refers to the athlete's belief that he or she can do something about a problem. Even athletes who know they should change their substance use will not if they believe that they cannot. Therefore the sports medicine professional conveys a sense of hope and optimism that positive change is possible.

Brief Intervention

brief intervention—A form of counseling conducted over a few sessions in which awareness of a problem is raised, changing the problem behavior is advised, options for making the change are provided, and personal responsibility for making the change is emphasized. The counselor actively supports the athlete's motivation to change through empathy and therapeutic optimism.

Many problems, especially when detected early, do not require referral to a specialist. **Brief intervention** refers to a form of counseling conducted over one or a few sessions. It is aimed at athletes who use substances in a hazardous way but have not yet developed problems and at athletes who have mild to moderate abuse problems (see figure 11.1). Athletes with severe problems or dependence usually require specialized treatment. The components of effective brief interventions can easily be remembered with the FRAMES mnemonic: feedback, responsibility, advice, menu, empathy, and self-efficacy (Miller & Rollnick, 1991). While all these components are useful, they are not necessarily applied in the same order as in the mnemonic.

Feedback

After the assessment, provide feedback from the screening test, history, physical exam, and laboratory tests. When normative scores and lab values are available, these should be presented and compared with the individual's score. For example:

- *One of your liver enzymes known as GGT was elevated to 128, and the normal range is 0 to 30 (show athlete the actual laboratory report). This occurs when the liver is exposed to too much alcohol.*
- *The AUDIT is a test that screens for alcohol problems. Your score on the AUDIT was 23, and the cut-off for low-risk drinking is 8.*

The strategy of feedback is to present the athlete with the facts in a nonjudgmental fashion along with information that allows the athlete to understand the personal implications of those facts. Scare tactics are avoided, which may increase the athlete's defensiveness. Rather, the discrepancy between the "normal" range and the athlete's status helps to build motivation for change. The athlete's response to the feedback should be elicited and responded to empathically:

- *What do you think about this?*
- *How are you feeling about this information?*
- *You seem uncomfortable. This is not easy for you to hear.*

Responsibility

Both the sports medicine professional and athlete must be clear that the athlete is responsible for changing or not changing. Emphasizing responsibility is also a good technique for diffusing resistance because the sports medicine professional acknowledges that the locus of control for changing resides in the athlete. For example:

- *It's up to you whether you change or not. I hope that you do, and if you decide to, I will do everything in my power to help you. But no one can make you change if you don't want to.*

Advice

Advise the athlete to make a change. For example:

- *I would like you to stop drinking altogether for the next two weeks so I can recheck you and see what effect that may have on recovering your muscle strength.*
- *I would like you to limit your drinking to no more than two drinks a day. When I see you next, we will talk about how that goes.*
- *I would like you to see a specialist in drug problems for your cocaine problem.*

Menu of Options

Whenever possible, offer the athlete a choice of goals or strategies from which to choose. Offering a menu of options enlists the athlete as a partner in the decision making, which reduces the athlete's resistance to change. Here are two examples of how you can do this:

• *There are a number of options we can try to help you stop drinking. You can simply try it on your own. You can attend some AA meetings. You can use a self-guided manual that will help you track your tendencies to drink and come up with alternatives to drinking.*

• *You can stop drinking altogether or you could limit yourself to no more than two drinks a day.*

Empathy

Empathy remains the cornerstone of all counseling. It is a two-step process. First, the sports medicine professional should strive to understand the athlete's point of view and feelings about using substances and related problems. Then the sports medicine professional communicates that understanding to the athlete. Athletes who feel understood and trust their treatment team are most likely to accept and benefit from the treatment team's interventions.

Self-Efficacy

Self-efficacy refers to the athlete's belief that change is possible. Athletes will not change if they do not think they can. Therefore, the sports medicine professional should provide encouragement and support the athlete's efforts to change. Probably all athletes have had the experience of setting training and performance goals that they achieved. By reminding athletes of past successes, their sense of self-efficacy can be enhanced.

self-efficacy—
The athlete's belief in his or her ability to make a change or complete a task successfully.

Referral

Although brief interventions can be done in one or more visits, treatment often takes place over time. Frustration and burnout can occur from trying to accomplish too much too fast. When brief interventions are not successful, referral to specialized treatment is indicated (see figure 11.1). Referral to specialized treatment is indicated for moderate to severe problem use, dependent use, or problems complicated by significant psychiatric or medical comorbidities. After a referral is made, the sports medicine professional should maintain contact with the addiction specialist—with the athlete's consent—to determine whether the athlete followed the recommendation and to track the athlete's progress in treatment. The sports medicine professional can make better referrals if he or she is familiar with the various levels of specialized care for substance problems.

Levels of Specialized Care

The following levels of care are listed in order of increasing intensity of service.

• *Outpatient assessment* services conduct an initial consultation and evaluation to determine the appropriate level and type of care for each person. Many HMOs have a center for diagnosis and referral (CDR), which provides assessment services for patients with substance problems.

• *Traditional outpatient care* consists of one to three hours a week of individual, group, or family therapy. Athletes may enter this level of care initially or transfer to this level after completing a more intensive level of care.

- *Intensive outpatient* and partial hospital care usually involve patients in a minimum of 3.5 hours a day of treatment for three to seven days a week for approximately four weeks. Programs provide education; individual, group, and family therapies; and a milieu in which patients and staff can interact less formally during a meal or break. Patients typically sleep at home.

- *Residential care* allows patients to spend 24 hours a day in a protected, safe setting in addition to providing the same services as in partial hospital care. Subacute detoxification using supportive care and oral medications is often available. Duration of care typically varies from one to four weeks.

- *Inpatient care* is hospital-based treatment for acute detoxification. Such care is indicated when detoxification either requires intravenous medication or is complicated by serious psychiatric or other medical illness.

- *Long-term residential care* is more intensive than inpatient and short-term residential care only in terms of duration, which typically ranges from 3 to 12 months.

Referral to Self-Help Groups

Sports medicine professionals should familiarize themselves with various groups that offer support for athletes with substance problems. Addresses of several organizations are included so that you can send for descriptive literature of the various programs. Many of the organizations also maintain home pages on the World Wide Web. Relevant groups are very helpful to recommend to athletes as part of their menu of options to help them change.

Alcoholics Anonymous and Al-Anon

Alcoholics Anonymous (AA) was founded in 1935. It has spiritual, not religious, principles of accepting powerlessness over alcohol and seeking help from a "higher power" as the individual understands it (Alcoholics Anonymous, 1976). AA is based on 12 steps and 12 traditions. The only requirement for attending meetings is a desire to stop drinking. The contact number for AA is available in most local phone books. Al-Anon is a 12-step group designed for the support of significant others who are affected by the alcoholic.

> Alcoholics Anonymous
> P.O. Box 459, Grand Central Station
> New York, NY 10163
> (212) 686-1100

> Al-Anon Family Group Headquarters, Inc.
> 1600 Corporate Landing Parkway
> Virginia Beach, VA 23454-5617
> (800) 356-9996

Narcotics Anonymous

Narcotics Anonymous (NA) is a 12-step program that is often preferred by individuals whose primary or preferred drug is not alcohol. Nar-Anon, modeled after Al-Anon, is the corresponding group for family members and concerned others.

> Narcotics Anonymous
> World Service Office, Inc.
> P.O. Box 999
> Van Nuys, CA 91406
> (818) 780-3951

Cocaine Anonymous

Cocaine Anonymous (CA) is a 12-step program specific to cocaine users. Because this group has fewer meetings, people often go to AA and NA for primary support.

Cocaine Anonymous
3740 Overland Ave., Suite H
P.O. Box 2000
Los Angeles, CA 90034
(800) 347-8998

Rational Recovery and Secular Organization for Sobriety

Rational Recovery (RR) and Secular Organization for Sobriety (SOS) are abstinence-oriented alternatives to 12-steps groups that do not emphasize spiritual principles or reliance on a higher power.

Rational Recovery
P.O. Box 800
Lotus, CA 95651
(916) 621-4374

Secular Organization for Sobriety
5521 Grosvenor Blvd.
Los Angeles, CA 90066
(310) 821-8430

Moderation Management

Moderation Management (MM) is a support group for problem drinkers who desire to drink within moderate limits (Kishline, 1994). MM is not intended for people with alcohol dependence or alcoholism.

Moderation Management
P.O. Box 6005
Ann Arbor, MI 48106
(734) 677-6007

CASE STUDY

Alan is a 21-year-old college junior who four weeks earlier underwent surgical repair of a knee injury after a skiing accident. He attends the sports medicine clinic two to three times a week for rehabilitation but sometimes misses his appointments without calling. He complains of severe pain and asks the athletic trainer to request more pain pills from the doctor on his behalf. His physical exam is inconsistent in that he complains strongly of pain with certain maneuvers but then is observed at a distance exercising the same motion without so much distress. At one midday appointment, there is an odor of alcohol on his breath. When asked if he's been drinking, he denies it. However, he seems upset and wants to talk about a recent breakup with his girlfriend.

QUESTIONS FOR ANALYSIS

1. How could you use a discussion about the athlete's girlfriend to uncover information about Alan's use of substances?

2. How would you determine whether Alan used alcohol inappropriately on just this one occasion because he was upset about his girlfriend (hazardous use) or whether he has recurrent problems from drinking (substance abuse)?

3. You choose to wait until the next appointment, when Alan does not smell of alcohol, to ask questions about his alcohol use. He now admits, with some

embarrassment, to having two drinks before coming in last time. In response to the F-Q-Max questions, he says he typically has six drinks a day on weekends and scores negative on the CAGE questions. How would you characterize his pattern of use (at-risk use, problem use, dependent use)? What would your counseling goals be? How would you determine what stage of change Alan was in?

4. Alan does not perceive that his drinking is a problem, nor does he see any need to reduce it within moderate drinking guidelines. He does say that his girlfriend thought he drank too much. He denies driving after drinking or immediately before his skiing accident. However, he did drink heavily on the night before his skiing accident. How might you use the FRAMES mnemonic to guide your counseling intervention?

5. How would you determine whether Alan is abusing or dependent on opioids?

SUMMARY

Knowledge of the clinical manifestations of substance abuse and dependence helps sports medicine professionals identify and assess athletes with substance-related problems. The core signs and symptoms of substance use disorders are impaired control, continued use despite adverse consequences, tolerance, and withdrawal. Abuse is defined as the continued use of a substance despite adverse consequences. Physical dependence refers to the presence of withdrawal symptoms and sometimes tolerance. Substance dependence is a more severe problem than abuse and is defined as impaired control and adverse consequences, with or without tolerance and withdrawal. Relatively simple screening tests for abuse and dependence are available to assist the sports medicine professional. When the screening tests are positive, further assessment is indicated. The physical and laboratory exams are done by the physician and may provide further information about the extent and severity of the problem. The physician also determines whether medical detoxification is needed. Finally, the athlete's concerns about, and perceptions of, the problem and the athlete's motivation to change are assessed.

The assessment guides the treatment goals and type of counseling to be provided. Abstinence from the problematic substance, as well as from other addictive substances, is usually the treatment goal of choice. However, athletes who drink too much alcohol (exceeding the 0-3-4-7-14 rule) without evidence of problems or athletes with only mild alcohol problems may appropriately be counseled with the goal of moderate use. When substance-related problems are mild to moderate and the athlete is motivated to change, the sports medicine team can proceed with brief intervention techniques. If problems are moderate to severe or if there is evidence of dependence, referral to specialized treatment is indicated. Motivational counseling, based on a stages-of-change model, can be employed by the sports medicine team when athletes are resistant either to changing their substance-using behavior or to seeing a specialist in addictions treatment.

Although a number of counseling techniques are presented, the FRAMES mnemonic reminds the sports medicine professional that effective interventions often include (1) providing nonjudgmental *feedback* from the assessment, (2) emphasizing the athlete's *responsibility* for any change to occur, (3) giving clear *advice* about the type of change that would be most helpful, (4) offering a *menu* of options for how treatment goals can be achieved, (5) conducting all the counseling with *empathy* for the athlete's situation and feelings, and (6) supporting the athlete's sense of *self-efficacy* that positive change can occur with appropriate treatment, efforts, and actions.

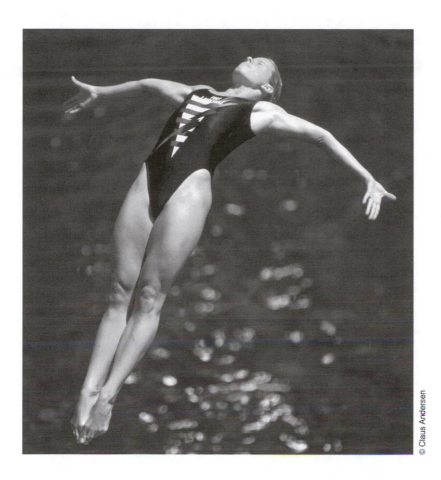

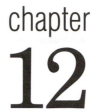

© Claus Andersen

Recognizing and Assisting Athletes With Eating Disorders

Trent A. Petrie, PhD, *University of North Texas*

Roberta Trattner Sherman, PhD, *Bloomington Hospital, Bloomington, Indiana*

CHAPTER OBJECTIVES

Describe the symptoms associated with the three major diagnostic categories of eating disorders: bulimia nervosa, anorexia nervosa, and eating disorders not otherwise specified (e.g., binge eating)

Identify the warning signs associated with disordered eating behaviors and attitudes

Understand the prevalence of eating disorders and related behaviors

Illustrate how eating disorders are multidimensional problems that require assistance on many levels, such as emotional, nutritional, and physical

Describe how variables such as sex, age, and sport environment may be risk factors

OPENING CASE STUDY

After competing as a diver for two years at a junior college in her community, 20-year-old Jill was offered a scholarship to attend a National Collegiate Athletic Association (NCAA) Division I university that was located in another state. The university coach had been very impressed with Jill's accomplishments at the junior college and hoped she would have an immediate and positive impact on the diving program. Although excited about the opportunity, Jill was unsettled about leaving her family and the community in which she had grown up and was inwardly unsure about her ability to compete at this level.

During the spring and summer before attending the university, Jill's father became ill and subsequently passed away. The stress and emotional strain of the illness coupled with the time required to attend to her family's needs left little time for Jill to train or focus on her diving. As a result, Jill was neither at her physical nor mental best when she left for school. During the summer she gained about eight pounds (four kilograms), and because she had been unable to dive for much of the summer, she began to have even more doubts about her ability to compete. She was not comfortable with her current weight and hoped that she would have time once she arrived at school to get back into shape before practices officially began.

Although her academic transition to the university was going smoothly, Jill was overwhelmed by the demands of a Division I training regimen. Only four weeks into the semester, she found herself quite lonely being away from home and family and with few friends in whom she could confide. Although she was working hard in practices, she had been unable to lose all the weight she wanted and was becoming increasingly self-conscious about how she looked in her swimming suit. In addition, she was unable to consistently perform her dives and regain the outward confidence she had in junior college. In an effort to be helpful, an assistant coach suggested that her performances and scores might improve if she could lose a little more weight and look a little leaner.

During the next two months, Jill made a concerted effort to lose weight to improve her diving. She maintained a very strict, low-calorie, low-fat diet and exercised in addition to scheduled workouts. Although she experienced initial success in following this regimen and losing weight, she found it increasingly difficult to eat so little every day. She began to binge-eat every few days in response to her physical hunger or to her feelings of loneliness and low self-esteem. As the tendency to alternate between fasting and bingeing increased, she became increasingly disgusted with herself and felt guilty about her inability to stick to her diet. In response, she began to exercise even more and at times made herself throw up after eating uncontrollably. By the end of her first semester in school, Jill felt depressed and out of control.

Unfortunately, Jill's experiences as described in the case study are not uncommon for college-aged women in the United States. Although only a small percentage develop diagnosable eating disorders such as anorexia nervosa or bulimia nervosa (American Psychiatric Association [APA], 1994), large numbers of women experience a broad range of disordered eating attitudes and behaviors, such as high levels of body dissatisfaction, excessive exercising to lose weight, binge eating, strict dieting, and purging (e.g., vomiting). For example, recent research has shown that over 60 percent of female undergraduates could be categorized as having one of these intermediate (i.e., subclinical) forms of disordered eating (Mintz & Betz, 1988). Although men do suffer from these problems too, women are approximately 10 times more likely to develop an eating disorder (APA, 1994).

Athletes are a subgroup who have been identified as at potentially increased risk for the development of eating disorders. Athletes experience many of the same general sociocultural pressures that place nonathlete women at risk for developing eating disorders (e.g., media emphasis on thinness and beauty). In addition, demands exist within the sport environment that may increase their risk, such as the following (Swoap & Murphy, 1995):

- Coaches' expectations concerning weight
- Participating in sports that have specific weight requirements, demand low percentage body fat for performance, or value thin body physiques
- Peer pressure to use pathogenic weight control techniques

The intense exercise, dietary restraint, and perfectionism common among high-performance athletes also may be risk factors for some in the development of eating disorders (e.g., Davis, Kennedy, Ravelski, & Dionne, 1994; Wilson & Eldredge, 1992). Reviews of eating disorder research with athletes have suggested prevalence rates of diagnosable and subclinical disorders comparable with, and in some cases greater than, those of nonathletes (e.g., Wilmore, 1991).

The purpose of this chapter is to provide a general introduction to the topic of eating disorders in athletes and to describe some of the factors that may place athletes at risk for such problems. In addition, models for prevention and remediation based within multiprofessional treatment teams are presented. Before beginning, however, we address the chapter's limitations. First, eating disorders are multidimensional problems and, as such, it is impossible to cover all related issues or adequately describe all avenues of treatment. Instead, this chapter provides an overview of the key social and psychological factors in the identification and treatment of athletes with eating disorders and directs the reader to other detailed sources when appropriate. Second, although eating disorders occur in both sexes, considerably more is known about these problems with respect to women's functioning and development. Thus the primary, though not sole, focus of the discussion is on female athletes and their experiences.

DESCRIPTION AND PREVALENCE OF EATING DISORDERS

In this section we present information regarding the diagnostic criteria of bulimia nervosa and anorexia nervosa and discuss the prevalence of these disorders, with a focus on findings from athlete populations. In addition, we introduce the concept of subclinical disorders and address how these problems may be more prevalent and equally problematic as the diagnosable eating disorders.

Clinical Eating Disorders

Eating disorders are psychiatric disorders that affect individuals' psychological, physical, nutritional, interpersonal, and emotional functioning and are characterized by dysfunctional eating patterns (e.g., food restriction) and disturbances or distortions about body size and shape. The *Diagnostic and Statistical Manual of Mental Disorders* (DSM-IV; APA, 1994) provides two specific diagnostic categories: anorexia nervosa (see table 12.1) and bulimia nervosa (see table 12.2).

In considering the introductory case example, it is clear that Jill is experiencing the symptoms associated with bulimia nervosa. She is binge-eating frequently and then engaging in compensatory behaviors (i.e., vomiting and excessive exercise) to prevent weight gain, and her self-worth is strongly influenced by her current body size and her perceptions about appearance. Her binge-eating behaviors seem to have been triggered by her initial strict dieting—a common sequence—and maintained by the continued food deprivation, social isolation, and negative self-evaluation. She feels out of control and is obviously in need of assistance.

Table 12.1   DSM-IV Criteria for Anorexia Nervosa

A. Refusal to maintain body weight at or above a minimally normal weight for age and height (e.g., at least 85% of expected body weight).

B. Intense fear of gaining weight or becoming fat, even though underweight.

C. Disturbance in the way in which one's body weight or shape is experienced, undue influence of body weight or shape on self-evaluation, or denial of the seriousness of the current low body weight.

D. In postmenarcheal females, amenorrhea, i.e., the absence of at least three consecutive menstrual cycles. (A woman is considered to have amenorrhea if her periods occur only following hormone, e.g., estrogen administration.)

Specify: Restricting type (during the current episode of anorexia nervosa, the person has not regularly engaged in binge eating or purging behavior) or binge eating/purging type (during the current episode of anorexia nervosa, the person has regularly engaged in binge eating or purging behavior).

Reprinted from APA (1994). *Diagnostic and statistical manual of mental disorders* (4th ed., pp. 544-545). Washington, DC: Author.

Table 12.2   DSM-IV Criteria for Bulimia Nervosa

A. Recurrent episodes of binge eating. An episode of binge eating is characterized by both of the following:

   (i)   eating, in a discrete period of time (e.g., within any two-hour period), an amount of food that is definitely larger than most people would eat during a similar period of time and under similar circumstances, and

   (ii) a sense of lack of control over eating during the episode (e.g., a feeling that one cannot stop eating or control what or how much one is eating).

B. Recurrent inappropriate compensatory behavior in order to prevent weight gain, such as self-induced vomiting; misuse of laxatives, diuretics, enemas, or other medications; fasting; or excessive exercise.

C. The binge eating and inappropriate compensatory behaviors both occur, on average, at least twice a week for three months.

D. Self-evaluation is unduly influenced by body shape and weight.

E. The disturbance does not occur exclusively during episodes of anorexia nervosa.

Specify: Purging type (during the current episode of bulimia nervosa, the person has regularly engaged in self-induced vomiting or the misuse of laxatives, diuretics, or enemas) or nonpurging type (during the current episode of bulimia nervosa, the person has used other inappropriate compensatory behaviors, such as fasting or excessive exercise, but has not regularly engaged in self-induced vomiting or the misuse of laxatives, diuretics, or enemas).

Reprinted from APA (1994). *Diagnostic and statistical manual of mental disorders* (4th ed., pp. 549-550). Washington, DC: Author.

In general, approximately 0.5 to 1.0 percent of adolescent women and 1.0 to 3.0 percent of young adult women suffer from anorexia nervosa or bulimia nervosa; rates for men are one tenth or less of those for women (APA, 1994). For athletes, however, the picture is less clear. Unfortunately few prevalence studies have been conducted, and conflicting findings have emerged from those that have been conducted. In a survey of all NCAA member institutions (Dick, 1991), over 60 percent of the respondents reported having had at least one athlete with either bulimia nervosa or anorexia nervosa in the last two years. Of these reported incidents, 93 percent were from women's sports, particularly gymnastics, cross-country, swimming, and track (running events only). For men, incidents of eating disorders were found primarily in wrestling, cross-country, gymnastics, and track (running events only). Although eating disorders were most prevalent in these sports, they did occur across most other sports as well (Dick, 1991). More recent research has shown that female elite athletes in the United States and Europe suffer from diagnosable eating disorders at rates of less than 8 percent for bulimia and 1.5 percent for anorexia (Petrie & Stoever, 1993; Sundgot-Borgen, 1994).

Regardless of the frequency of these disorders, it is important to recognize the concomitant psychological, physiological, and physical costs. Individuals with these eating disorders often report body dissatisfaction, depression, low self-esteem, concerns about weight and appearance, lack of assertiveness, obsessive-compulsive tendencies, perfectionism, dietary restraint, anxiety, and lack of perceived control. Further, disruptions of physiological and physical functioning are common, including electrolyte imbalances and mineral deficiencies, reductions in metabolic rate, increased food efficiency, amenorrhea (in women), decreases in serum testosterone (in men), dehydration, loss of dental enamel, and cardiac arrhythmias.

Until well-controlled, epidemiological research is conducted, the exact prevalence of eating disorders in athletes will be unknown. Even so, it is clear that male and female athletes do suffer from clinical eating disorders and do so at rates that are at least comparable to, if not greater than, nonathletes. In addition, eating disorders appear to occur most frequently in sports that emphasize an aesthetic component (e.g., diving, gymnastics), have weight requirements (e.g., wrestling), or stress endurance (e.g., cross-country). Finally, it is important to remember that these disorders have psychological, emotional, and physical costs that are not obvious from simple prevalence rates.

Subclinical Eating Disorders

The DSM-IV (APA, 1994) provides a system for diagnosing anorexia or bulimia nervosa, yet many individuals who have disordered eating problems do not meet diagnostic criteria for these disorders because their symptoms are not sufficient in number or frequency. In fact, many more athletes experience **subclinical eating problems** than the actual clinical disorders. For example, in a sample of female collegiate gymnasts, over 60 percent were classified as having a subclinical eating problem, such as binge eating or excessive exercising, while fewer than 5 percent were viewed as at risk for bulimia (Petrie, 1993; Petrie & Stoever, 1993).

Fortunately, research concerning the prevalence of subclinical eating disorders has been substantial, and there appears to be more consistency across findings than has been reported in studies on bulimia and anorexia. Although the exact frequencies vary, substantial numbers of adolescent and collegiate female athletes use **pathogenic weight control behaviors**, though the tendency is to rely on excessive exercise and dieting or fasting more than on vomiting, laxatives, and diuretics. For example, Petrie and Stoever (1993) found that over 50 percent of their sample of female collegiate gymnasts exercised at least two hours per day specifically to burn calories, while 7.8 percent, 4.2 percent, and 3.3 percent reported using vomiting, laxatives, or diuretics, respectively, to control weight. In another sample of female gymnasts, Rosen and Hough (1988) reported that all athletes were dieting, but only 26 percent, 12 percent, and 7 percent were using vomiting, diuretics, or laxatives, respectively, to control their weight. Athletes also binge-eat, though the prevalence of those doing so at least twice a week may be less than 20 percent (Rosen, McKeag,

subclinical eating problems— Problems associated with eating that do not meet DSM-IV diagnostic criteria for bulimia nervosa or anorexia nervosa but that are severe in their own right and can be the focus of psychological treatment. Such problems may include excessive dieting or fasting, extreme body dissatisfaction or disparagement, binge eating, compulsive exercising, and purging (i.e., using vomiting, laxatives, diuretics) to lose weight.

pathogenic weight control behaviors— Those approaches to weight control, including excessive exercise, excessive dieting, fasting, vomiting, or laxative and diuretic use, that are associated with the development of clinical eating disorders.

Hough, & Curley, 1986). As in the case of women, excessive exercising and dieting appear to be the two most common subclinical behaviors for men (Black & Burckes-Miller, 1988). This lower level of binge eating and focus on exercise is consistent with the idea that sociocultural beauty ideals have shifted from anorexic thinness toward a form characterized by strength, health, and fitness.

In addition to these more general forms of subclinical eating disorders, a disorder specific to the athletic experience has been suggested. Anorexia athletica (Sundgot-Borgen, 1993) is characterized by weight loss, which is brought about by severe restrictions in dietary intake, and intense fears associated with gaining weight and becoming fat. The athlete with this disorder also may demonstrate features such as menstrual irregularities and binge eating (see table 12.3 for a complete list of the criteria). Recent research has suggested that approximately 8 percent of elite female athletes may suffer from this disorder (Sundgot-Borgen, 1994).

It is important to realize that these subclinical eating disorders are serious in themselves. Pathogenic weight control methods (e.g., vomiting, laxatives), excessive exercising, binge eating, and dieting or fasting are associated with many of the same psychological, physiological, and physical disturbances found with clinically diagnosable eating disorders. Thus an athlete does not have to be suffering from a clinical disorder to experience significant psychological and physical distress and need treatment. Finally, it is important to note that restrictive dieting or fasting can be associated with the development of binge eating, and excessive physical activity or exercise has been related to eating disorders (e.g., Davis et al., 1994). Although controlled longitudinal studies have not been conducted to confirm these associations, nondiagnosable eating problems such as these may serve as precursors to the development of bulimia or anorexia for some individuals.

EATING DISORDER WARNING SIGNS

Although many of the symptoms associated with eating disorders, such as extreme weight loss or binge eating in the presence of friends and family, may be noticeable, many others are not as obvious or may be hidden by the athlete. For example, vari-

---

Table 12.3 Criteria for Anorexia Athletica

1. Weight loss (> 5% of expected body weight)   +
2. Delayed puberty (no menstrual bleeding at age 16, primary amenorrhea)   [+]
3. Menstrual dysfunction (primary or secondary amenorrhea or oligomenorrhea)   [+]
4. Gastrointestinal complaints   +
5. Absence of medical illness or affective disorder explaining weight reduction   +
6. Disturbance in body image (as defined in DSM-IV)   [+]
7. Excessive fear of becoming obese   +
8. Restriction of caloric intake (e.g., < 1200 calories)   +
9. Use of purging methods (vomiting, laxatives, diuretics)   [+]
10. Binge eating (as defined in DSM-IV)   [+]
11. Compulsive exercising (as defined in DSM-IV)   [+]

+ = criteria that are necessary for diagnosis;
[+] = at least one of these criteria is necessary for diagnosis.

ous purging behaviors (e.g., vomiting) are likely done in private to avoid detection. Still other behaviors, such as exercising and fasting or dieting, may go undetected because within the sport environment they are seen as "normal" or rewarded as a sign of the athlete's dedication. Given that many of the eating disorder diagnostic criteria are not easily seen, it is important to pay attention to other signs or behaviors that may indicate either a clinical or subclinical problem. Table 12.4 lists several important characteristics to consider.

In considering these warning signs, you should not automatically assume that the presence of one is indicative of an eating disorder. It is important, however, not to ignore the existence of any signs because early identification is important. If sports medicine professionals have concerns about athletes who are evidencing one or more of these signs, they should talk with a professional (e.g., psychologist) who is trained in the treatment of eating disorders. Although general suggestions for assisting athletes with eating disorders are offered in this chapter, discussing specific cases with professionals in your own community will generally be the best course of action. This approach allows sports medicine professionals to individualize their assessment and treatment of athletes within their own sport environments.

WHY ARE ATHLETES AT RISK?

The development of eating disorders is caused by many factors, including family influences, physiological functioning (e.g., levels of brain neurotransmitters), personality, psychological functioning, and environmental or social factors. Although all have received attention and are important for understanding eating disorders, social or environmental factors may be most relevant to a discussion of eating disorders in athletes. In general, women are subjected to societal pressures, often in the form of media messages, to behave in certain ways (e.g., diet) and to achieve a certain body shape and look (e.g., physically fit, firm). Men, too, appear to be exposed to societal pressures about how they should look and behave, though the media messages are centered more around issues of gaining health and becoming physically fit than losing weight or achieving some beauty ideal (Petrie et al., 1996). Tragically, these daily

---

Table 12.4   Warning Signs and Behaviors Associated With Eating Disorders

1. Excessive concern with or self-deprecating comments about body size and shape

2. Noticeable fluctuations (gain or loss) in weight

3. Changes in "normal" (for that person) eating behaviors: eating less, becoming preoccupied with food (e.g., avoiding sugars or red meats) and caloric content, fasting for extended periods of time (e.g., one or more days), eating more or binge-eating, eating secretively, not eating with teammates during planned meals, stealing food

4. Excessive exercising (e.g., running after practices when not required)

5. Depressed mood, low self-esteem, or both

6. Use of diet pills, laxatives, diuretics, or syrup of ipecac

7. Going to the bathroom frequently after meals

8. Fear about gaining weight or becoming fat even when weight is normal or below normal

9. Bloodshot eyes, smell of vomitus, nicks or cuts on knuckles or fingers after visiting bathroom

messages about how one should look often run counter to what is physically and physiologically possible, particularly for women. Indeed, media messages about body size and shape are quite discrepant from women's normal sizes, presenting an "ideal" that is thinner and has smaller hips than typical. While the differences in women's real and ideal body sizes and shapes have increased, so have the number of messages women receive to exercise and diet to achieve this ideal. Women are constantly being told to achieve a body size that most cannot achieve and are being encouraged to do so through restrictive diets and excessive exercise. It is no wonder that so many women report being dissatisfied with their bodies and use various pathogenic weight control measures.

Female and male athletes are not immune to these general societal pressures. In fact, the sport environment may present additional pressures that contribute to the development of disordered eating for some athletes. Swoap and Murphy (1995) suggested that several factors encourage a potentially unhealthy focus on weight and body shape, including weight restrictions, judging criteria that emphasize thin and stereotypically attractive body builds, performance demands that encourage very low percentage body fat, coaches applying pressure to lose weight, and peer pressure to try pathogenic weight loss techniques. Indeed, this focus on weight is often associated with dietary restraint and increased exercise. When such conditions exist, Wilson and Eldredge (1992) suggest one of two outcomes: (1) the development of eating disorders, which occurs when other **psychopathology** is present, or (2) normative dieting and discontent and/or abnormal weight control behaviors, which occur in the absence of predisposing psychopathology. These two outcomes are what we have labeled clinical and subclinical eating disorders.

Although all athletes experience competitive pressures and have performance demands, differences exist in the extent to which the factors proposed by Swoap and Murphy (1995) are present. For example, athletes who compete in sports that require a certain weight (e.g., wrestling) or in which appearance or body shape plays a role in determining outcome (e.g., gymnastics or diving) may be more likely to experience such pressures than those who compete in sports with no set weight requirements or in which body shape is less central in determining success (e.g., basketball or soccer). Indeed, recent research has suggested that female athletes in such "lean sports" are more concerned with dieting, preoccupied with their weight, and driven to reach a thin ideal than female athletes from nonlean sports (e.g., Davis & Cowles, 1989; Petrie, 1996). This finding also has been demonstrated with male athletes (Enns, Drewnowski, & Grinker, 1987), though not consistently across studies (Petrie, 1996).

General societal pressures as well as those specific to sport interact to increase some athletes' use of exercise and strict dieting or fasting to control their weight. These sociocultural pressures are important, but not sufficient, conditions to explain the development of eating disorders. The presence of other predisposing factors—such as unstable family environments, life stress, perfectionism and obsessive-compulsive tendencies, and depression—in combination with these sociocultural pressures increases the likelihood of athletes developing clinical disorders. Without such predisposing factors, athletes may experience only dietary discontent or the varied use of pathogenic weight control behaviors. Research suggests that athletes who participate in lean-sport environments, in which the social pressures previously outlined are most prevalent, are more likely to focus on their weight and dieting than athletes from nonlean sports.

psychopathology—Ways of thinking, feeling, or behaving that are maladaptive, interfering, or disturbing to a person or those around him or her.

PROVIDING ASSISTANCE

As mentioned previously, eating disorders are multidimensional problems that affect an individual's physical, psychological, interpersonal, and emotional well-being.

Eating disorders, even for nonathletes, require a variety of professionals to provide assistance, including psychologists, physicians, physical therapists, and dietitians. In working with athletes, sports medicine professionals and coaches become an integral part of the sport management team (Thompson, 1987). In this section we discuss the roles that each of these professionals can play in providing assistance to the athlete with an eating disorder.

The sport management team plays two quite different roles, depending on whether the focus is on **preventive interventions** or **remedial interventions**. In this section both approaches are discussed. First, primary issues involved in prevention are considered, then the roles of the sport management team members in remediation are described.

Prevention

Special approaches are needed to prevent eating disorders in athletes due to the unique needs, issues, pressures, and problems within the sport environment. Because athletic performance is a primary concern in the world of sport, it is easy to become focused on factors that are believed to enhance performance. In many sports, athletes, coaches, and other sport personnel believe that lowering body fat composition and body weight will result in enhanced athletic performance. Although there is some evidence for this relationship (Wilmore & Costill, 1987), other researchers have not found support for this purported connection (e.g., Sherman, Thompson, & Rose, 1996). Yet the relationship between decreased body fat and increased performance has often been viewed as an indisputable fact among many in the athletic community. Consequently, when an athlete is not performing well, it is common for weight loss or a decrease in body fat to be the suggested solution. In response, athletes all too often severely restrict their caloric intake, which may result in the development of the more serious eating disturbances that we have discussed previously. The strong relationship that exists between dieting and the development of eating disorders means that issues regarding weight and dieting are going to be particularly important in any prevention program.

Efforts at prevention must make health the primary focus. Although athletic performance is important, an individual's health should not be compromised to enhance performance. The sport world had a similar ethical dilemma several years ago when steroids were being used by some athletes and condoned by their coaches. Steroids make athletes bigger, stronger, faster, and more aggressive—characteristics associated with superior performance in many sports. However, the dangers of steroid use are so alarming that sport governing bodies began drug testing to ensure that athletes do not use these drugs (American College of Sports Medicine, 1987). Perhaps a similarly strong statement needs to be made regarding dieting and the dangers it can cause for athletes when performance is placed above potential health risks.

It is important that communication among members of the sport management team remains open and that the message given to athletes by all involved is consistent. A way to facilitate this process is to have one member of the sport management team serve as its primary coordinator. Because the athletic trainer usually has easiest access to other sport management team members and often knows the athletes best, the athletic trainer is often in the best position to serve as primary coordinator in preventive interventions. Although the functions of the sport management team overlap somewhat, each professional has certain primary roles in the area of prevention. We discuss these next and describe the ways in which the athletic trainer can facilitate communication and coordinate activities.

Athletic Trainer

The athletic trainer often knows the athlete better than any other individual within the sport environment. In addition, athletes often are more comfortable talking with

preventive interventions— Interventions whose goal is to avoid the onset of eating problems through education or early identification.

remedial interventions— Interventions in which the focus is relief from or dissipation of eating disorder symptoms that already are present.

athletic trainers about their problems than they are with their coaches. In fact, the athletic trainer may be in the best position to notice when an athlete is experiencing any physical or psychological problems (e.g., stress, depression). Thus the athletic trainer is in a unique and valuable position regarding the athlete's well-being and likely is able to determine whether the athlete's needs and concerns are being addressed by any prevention program.

For the most part, athletic trainers follow the athlete's physical condition on a regular basis. In so doing, the athletic trainer is more concerned about the athlete's health than his or her performance. Therefore any concerns expressed by the athletic trainer regarding weight are more likely to be seen as a health issue than a performance issue. Part of monitoring an athlete's health means obtaining a baseline of certain physical attributes at the beginning of a season and following them throughout the year to determine whether any problems arise. This monitoring can include the occasional weighing of an athlete, such as at the beginning of the season and when there is a concern about the athlete's health that might be reflected in his or her weight (e.g., dehydration after intense summertime workouts). However, weighing just for its own sake is not recommended. There should be a legitimate health concern, and the athlete should be informed of the purpose of the weighing. Athletes often become anxious when no one tells them why they are being weighed and what is to be done with the results. If this information will not directly benefit the athlete or be helpful in monitoring the athlete's health, then weighing should be avoided as a means of preventing future eating problems.

When weighing is necessary or has been determined to be beneficial, the athletic trainer is an appropriate person for that task. Any weighing, even if only once a year, should be handled in a sensitive manner. To assist athletic trainers in sensitively weighing athletes, the following guidelines are offered. First, privately ask the athlete whether he or she minds being weighed. The weighing itself also should be done privately. Remember that athletes who are most at risk for developing an eating disorder are also likely to be highly sensitive about their bodies and weight. Some athletes prefer not to know their weight, and in many cases this is not an unreasonable request. Any athlete who does not want to know his or her own weight is a person who realizes that this knowledge might lead to an unhealthy focus. In fact, difficulty with knowing one's weight can be indicative of an eating problem, and the trainer should be alert to other warning signs or behaviors. If the athlete's weight is within healthy limits, it is reasonable to comply with his or her request. If weighing is necessary, the athlete can simply be weighed "blind," that is, turned away from the scale readout. Remember that sensitive handling of weighing can be instrumental in preventing the onset of an eating disorder in an athlete predisposed to develop one.

If an athlete refuses to participate in a necessary weigh-in, it is important not to make a big deal about it at that moment or get into a power struggle with the athlete. Instead, find a few private moments when you can talk to the athlete about his or her refusal to participate. It may simply be that the athlete does not want to be part of a group weigh-in and would be happy to oblige if the weigh-in can be done privately. On the other hand, it may be that the athlete's refusal reflects more serious weight- or control-related problems. If the latter is suspected, as a member of the sport management team, the athletic trainer may want to consult with the sports physician and sport psychologist to determine the best way to intervene, given this athlete's personality and the demands of the sport environment.

Coach

The coach probably has more influence with the athlete than anyone else. Everything a coach says and does can have a tremendous impact on the athlete. Coaches therefore need to be accurately informed about nutrition, body composition, and performance. Otherwise, they are likely to contribute to the many myths about body composition and weight that exist in our culture in general and in the sport environment in particular. Athletic trainers can facilitate this education by providing the coach with reading materials or by talking with the coach about these issues and how they apply to the athletes under their care.

It is especially important for coaches to de-emphasize weight or, at the very least, not emphasize it. In some athletic programs, coaches are now completely removed from issues regarding weight. Some universities bar coaches from weighing athletes, from setting requirements regarding an athlete's weight, and in some cases from even being informed about the athlete's weight. This is a positive step and one that will allow the coach to focus on other aspects of the athlete's development. Again, weight should be considered only as a health concern and should be handled by the sports medicine professional, not the coaching staff. If, however, a coach forces the issue and requires team weigh-ins or takes body fat measurements him- or herself (e.g., by using calipers), members of the sport management team should intervene. Initially, members might talk with the coach about the potential problems with his or her behavior and help to educate the coach about more effective ways to work with athletes to help them achieve their best performances. If the coach is still undeterred, assistance from supportive upper-level athletic department administrators may be needed to stop the behavior.

If athletes are not performing as well as coaches think they should, it is too easy for coaches to assume that weight or fat loss would enhance performance. Athletes generally have control over their effort but may have far less control over their weight due to their genetic makeup. Unfortunately, some coaches do not understand this fact and assume that weight "problems" are the result of a lack of willpower. Coaches and athletes need to understand that rather than highlighting weight, it is more helpful to focus on physical conditioning, skill attainment, and strength development and to emphasize effort over outcome. Coaches also can focus on emotional and mental components, where considerable potential for enhanced performance exists. Mental attitude is now recognized by most to be a key element in an athlete's success. By stressing mental attitude, the coach in essence focuses on the athlete as a complete person rather than simply a physical body.

Many athletes are reticent about sharing their concerns with their coaches for fear of upsetting them. Apprehension about upsetting a coach comes about for various reasons, including a need to please others, fear of being seen as a failure or source of disappointment, and loss of playing time. If athletes have eating, weight, or emotional concerns and are worried about upsetting their coach, the athletic trainer can serve as the intermediary. Athletic trainers can give good advice to athletes about how to talk with their coach and at times may even help arrange and facilitate meetings between coach and athlete. Assistance in establishing open communication and discussion of minor concerns can be essential for preventing the development of more serious problems. In offering this recommendation, we are not suggesting that the athletic trainer take responsibility for adult athletes and talk with the coach for them. Instead, the trainer should act as a consultant for the athlete, offering advice and guidance on how the athlete can talk with the coach. In those instances where the athlete is a minor, then the athletic trainer may take a more active role in speaking with the coach and parents about whatever concerns exist.

Dietitian

Many athletic programs now use the services of a registered dietitian, and this is an encouraging trend. The athletic trainer can be instrumental in establishing contact with a dietitian and in facilitating his or her involvement with the team. The athletic trainer is often in the best position to discuss with coaches the benefits of using a dietitian and help them understand the importance of the information a dietitian can provide and how this information ultimately relates to improved performance.

Many coaches may be reluctant to devote time or financial resources to a dietitian if the benefits of such work are not clearly outlined.

On some teams a dietitian meets with team members to provide information regarding the nutrients they need to perform their best. Dietitians also may inform team members about the relationship between good health and good nutrition and alert them to the hazards of dieting. This approach focuses more on the nutritional needs of athletes than on the foods they should avoid. Food is viewed as a part of a healthy lifestyle rather than as an enemy to be avoided. In some programs dietitians are available to work with athletes on an individual basis and are instrumental in helping the athlete put together an individualized meal plan. Surprisingly, many athletes do not know what they need to eat to be healthy. An individualized meal plan can be extremely helpful for those who do not know where to begin. There are so many myths and untruths about food and nutrition that it is not unusual for even a seasoned athlete to be confused about what a healthy eating regimen should look like (see Stanton, 1994, and Wilmore & Costill, 1992, for additional information on nutrition and performance).

In addition to setting up meal plans, the dietitian is qualified to help determine an ideal weight range for an athlete. Notice that we say *weight range* rather than *ideal weight*. It is normal for an individual's weight to fluctuate somewhat. Setting a single ideal weight is too rigid and unrealistic. Actually, it is more important to set an exercise regimen and a healthy meal plan for each individual than to focus on weight at all. If athletes follow the plan, then the weight at which their bodies naturally level out is the weight at which their bodies will probably work best. It only makes sense that an adequately nourished body performs better than one that is not. The dietitian also is an appropriate professional to weigh an athlete if weighing needs to be done and the trainer is not available. The same previously discussed guidelines for the athletic trainer regarding sensitive weighing also apply to the dietitian.

Psychologist

In some athletic programs sport psychologists are actively involved with the athletes or at least are available for consultation. The psychologist has an important role in prevention by helping assess the mood of the athletes, the emotional climate of the team, and the general atmosphere within which the athlete must practice and compete. Athletes learn from one another. If one athlete begins a diet, others may follow. Athletes are competitive, and that competitiveness is often helpful to them in sport. However, if a competitive environment regarding weight exists on a team, an astute psychologist can intervene and help change the environment to avoid a "contagion" effect, that is, a spreading of eating disturbances from one athlete to another.

Psychologists are also more likely to be cognizant of the individual differences that exist within a group of athletes. Those differences may be physiological in nature, such as weight, yet there also are psychological or emotional differences that may predispose an athlete to an eating problem. By attending to an athlete's uniqueness, the psychologist can ensure that inappropriate or unrealistic expectations for the individual, whether these relate to weight, weight loss, sport performance, or any other aspect of the person that might be of interest, are minimized. Additionally, if a psychologist is alerted to individual mood or esteem problems early on, these might be resolved through counseling before the athlete needs to resort to more serious outlets, including the development of an eating problem.

The psychologist often has to rely on the other sports medicine professionals to serve as the eyes and ears within the sport environment or for an individual athlete. For example, if the sports medicine professional notices that an athlete has been "down" and has had difficulty concentrating for several days, he or she might share that observation with the psychologist, who can then talk with the athlete.

Given the strong bond that generally exists between sports medicine professionals and athletes, sports medicine professionals also can serve as a safe link between the athlete and psychologist. For example, a familiar and friendly face is often helpful to athletes when they attend their first counseling session. For this reason, sports medicine professionals might offer to initially accompany their athletes.

Sports Physician

Typically, every athlete is examined by a physician at least once in a season. Physicians who are attuned to the early signs of an eating problem can be instrumental in getting an athlete assistance before a full clinical disorder develops. Within the context of a general physical exam, it is certainly appropriate for the physician to ask about the athlete's appetite, eating patterns, sleep patterns, and general emotional well-being. This communicates to the athletes that eating is a part of good health and that the physician is concerned about all aspects of the individual.

The menstrual functioning of all female athletes is extremely important for the physician to inquire about and to monitor. Amenorrhea can lead to skeletal system injuries and should not be an accepted part of being an athlete. Because amenorrhea is a common symptom of eating disorders, it is imperative that physicians be aware of their female athletes' menstrual status. If physicians do not have regular contact with an athlete, athletic trainers can assume this role and consult with the team physician if a problem is noted.

Physical Therapist

In some instances, particularly those involving injury and physical rehabilitation, physical therapists have ongoing contact with athletes or sport teams. The physical therapist can perform many of the same functions an athletic trainer might, including monitoring the athlete's physical and psychological health, maintaining contact with the team's sport psychologist concerning the athlete, making sensitive referrals to other sport management team members when necessary, and conducting weighings when indicated for reasons of health. The guidelines concerning weighings outlined previously for athletic trainers apply to physical therapists as well.

Because physical therapists are likely to work with athletes in the select situation of injury rehabilitation, it is important to be aware of the psychological reactions athletes may experience when injured and how these reactions relate to eating disorders. Although not all athletes respond in this manner, it is not uncommon for those who are injured to be angry, confused, anxious, or depressed. Such reactions, if not addressed in a proactive and supportive manner, may precipitate the development of eating problems or even clinical eating disorders. For many athletes, particularly female athletes, participation in athletics serves as a primary mechanism through which weight and body shape are regulated. When injured and unable to maintain the same level of physical involvement and fitness, athletes may gain weight or feel anxious about perceived weight gain or changes in body composition (e.g., losing muscular definition). In addition, if athletes feel angry or depressed in response to their injuries, they may binge-eat as a means of coping. Thus, it becomes important for the physical therapist to be attuned to any changes in athletes' eating-related behaviors or attitudes toward their bodies. Such changes may indicate clinical or subclinical eating problems that may best be addressed by an eating disorder specialist.

Prevention Summary

The sport management team serves several critical functions in the prevention of eating disorders in athletes. First, through his or her relationship with the coach, the athletic trainer in particular is in an excellent position to make sure that time is made during practices for meetings with dietitians, psychologists, or physicians. Each member of the sport management team has valuable information to offer the athletes and coaching staff, yet time and access must be established for that to occur. In addition to the information provided by sport management team members, published materials are available that may be useful. For example, the NCAA (1989) has produced a set of videos and accompanying educational materials on eating disorders in sport. Remember, education is a key to any prevention program. Second, because athletic trainers are likely to have the most contact with the athletes, they are in a key position to monitor the athletes' functioning and notice many of the warning signs and behaviors of eating disorders. When such problems are noted, other professionals within the sport management team can be informed. Early identification of minor concerns is another key component of prevention. Finally, the athletic trainer generally knows the athlete better than most other members of the sport management team and is likely to be the one approached by the athlete when minor concerns arise. In this position the trainer can help the athlete access whatever services or people are needed, be it talking with the coach, meeting with the dietitian, or setting up an appointment with the psychologist or sports physician.

These suggestions and comments about eating disorders are not confined to sports medicine professionals who work with college-aged or older athletes. Eating disorders and concerns are present in grade school and adolescent athletes as well. In fact, many of the ideas about weight and performance may develop during early athletic experiences. Thus it becomes crucial for sports medicine professionals who work with young athletes to educate them about proper nutrition, weight, eating disorders, and performance. Early education about these issues may play a central role in reducing the later development of more severe eating problems.

Remedial Interventions

Once a member of the sport management team suspects that an athlete has an eating problem (e.g., exhibits several warning signs or behaviors), it is appropriate for that athlete to be evaluated by an eating disorder specialist to determine the extent of the problem and the need for treatment. However, approaching such an athlete to make a referral for an evaluation is, at best, difficult. The difficulty resides in the fact that most anorexic individuals are not able to see that they have a problem and simply deny its existence. Similarly, athletes with bulimia are likely to feel embarrassed and therefore deny their eating problem, in part out of fear of rejection or disapproval by others. In addition, athletes may fear that treatment will mean weight gain, which they believe will lead to negative consequences, not the least of which is decreased sport performance. Many athletes also fear that identification of the disorder will affect their playing time or their status or place on a team. Thus, approaching an athlete requires great care and sensitivity.

A thorough discussion of how to approach the athlete has been described elsewhere (Thompson & Sherman, 1993) as well as in chapter 8 and will not be recounted here. Suffice it to say that the best person to approach the athlete suspected of having an eating disorder is the individual who has the best rapport with the athlete. If no one on the sport management team feels especially close to the athlete, the individual who feels most comfortable talking about emotional problems and has a comfortable interpersonal style is usually the best choice. In some instances the athlete may be most comfortable talking with someone of the same sex. For example, female athletes may feel less threatened or embarrassed if they are approached by a female member of the sport management team. Although such preferences should be taken into account whenever possible, don't allow them to forestall talking to the athlete.

As previously mentioned, the athlete should be approached as soon as a problem has been identified because problems are always easier to treat when they are identified at an early stage. Regardless of who talks with the athlete, the best approach is to express concern for the athlete's physical and psychological well-being. Affected athletes need to know that their health and happiness are of foremost concern and that sport management team members are not there to criticize or embarrass them. Given that many, if not most, individuals with eating disorders have low self-esteem, it is easy for them to feel that they are being criticized. Thus, again, care and sensitivity are of paramount importance in approaching the individual. Even though the athlete's eating symptoms are important, it is recommended that eating behaviors not be the primary focus of this initial discussion. Rather, the eating symptoms are a concern only because they might reflect problems with the athlete's physical and psychological health.

If an athlete is evaluated and ascertained to have an eating disorder, the actual treatment of the problem should be provided by an eating disorder specialist (e.g., psychologist). The sport management team, however, will still be involved in the athlete's life, and therefore all members of the team need to recognize the roles they can play in helping the athlete recover.

Athletic Trainer

Athletic trainers are instrumental in the rehabilitation and reconditioning of an athlete's injury. Although eating disorders are not usually as easy to identify as a broken bone, they nevertheless affect the athlete's life in many similar ways. Athletic trainers therefore serve many of the same functions when caring for an athlete with an eating disorder as they do for an athlete with a physical injury.

One of the most difficult decisions to make is whether or not the affected athlete should continue training or competing while symptomatic. The athletic trainer is often the one who is best able to understand the physical and health concerns of the athlete, but who also understands the athlete's desire to remain a part of his or her sport and a part of the team. If the eating disorder specialist believes that training and competition are injurious to the athlete's health, the athletic trainer can help serve as a link for the athlete to the sport world as the athlete progresses in treatment. The athletic trainer can help the athlete feel part of the team by having regular contact with the athlete and by helping arrange for the athlete to participate in team meetings and other activities not directly involving training or competition.

If training and competition do not compromise the athlete's health and do not interfere with treatment, some athletes can remain involved with their sport; it should be the athlete's choice. If there is a conflict between attending treatment and attending practice, however, treatment must always come first. The athletic trainer can be an advocate and help ensure that an athlete who misses practice for treatment is not admonished or punished in any way.

Some athletes want to continue training because their sport is a part of their identity and a source of self-esteem. Other athletes may feel burned out or overwhelmed or just need a reason to take a break from a part of their life—feelings they may have been afraid to mention to others previously. These athletes find their eating problem a convenient opportunity to leave a sport with a "legitimate excuse." If the athlete chooses to continue with training and competition, the athletic trainer must closely monitor the athlete's physical and psychological response to training. An alert athletic trainer is usually the first to notice how an athlete is responding to training because it is the athletic trainer who is actually there with the athlete during training. Physicians and psychologists usually have to rely on self-reports, and individuals with eating disorders are often not the best or most objective observers of their own behavior. The firsthand reports from an alert athletic trainer are an invaluable contribution to the entire sport management team. It is extremely important that communication among team members remain open and that all are consistent in their focus on health as the primary concern and objective.

In some instances, athletes with an eating disorder may consider discontinuing participation in sport altogether. If such a decision is being considered, the athletic trainer might act as an initial sounding board for athletes as they talk through their options. In the end, though, we recommend that the athletic trainer facilitate a referral to a sport psychologist so that the athlete has someone outside the immediate sport environment with whom to talk. Having an objective and neutral professional, whose emphasis is the health and happiness of the athlete, can be crucial for the athlete when making such an important life decision. Coaches and athletic departments may have a difficult time remaining unbiased because they often have strong investments in the individual remaining an athlete. In addition, taking the time to talk with the sport psychologist will ensure that any decision is not made impulsively. Although terminating sport participation may be the healthiest resolution for many athletes, others may experience severe emotional distress as a result of such a decision. Thus it is important for the athlete to have considerable support as he or she makes the decision about future involvement in sport.

When appropriate and requested by the eating disorder specialist, the athletic trainer is in the best position to actually monitor some of the athlete's eating. As the athlete returns to competition and participates in training tables or eats with the team on road trips, the athletic trainer is able to see how well the athlete is responding to the meal plan set by the dietitian. Likewise, the athletic trainer is often the best person to monitor the athlete's weight when such information is needed.

Coach

Because the coach is one of the most influential people in the athlete's life, the manner in which the coach responds to the athlete's need for referral, treatment, and aftercare is of utmost importance. If the coach does not support treatment, it probably will not happen. Supportive coaches need to communicate their concern for the athlete's well-being by prohibiting training until the athlete complies at least with an evaluation and follows up with treatment, if recommended. This stance conveys to the athlete that his or her physical and psychological well-being and treatment are the first priority. Sports medicine professionals may be in a position to convince a reluctant coach that athletes perform better once they are healthier and happier. As treatment progresses, the coach can contact the eating disorder specialist (directly or through another sports medicine professional) to receive input as to when it is safe for the athlete to return to training or competition.

The coach and all sport management team members must understand the athlete's need for confidentiality regarding treatment. Confidentiality means that information about the athlete's condition and treatment are shared only with the athlete's permission. If the athlete does not want information shared, it should not be provided to anyone. Confidentiality is not only the individual's right; it is necessary for successful treatment. The affected individual must feel free to talk about private and personal issues in order to recover. Additionally, mental health professionals working with the athlete are ethically bound to maintain the individual's confidentiality. They cannot release information about an adult athlete (18 years or older) to anyone—even parents—without the athlete's permission. For minor athletes (17 years or younger), however, parents and other individuals (e.g., teachers) may have the right to know about the athlete's status and his or her treatment. In such cases, it is important to discuss confidentiality at the beginning of treatment with parents and the minor athlete; all parties should understand how and when information will be shared. In doing so, it is important to remember that the health and well-being of the athlete are the primary concern. Coaches, however, are not bound by the same ethical guidelines and may need to be instructed regarding the importance of confidentiality. Some athletes may prefer that information not be shared with coaches or other sport personnel. In this event, sport personnel must accept this without reprisal. In our experiences, athletes generally do not refuse the sharing of necessary information with appropriate sport management team personnel if they are approached in a sensitive and caring manner, that is, by involving the athlete in the process and fully explaining how and why the information is to be shared before doing so.

The coach also will have the task of explaining to other team members why an affected athlete is not training or competing. Again, confidentiality and privacy have to be considered. The athlete in question must have a say as to how this is handled. If the athlete wants no information to be given to the team regarding his or her disorder or absence from training or competition, the coach should comply. If the athlete does not want others to know his or her condition, the coach can simply state that "I don't have any information that I can share with you." A coach who takes this approach is also communicating to team members that he or she can be trusted with confidential matters. Team members respect this, and it also makes it easier for other athletes to talk with their coach if they should encounter a problem in the future.

Dietitian

Any athlete with an eating disorder should work with a dietitian, ideally one who is especially knowledgeable about eating problems. Whenever possible, the dietitian should have an appreciation for sport and the important role it plays in the lives of many athletes. The dietitian helps educate the athlete about nutritional needs, especially how those needs change under conditions of training and competition. This education can also include how good nutrition improves athletic performance because this information may help motivate some athletes to improve their nutritional intake. The dietitian's role might include meal planning, nutritional counseling, helping to set a target range for weight or body composition (e.g., percentage body fat), and weighing the athlete when appropriate. A primary treatment goal is to restore normal eating patterns, and learning to eat regularly and healthfully and to plan nutritious meals is essential in accomplishing this goal.

Psychologist

A sport psychologist who is a member of the sport management team and who is also trained in the treatment of eating disorders is the best person to intervene. Usually, however, an eating disorder specialist is not already a part of the sport management team. The role of the sport psychologist then is to assist in arranging the best and most appropriate referral for treatment. It is beyond the scope of this chapter to address treatment approaches. However, the most important factor is to find an eating disorder treatment specialist who, if possible, has knowledge of sports environments and experience working with athletes. If this professional is not a member of the sport management team, the team or sport psychologist can become the primary liaison between the eating disorder specialist and the sport management team. Psychologists and other mental health professionals are familiar with the need for confidentiality and can speak with the athlete about what information may be shared with whom. Highly visible athletes might receive calls from the media regarding an absence from competition. Family members may also want more information than the athlete would like provided. The sport psychologist can help provide assistance in these matters and instruct the rest of the sport management team about how to handle confidentiality. Again, confidentiality (and its limits) should be discussed at the beginning of any intervention. In addition, when communication with other sport management team members is necessary and approved, athletes always should be informed about the content and purpose of the communication.

Physician

Because eating disorders can have so many physical ramifications, the team physician plays an important role in monitoring the athlete's health. Some of the medical complications have been mentioned earlier, but more detailed information is available elsewhere (see Mitchell, 1986a, 1986b). The most frequent difficulties can also be monitored in part by the athletic trainer. Although medications should not be the sole or even the primary treatment for an eating disorder, many patients with eating disorders have benefited from some psychotropic medications (see Garfinkel & Garner, 1987). In addition to making decisions concerning medication, the physician treats any physical complications. The athletic trainer is once again a valuable resource to the physician, both in terms of alerting the physician to symptoms and monitoring the ongoing progress of any medical treatments.

Physical Therapist

The role of the physical therapist may be very similar to that of the athletic trainer, particularly if the therapist has ongoing or daily contact with the athlete. As mentioned in the section on prevention, physical therapists' involvements with athletes often concern injury and physical rehabilitation. If an athlete is injured and also suffers from a clinical or subclinical eating disorder, physical therapists must consider certain issues. First, they must consider the nature of the relationship between the athletic injury and the presence of the eating disorder. As discussed previously, disruption of athletic participation may precipitate the development of eating concerns. In such situations, resuming athletic participation may result in the lessening or ending of the problem. Even so, the fact that eating problems emerge under this stressful situation is reason enough to make a referral to an eating disorder specialist so as to minimize the possibility of problems arising in the future. Second, even when the athlete physically recovers from the injury, the ramifications of returning to athletic participation in the presence of the eating problem must be considered. As discussed in the section on athletic trainers, there are several factors to consider when making this decision and several things a physical therapist (or athletic trainer) can do to facilitate the athlete's continued involvement with the team. Keeping athletes connected with and involved in the sport environment can be an integral part of helping them maintain a positive attitude during treatment and rehabilitation.

Remedial Intervention Summary

Although the treatment of eating disorders should be conducted by specialists, the sports medicine professional still can play a critical role in the athlete's recovery. The sports medicine professional is in the position to talk with the athlete about what is happening and help him or her understand the importance of treatment, ensure that the athlete has access to specialists, and help the athlete continue to feel a part of the team. In addition, sports medicine professionals, particularly athletic trainers, can play an invaluable role because of their daily contact with the athlete. The athletic trainer can be involved in monitoring the athlete's performances, eating behaviors (e.g., how well the athlete is following established meal plans), mood states, and weight, when appropriate. Sharing such information with the eating disorder specialist, physician, or dietitian allows these professionals to determine whether the treatment is working and to make changes as necessary. Finally, the athletic trainer can work with the coach to help him or her understand the multidimensional nature of eating disorders and the necessity for treatment. Because eating disorders are not as obvious as many physical injuries, some coaches may be less understanding about the need to restrict involvement in practices and competitions or to seek treatment.

Shannon is in her first year as a student athletic trainer at a Division I university. She has been assigned to the women's swimming team, which has a new coach who was brought in because of his success in developing winning programs. The coach has the reputation of being personable with athletic trainers and other personnel, but with his swimmers he is known to be demanding and, in some cases, belittling. As the season starts, one of Shannon's tasks is to assist the coach in weekly weigh-ins. On Mondays before practice begins, the coach brings together all the athletes to be weighed in a large open room. During these sessions, the coach publicly announces each swimmer's weight (which Shannon is supposed to record) and then comments on whether he believes the athlete is "too fat." He assigns early morning running sessions to athletes who he believes weigh too much and encourages them to restrict their food intake. Privately he tells Shannon that this peer pressure is the best way to keep the swimmers thin and lean, which is necessary to be successful.

As the season progresses, Shannon begins to notice changes in some of the athletes. All the swimmers dread the weigh-ins, but some seem to be affected even more strongly. She notices that a few of the women are sluggish in practices, seem overly tired, look gaunt, or have lost weight that they really did not need to lose. In addition, at training table, these women only pick at their food, generally eating only a few vegetables and soda crackers. A week later, one of these women privately approaches Shannon in the training room before the Monday weigh-in. She is crying and visibly upset at the prospect of being weighed that day. She "confesses" that over the weekend she had broken down and eaten a lot of food. She is scared about what she will weigh and what her coach will say.

QUESTIONS FOR ANALYSIS

1. What problems exist in the way the coach is handling the weight and health of his athletes? On what myths might the coach be basing his behavior?

2. What might Shannon do to intervene on behalf of the team now that she is aware of how the coach's behavior is affecting the team?

3. How might Shannon assist the individual athlete who has approached her privately?

4. How should Shannon have responded to the coach when he suggested public and weekly weigh-ins?

Jody had been running ever since she could remember. Her father was a high school track coach and an avid runner himself. When she was younger, she used to attend the high school meets that her father coached and wanted to be like his star athletes when she grew up. Even so, when she began running, she did it just for fun. By junior high, though, she was a standout on her school team. Once she got to high school, she got extremely serious about her running. She spent a lot of time training with her father above and beyond her regular school practices. She was a natural runner, and she enjoyed the time that she and her dad shared together in her sport. He obviously took great pride in his daughter's accomplishments, and together they kept records of her best times and watched her improvements over her four years in high school. By her junior year in high school, several college track teams were showing interest in recruiting her. She was offered track scholarships from four different colleges and finally decided on attending an NCAA Division I university. She wanted to a attend a school where she could run outdoors year round. She had never liked having to retreat to indoor running during

CASE STUDY I

CASE STUDY II

some New England winters at home, so she chose to attend a university in a warmer climate.

The summer before college, Jody really intensified her training workouts. She wanted to be prepared for collegiate competition. Her father was her coach for that summer, and both became anxious at the prospects of her upcoming year at college. When Jody arrived at college, she was initially homesick and called home frequently. Over the next few months, she began to make some friends and got closer to some other athletes on the team. But whenever she got really lonely, she would go out for a long run and come home so exhausted that she would forget how lonely she had been. Despite all her efforts, however, her times were not improving. Having come from a situation where she was the big fish in a small pond, Jody now found herself just another fish in a very big pond. The level of ability and competition at the college level was overwhelming. Not knowing what else to try to improve her time, Jody started a very strict diet in hopes that shedding a few pounds would help her shed a few seconds off her racing times.

At first, Jody was energized by her new diet and regained the determination to improve her running. Within a few months, however, she began to look pale and feel depressed. She was becoming more socially isolated and spent most of her free time worrying about her eating, weight, and running. When her diet stopped producing weight loss, Jody decided to vomit after eating meals. She had heard about this but had never felt that she needed to try it before. But as her energy level and self-esteem began to plummet, Jody felt desperate to try anything to get back in control of her running and her life.

The team's athletic trainer had noticed that Jody had been looking pale and lifeless and wondered whether she was feeling okay. One hot afternoon when the team was running stadium steps, Jody began to feel very dizzy and had to stop. She was dehydrated and felt as if she was going to faint. The athletic trainer talked with her and learned that she had been without her menstrual cycle for the past eight months. Jody also admitted that she was having difficulty sleeping and difficulty concentrating on her school work. Although she said her eating was fine, the athletic trainer saw enough signs to wonder whether that was true. The athletic trainer knew that an upcoming meet was especially important to Jody because her father was going to fly out to attend. She wanted him to be proud of her. The pressure she was putting on herself was obvious to everyone but Jody.

Questions for Analysis

1. What are the signs and symptoms of Jody's eating problem?

2. How might the athletic trainer intervene to assist Jody?

3. What life events or pressures might have contributed to Jody's eating problems?

4. What could the athletic trainer have done differently to intervene sooner?

CASE STUDY III

John was a member of the school's wrestling team and was just beginning his junior year. He had not wrestled much the past two years because he was not able to get down to the weight his coach wanted. This year, however, he was hopeful because he had shed 15 pounds (7 kilograms) during the summer and was below the weight his coach wanted. Besides, the teammate who had wrestled at that weight had transferred to another school so there was an opening.

During preseason physicals the sports physician and athletic trainer commented on his weight loss. When asked how he accomplished it, John seemed to become embarrassed and tried to change the subject. At that time John seemed healthy, so no additional comments were made.

As the season progressed, though, the athletic trainer noticed that John had lost some additional weight (about three pounds, or a kilogram) and seemed fatigued during many of his practices. This weight loss and loss of energy seemed odd because the athletic trainer had seen John eat; he ate as much as anyone on the team. In fact, some of his teammates said that they wished they could eat like him and still lose weight. When the athletic trainer tried to talk with John about his performances in practice, John brushed off the concern, stating that he was just tired from staying up late to study.

Although John was wrestling at his lower weight, he was not as successful as he had expected: His record was 3-5 when he had hoped for 6-2. At an away tournament the following weekend, John lost his two matches, which kept the team from victory. At dinner that evening, John seemed depressed and withdrawn. After dinner, John excused himself to go to the bathroom. A few minutes later, the athletic trainer, who was concerned about John, followed him to the bathroom. When the athletic trainer entered, he heard what sounded like someone throwing up. No one else was in the rest room, so it had to be John.

Questions for Analysis

1. What are some of the signs and symptoms of John's eating problem?

2. How and when should the athletic trainer confront John? What consideration should the athletic trainer give to the fact that John is male?

3. How could the athletic trainer and sports physician have intervened earlier in the season?

4. If John admits that he has an eating problem, what individuals from the sport management team would you recommend work with John? What roles should these professionals take?

SUMMARY

Eating disorders are multidimensional problems that affect most areas of an individual's functioning. Female athletes, like women in general, experience these disorders at a much higher rate than men. Factors specific to the sport environment, such as weight restrictions or pressures from coaches, can add to the societal pressures that many individuals experience to achieve a certain body size and look. These combined pressures can increase an athlete's risk of developing eating disorders. Although the exact prevalence is not clear, substantial numbers of female athletes suffer from clinical eating disorders and display many subclinical symptoms, such as body dissatisfaction, binge eating, dieting, and excessive exercising. These disorders are associated with psychological and physical complications that can be severe and disruptive. Sports medicine professionals should be aware of these problems and familiar with the signs and behaviors that often serve as indicators of more severe problems.

Sports medicine professionals should also be aware of the issues related to treatment and the roles they can play as part of a sport management team. In prevention, sports medicine professionals play key roles in making time available during practices for information to be shared with athletes and coaches, in monitoring the athletes' day-to-day behaviors, and in helping athletes access people and services when minor concerns arise. When an eating disorder is found, the sports medicine professional's role still remains important, even though treatment is generally handled by specialists. The sports medicine professional, due to his or her contact with the athlete and coaching staff, can assist the athlete in continuing to feel a part of the team as the athlete undergoes treatment, monitor the athlete's performances and behaviors and share the information with other sport management team members who are directly involved in providing treatment, and educate the coaches about eating disorders and the importance of the athlete's seeking treatment. These roles all are crucial to the athlete's recovery.

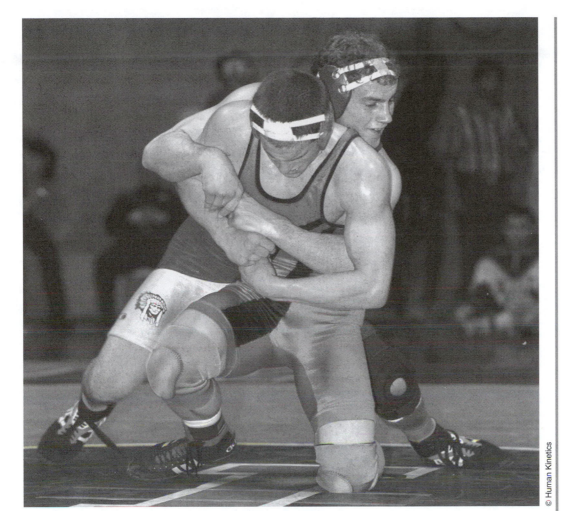

chapter 13

Counseling Athletes With Nutritional Concerns

Susan M. Kleiner, PhD, RD, *University of Washington*

CHAPTER OBJECTIVES

Understand the basic principles of nutrition assessment, evaluation, and counseling

Identify the tools and techniques most suitable for the nutrition assessment, evaluation, and counseling of athletes by sports medicine professionals

Learn how to influence the diets and food behaviors of athletes in a counseling setting

An athlete's diet affects his or her health and physical performance, now and in the future. According to the National Center for Health Statistics, of the 10 leading causes of death, five—coronary heart disease, generalized atherosclerosis, stroke, some types of cancer, and diabetes—have been associated with dietary excesses or imbalances, and another three—cirrhosis of the liver, accidents, and suicides—are often the result of excessive alcohol intake. Together, these eight conditions account for as many as 70 percent of all U.S. deaths each year (USDHHS, 1988).

The relationship between nutrition and exercise is clear and can be reduced to two major factors (Hedquist, 1993):

- Exercise increases the rate of utilization of energy substrate and certain nutrients with a concomitant rise in heat production.

- The increase in heat production results in a greater loss of body water (and associated minerals) via sweat in the body's attempt to maintain normal body temperature.

By following good nutritional practices, athletes not only have a better chance of maintaining health and improving their performance, but if they do become injured, an appropriate diet can assist with the process of returning them to the playing field as quickly as possible.

Athletes' nutritional needs are based on their age, lifestyle, health status, level of physical activity, physical conditioning, and type of sport. Athletes are prey to nutritional faddism and misinformation. The diets of many athletes are inadequate because of their overly restrictive eating habits and obsessions with body weight and food (Storlie, 1991). Making sure that athletes get appropriate nutrition advice and then learn to apply the information correctly is a task that must be approached with care. Sports physicians and athletic trainers usually play more of a counseling role with athletes than physical therapists. But the physical therapist may be the person who hears a complaint or a question regarding nutrition and must be well-informed enough to either answer the question appropriately or refer the athlete in the proper direction.

Young athletes must be introduced to basic nutrition principles as early as possible. Since it is unlikely that most athletes have contact with a dietitian, it is imperative that athletic trainers, physical therapists, coaches, and sports physicians develop the skills to counsel athletes in healthy dietary practices. In most cases, physicians, physical therapists, athletic trainers, and coaches may identify a nutritional concern through general daily communication or a primary screening process. But the most likely professional to do nutrition counseling is the athletic trainer or the physician. All the professionals must be informed of the athlete's progress since it can often take a team approach to solve the dietary concern.

As a sports medicine professional, you play an important role in helping athletes learn appropriate nutritional behaviors. Accomplishing this task requires an understanding of the **physiological** as well as **psychosocial** influences that affect athletes' dietary practices. Practical skills in counseling and education are needed to motivate athletes to modify their food choices and eating habits. The purpose of this chapter is to introduce you to the basic principles of nutrition assessment, evaluation, and counseling. Then, by giving you the tools to apply these principles and to appropriately evaluate dietary information, you can positively influence the nutritional practices of athletes in a counseling setting.

The publication of the Dietary Guidelines for Americans (see figure 13.1) has given us a dietary model to follow while counseling athletes (USDA, 1995). While all people have individual **nutritional requirements**, these guidelines offer general **dietary recommendations** that can be applied to the majority of people. For some athletes, the guidelines may serve as minimum dietary recommendations. The dietary guidelines emphasize the positive, rather than negative, aspects of eating be-

physiological— Pertaining to the functional processes in an organism.

psychosocial— Pertaining to or involving both mental and behavioral aspects and the influence of society.

nutritional requirements— The nutrient amount required by the body to maintain health and growth.

U.S. Dietary Guidelines

• **Eat a variety of foods.**

3–5 servings vegetables (especially dark green and yellow)

2–4 servings fruits (especially citrus)

6–11 servings breads, cereals, rice, pasta

2–3 servings milk, yogurt, cheese

2–3 servings meats, poultry, fish, dry beans and peas, eggs, nuts

• **Balance the food you can eat with physical activity; maintain or improve your weight.**

• **Choose a diet with plenty of grain products, vegetables, and fruits.**

1 serving grain = 1 slice bread, 1/2 bun, bagel, English muffin, 1 oz. cold cereal, 1/2 cup cooked cereal, rice, pasta, grains

1 serving grain, vegetable/fruit = 1 cup raw, 1/2 cup cooked, 1 medium piece

• **Choose a diet low in fat, saturated fat, and cholesterol.**

Less than 30% of daily calories from fat

Less than 10% of daily calories from saturated fat

Less than or equal to 100 mg cholesterol per day

• **Choose a diet moderate in sugars.**

Examples of sugars include table sugar, brown sugar, raw sugar, glucose, fructose, maltose, lactose, honey, syrup, corn sweetener, high-fructose corn syrup, molasses, fruit juice concentrate.

• **Choose a diet moderate in salt and sodium.**

2,400 mg of sodium daily is a reasonable guideline for dietary intake.

• **If you drink alcoholic beverages, do so in moderation.**

Less than 1 drink/day for women, less than 2 drinks/day for men; children and adolescents should not drink alcohol

1 drink = 12 oz. beer, 5 oz. wine, 1.5 oz. liquor (80 proof)

Figure 13.1 Dietary Guidelines for Americans (USDA, 1995).

dietary recommendations—*The nutrient amount recommended when other factors, such as nutrient bioavailability, food supply, health status, and cooking losses, are taken into consideration along with nutrient requirements.*

havior. Instead of stating to "avoid" or "do not eat" certain foods, the guidelines suggest that all foods can be eaten, but in moderation. This positive approach is more successful in promoting behavioral change.

BASIC PRINCIPLES OF NUTRITION ASSESSMENT AND SCREENING

An effective nutrition care plan for athletes is based on the four principles of classical nutrition assessment:

- Anthropometric studies
- Dietary studies
- Biochemical studies
- Clinical studies

Nutrition and physical performance indicators are integrated to determine the physiological needs of the athlete, then they are compared with food intake. Additional factors that will affect the athlete's dietary choices, such as level of motivation, social pressures, beliefs, competitive goals, work and school schedules, must be considered before attempting to counsel the athlete about dietary change (Storlie, 1991).

Nutrition assessments or screening of athletes should be done at the beginning of each season. Since many athletes participate in several different sports, they may be evaluated several times during the school year. This is an appropriate approach. The individual who performs the screening may differ, depending on the structure of the institution; however, the athletic trainer or sports physician is most likely to conduct the screening and assessment.

All members of the sports medicine team must ultimately be involved in any dietary intervention. Unless all members work together to support the athlete and encourage the recommended changes, the likelihood of a successful outcome is reduced. Coaches see the athletes on a regular basis, so they need to be aware of the dietary recommendations, to observe the athletes, and to answer simple nutrition questions or refer the athlete back to the athletic trainer or sports physician. Physical therapists see athletes on a more intimate basis, where athletes may feel less threatened and more willing to divulge information they otherwise may not share with other sports medicine professionals. All the professionals must be "on the same page" and support a consistent message to the athlete to help ensure a positive outcome.

Storlie (1991) described a conceptual framework for conducting nutrition assessments of athletes (see figure 13.2). Since most athletes have several different diet and training schedules, such as in-season, competitive season, and off-season training regimens, it is important to include the various diet and training modalities as part of the nutrition assessment. This model promotes a comprehensive approach to nutrition assessment. In practice, circumstances may hinder the collection of such detailed information. Nevertheless, a best effort is better than no effort at all.

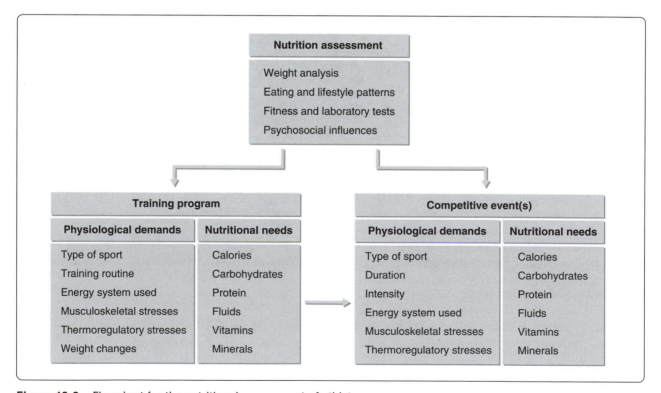

Figure 13.2   Flowchart for the nutritional assessment of athletes.

From Storlie, J. Nutrition Assessment of Athletes: A model for intergrating nutrition and physical performance indicators. *International Journal of Sport Nutrition* 1991, 1, 192-204.

Depending on the individual athlete's situation, different types of data collection techniques may be used. Whether nutrition assessments are conducted in a primary care setting or away from a medical facility (e.g., school, athletic facility), we need practical and reliable methods to quickly assess an athlete's nutritional status and to solve common problems. Common nutritional problems should be addressed directly so that athletes understand the importance of the diagnosis and recommended intervention. Preventive nutrition assessment and counseling should also be carried out on a regular basis by a designated professional who has good rapport with the athletes.

When uncommon or more complicated disorders are detected (such as **hypoglycemia**, **diabetes**, eating disorders), athletes should be referred to specialists. Referrals to specialists such as **registered dietitians**, psychologists, and specialized physicians with experience working with athletes can complement the care of the primary physician, coach, or athletic trainer, resulting in improved compliance and outcome.

The following sections cover the parts of a nutrition assessment, which include determining the appropriate body weight and energy needs of athletes, what they are eating, their current state of health, and their emotional and lifestyle demands. Since different methods are appropriate for different environments, several collection methods and tools are discussed. After all this information is collected, it is analyzed and evaluated. It then becomes the foundation for the final dietary recommendations.

Anthropometric Weight Analysis

The body weight of an athlete plays a crucial role in physical performance and long-term health. The determination of an athlete's energy needs is based on his or her average daily energy expenditure and on whether the athlete needs to lose weight, maintain weight, or gain weight. Since body weight is generally a primary concern for athletes, it is most productive to begin the nutrition assessment by addressing and evaluating this issue thoroughly.

The determination of **optimal body weight** is a somewhat subjective process. Generally, three methods are applied and evaluated to determine an athlete's optimal body weight (Storlie, 1991):

- Personal goal weight
- Height/weight formula
- Percentage body fat prediction

The athlete's personal goal weight is an indicator both of the athlete's knowledge of his or her own body and the weight at which it performs and feels best and of his or her motivation and body image. The collection of anthropometric data such as current weight, height, and percentage body fat offers the tools to predict optimal body weight. These data can then be reviewed and applied to determine how the athlete's present weight deviates from both the predicted weight and the athlete's personal weight goal.

Weight Assessment Tools

There are a number of sources that thoroughly discuss the various protocols for anthropometric assessment (Manore 1993; McArdle, Katch, & Katch, 1994). Because the tools used for the assessment of an athlete's weight must be practical yet reliable, optimal body weight should be determined using both height/weight and percentage body fat assessment techniques.

An accepted rule-of-thumb technique for determining optimal body weight based on height uses the following calculation: For women, add 100 pounds (45.4 kilograms) for the first 5 feet (1.5 meters) of height plus 5 pounds (2.3 kilograms) for every inch

hypoglycemia— *Deficient glucose concentration in the blood, which may lead to nervousness, hypothermia, headache, confusion, and sometimes convulsions and coma.*

diabetes—*A disease characterized by high blood sugar levels that are caused by insufficient action of the hormone insulin.*

registered dietitian—*A person who has completed at least a bachelor's degree program approved by the American Dietetic Association, has participated in a supervised professional practice program, and has passed a national registration examination.*

optimal body weight—*The weight at which the body performs optimally, both mentally and physically, and promotes the greatest opportunity for health.*

(2.5 centimeters) over 5 feet. For men, add 106 pounds (48.1 kilograms) for the first 5 feet of height plus 6 pounds (2.7 kilograms) for every inch over 5 feet. This calculation may be somewhat inaccurate for the very lean individual because lean body mass is not considered as part of the predictive formula.

Using height/weight tables to predict optimal body weight can be misleading. These tables are developed based on average individuals, not athletes. Athletes tend to be less fat and more muscular than the average individual. A very lean, muscular bodybuilder or strength-training athlete may appear overweight when judged by a height/weight chart yet be far from overfat. Lean, small-boned endurance athletes may appear underweight according to height/weight tables, yet their weight is appropriate for their body structure and the requirements of their sport.

Guidelines for percentage body fat predictors can be found in table 13.1. Once an athlete's present body weight and percentage body fat is determined (generally by skinfold anthropometry), optimal body weight can be calculated from the following formula using the desired percentage body fat. Since predictive formulas for percentage body fat determination are based on lean body mass determinations, athletes who deviate from normal lean body mass distributions will have misleading results. This notion reinforces the need to use both height/weight and percentage body fat predictors in determining optimal body weight. Then, considering all three predictors (personal goal, height/weight goal, percentage body fat goal) the sports medicine professional and the athlete must work toward a realistic goal through negotiation and professional judgment.

Calculation of Optimal Body Composition

Once an athlete's present body weight and percentage body fat are determined, you can calculate how much body weight can be lost to maximize fat loss and minimize muscle loss, based on the desired percentage body fat. For example, if a 140-pound athlete with 18% body fat would like to have only 14% body fat, you would use the following calculations:

Present body weight: 140 pounds (63.5 kilograms)

Present body fat: 18 percent

Desired body fat: 14 percent

$140 \times .18 = 25.2$ pounds (11.4 kilograms) fat

$140 - 25.2 = 114.8$ pounds (52.1 kilograms) lean body mass

$114.8 \div .86 = 133.4$ pounds (60.6 kilograms) total at 14 percent body fat

---

Table 13.1 Guidelines for Acceptable Percent Body Fat Levels

	Male (%)	Female (%)
Essential	3	12
Recommended for athletic performance	5-10[a]	12-15[a]
Recommended for health and fitness	11-15[b]	15-20[b]
Average American adults	15-18	18-23
17-30 yrs	12-15	22-29
31-68 yrs	18-27	25-34
Excess	>20	>30

[a]Males: long-distance runners, wrestlers, gymnasts, basketball players, soccer players, swimmers, body builders, football backs, tennis players; Females: gymnasts, ballet dancers, long-distance runners.
[b]Males: baseball players, football linemen, weightlifters, weightmen in track and field; Females: other athletes

From Storlie, J. Nutrition Assessment of Athletes: A model for intergrating nutrition and physical performance indicators. *International Journal of Sport Nutrition* 1991, 1, 192-204.

Health Goals Versus Competitive Goals

The process of determining optimal body weight is generally a dynamic one. Body weight goals change with age and with sport. Athletes who participate in several different sports throughout the year may have different weight goals that are sport specific. Body weight goals fluctuate with on-season, competitive season, and off-season training. Athletes who participate in events with official weight classifications such as wrestling, boxing, and bodybuilding alter their weight goals frequently and repetitively. Sometimes the competitive goals of the athlete are potentially at odds with health goals. Yet an athlete may be determined to achieve what he or she believes is the competitive edge with rapid weight loss. Since performance is the ultimate goal of the athlete, counselors must keep this factor in mind when athletes desire to reach an unrealistic weight goal. Research has shown that rapid weight loss in wrestlers trying to compete in lower weight classes adversely affects their performance (Tipton, 1990). Bodybuilders who have been on rigid dietary regimens before competitive events are at risk of metabolic abnormalities that can affect their performance as they enter competition (Kleiner, Bazzarre, & Ainsworth, 1994; Kleiner, Bazzarre, & Litchford, 1990). Using this information may be the most helpful way to achieve a negotiated optimal body weight that can meet both performance and health goals. Finally, if the counselor suspects that eating disorders are present, this approach may not be appropriate, and assistance should be sought from an eating disorders specialist.

Determination of Calorie Requirements

After optimal body weight has been determined, approximate energy needs can be calculated. Daily **basal energy expenditure** (BEE) can be determined using the following formula using age (years), body mass (kilograms), and height (centimeters):

basal energy expenditure (BEE)—The minimal energy the body requires to support itself when resting and awake.

Women:

$$BEE = 655 + (9.6 \times mass) + (1.85 \times height) - (4.7 \times age)$$

Men:

$$BEE = 66.0 + (13.7 \times mass) + (5.0 \times height) - (6.8 \times age)$$

By interviewing the athlete about daily activities, the additional energy cost of these activities can be determined. Information about daily routines (eating, sleeping, shopping, reading, walking, stair climbing) as well as specific sports activities (type of activity, frequency, intensity, and duration) over a week's time are required to achieve accurate results. Using a table of energy expenditure (McArdle et al., 1994), the average daily activity level can be factored into the recommended calorie intake. The final step is to consider whether the athlete wants to gain, maintain, or lose weight. By adding or subtracting 500 to 1000 calories per day from the calculated energy requirement, athletes will gain or lose approximately one to two pounds (0.5 to 1 kilogram) per week. The 500- to 1000-calorie-per-day deficit should be designed as a combination of reduced nutritional intake and increased energy expenditure through exercise. Since 1600-1800 calories are required to consume adequate nutrients, total calories should not go below this level. As with the determination of optimal body weight, energy requirements are dynamic, based on the changing activity levels of athletes throughout their seasons. To maintain weight goals, periodic adjustments in calories must be made to reflect changes in training and competition.

Dietary Assessment: Eating and Lifestyle Patterns

Evaluating the diet of an athlete consists of understanding what the athlete eats, as well as why, where, when, and how the athlete eats. It includes everything that an athlete consumes, including all dietary supplements and sports nutrition products. The lifestyle routines and stresses that athletes face profoundly affect food selection, food preparation, and eating habits, which ultimately affect health and performance. It is critically important to collect information about the athlete's daily routines, such as training, work or school commitments, travel, and so on. With this information in mind, you and the athlete can design a program that fits the athlete's lifestyle and will really work.

All dietary assessment tools have strengths and weaknesses, yet the collection of food intake data is critical to the complete nutrition assessment of athletes. The collection of dietary data is also important for the development of an intervention and counseling strategy and a follow-up plan.

Examples of various dietary assessment tools follow. They can be applied as given here or can be adapted to specific groups by adding or deleting pertinent questions or sections. With athletes in particular, it may be appropriate to always include questions regarding the dietary pattern followed during in-season, off-season, or competitive season training schedules. Since each tool has its strengths and weaknesses, two or more tools may be used to provide more complete and accurate information about the dietary intake of an athlete.

Generic Nutrition Questionnaire

The generic nutrition questionnaire (see table 13.2) is a universal questionnaire. Counselors can select those questions that are appropriate for each situation then add others to elicit specific information required in their particular setting. If necessary, the questions can be phrased for the counselor to answer; otherwise, questions can be answered by the athlete.

24-Hour Recall

The 24-hour recall (see table 13.3) is a dietary assessment tool that provides a window on historical food intake during a specific time. It can be used for any age group. The recall is based on the premise that information about foods and beverages that were consumed during the previous 24-hour period represents the athlete's typical food intake and habits. This assumption is flawed if the previous 24-hour period was not a typical day for the athlete. It is therefore extremely important to determine whether the previous day's food intake was typical of the athlete's diet. The 24-hour recall is best used with a second dietary assessment tool. It can also be useful during follow-up visits to determine whether the athlete is adapting to dietary recommendations.

Food Frequency Form

The food frequency form (see table 13.4) is a checklist that elicits data regarding the kinds of food eaten and the frequency of intake over a period of time. It can help to confirm the adequacy or deficiency of an athlete's diet and is best used with a second dietary assessment tool.

Food Diary and the Food and Activity Record

The food diary (see table 13.5) is a self-recorded description of intake over a period of days (usually three to seven). Different from a recall, which is a historical record based on the athlete's memory of the past 24 hours, the food diary is recorded by the athlete immediately after he or she eats. The athlete is given instructions on how to complete the diary at the first visit and returns the diary at the follow-up visit. The food and activity record (see table 13.6) describes food intake, activity, and mood. Each of these tools can be used as it appears or can be adapted to specific situations.

Table 13.2   Generic Nutrition Questionnaire

Name: _____   Date: _____

	Follow-up Required

Data

I. Appetite

   a. How would you describe you appetite?

      ( ) Hearty   ( ) Moderate   ( ) Poor

   b. Do you enjoy eating?

      ( ) Yes   ( ) No   ( ) Sometimes

II. Eating pattern and attitudes about food

   a. Do you eat at approximately the same time every day?

      ( ) Yes   ( ) No   ( ) Sometimes

   b. Do you skip meals?

      ( ) Yes   ( ) No

      If yes, at what times?

      _____

   c. Are there any foods that you do not eat because you don't think they are good for you?

      ( ) Yes   ( ) No

      If yes, what?

      _____

   d. Do you usually eat anything between meals?

      ( ) Yes   ( ) No

      If yes, name the two or three snacks (including bedtime snacks) that you have most often.

      _____

      _____

   e. During one week, where do you eat most of your food?

      Home _____   School _____

      Work _____   Restaurant _____

      Other _____ (identify)

   f. Are there any foods that you regularly eat because you think that they are good for you?

      ( ) Yes   ( ) No

      If yes, what?

      _____

III. Food choices

   a. Are there any foods you can't eat?

      ( ) Yes   ( ) No

      If yes, what food(s)?

(continued)

Table 13.2 *(continued)*

Data	Follow-up Required

Data

What happens when you eat this food?

_____

_____

b. Are you allergic to any foods?

( ) Yes   ( ) No

If yes, what food(s)? _____

What happens when you eat this food?

_____

_____

c. Are there certain foods that you do not eat because you don't like them?

( ) Yes   ( ) No

If yes, what food(s)? _____

d. Are there certain foods that you avoid eating because of your religious beliefs?

( ) Yes   ( ) No

If yes, what food(s)? _____

e. Are there certain foods that you avoid eating because of your ethnic/cultural background?

( ) Yes   ( ) No

If yes, what food(s)? _____

f. Are there certain foods that you eat regularly because of your ethnic/cultural background?

( ) Yes   ( ) No

If yes, what food(s)? _____

g. How is your food usually prepared?

( ) Baked   ( ) Broiled   ( ) Fried

Other _____

h. Do you drink milk?

( ) Yes   ( ) No

If yes:

( ) Whole milk   ( ) Skim milk

( ) Other; specify _____

i. List five of your favorite foods:

_____

j. List five of your least favorite foods:

_____

IV. Weight history

a. Have you ever had any problems with weight?

( ) Yes   ( ) No

b. If yes, what?

(continued)

236

Table 13.2 *(continued)*

Data	Follow-up Required
( ) Underweight ( ) Overweight	

( ) Other _____

c. Are you now on a diet to lose weight?

( ) Yes   ( ) No

If yes, what kind? _____

_____

How long? _____

Who recommended it? _____

d. How do you feel about your weight?

( ) Too heavy   ( ) Too thin   ( ) Okay

e. Do you ever vomit to keep your weight down?

( ) Every day   ( ) 3-4 times/week

( ) Every week   ( ) Sometimes   ( ) Never

V. Supplements and medications

a. Are you now taking any vitamins or mineral supplements?

( ) Yes   ( ) No

If yes, what, now often, and what brand?

_____

b Do you regularly take any medications prescribed by your doctor?

( ) Yes   ( ) No

If yes, what? _____

c. Do you regularly take any "over-the-counter" medications?

( ) Yes   ( ) No

If yes, what? _____

VI. Smoking, alcohol, and substance use

a. Do you smoke?

( ) Yes   ( ) No

If yes, what, how many cigarettes per day?

_____

b. Do you drink any alcoholic beverages (liquor, wine, wine coolers, beer)?

( ) Yes   ( ) No

If yes, what do you drink and how often?

_____

_____

c. Do you smoke marijuana?

( ) Yes   ( ) No

If yes, how often?_____

d. How often do you use crack, cocaine, speed, or other street drugs?

( ) Every day   ( ) 3-4 times/week

( ) Every week   ( ) Sometimes   ( ) Never

(continued)

Table 13.2 *(continued)*

Data	Follow-up Required

Data

VII. Exercise

    a. How often do you exercise?

       ( ) Every day   ( ) 3-4 times/week

       ( ) Every week   ( ) Sometimes   ( ) Never

    b. List kinds of exercise you do most often _____

    c. How often do you get out of breath when you exercise?

       ( ) Every week   ( ) Sometimes   ( ) Never

VIII. Household information

    a. Indicate the person who does the following in your household:

    Plans the meals _____

    Buys the food _____

    Prepares the food _____

    b. How much is spent on food each week for your household?

       $ _____   ( ) Don't know

    For how many people? _____

    c. Are there periods in the month when there isn't enough money for food or you run out of food?

       ( ) Yes   ( ) No

    If yes, when and how long are these periods? _____

    _____

    d. Indicate the types of kitchen equipment you have in your home.

       ( ) Refrigerator   ( ) Working stove

       ( ) Hot plate   ( ) Piped water   ( ) Sink

IX. Food programs

    a. Are you receiving any of the following:

       ( ) Food stamps   ( ) WIC vouchers   ( ) Commodity foods

    b. Does your family use:

       ( ) Food co-ops   ( ) Food shelves

       ( ) Food pantries   ( ) Soup kitchens

       ( ) Free or reduced-price school lunch and/or breakfast

       ( ) Summer feeding program

    c. How many hot meals do you have each week?

       >7   7   6   <6

Modified from Simko, M.D., Cowell, C., and Gilbride, J.A.: *Nutrition assessment: a comprehensive guide for planning intervention*, Rockville, Md, 1984, Aspen Publishers.

Table 13.3 24-Hour Recall

Name: _____   Date of Birth: _____
month / date / year

ID# _____   Sex _____

Time	Place	Food	Amount	For Practitioner Use
				Summary

a. This is a typical day.   Yes _____   No _____

b. I take vitamin/mineral supplements.   Yes _____   No _____

   If yes, name the brand _____

c. I have been on a special diet during the past 3 months.   Yes _____   No _____

   If yes, the kind of special diet _____

Instructions:

1. Record time of day or night when you ate food or drank beverages (8 AM, 9 PM, etc.).

2. Indicate the place where you ate (home-kitchen, home-living room, restaurant, etc.).

3. Describe the specific food eaten or drunk during a 24-hour period, beginning with the first meal or snack (e.g., fried chicken, plain yogurt); use brand names.

4. Indicate the amount of food or beverage (e.g., ½ cup, 1 slice, 1 chicken leg, etc.).

Modified from Simko, M.D., Cowell, C., and Gilbride, J.A.: *Nutrition assessment: a comprehensive guide for planning intervention*, Rockville, Md, 1984, Aspen Publishers.

Table 13.4 Food Frequency Form

Client's Name: _____ Date: _____

Interviewer: _____

Food	Don't eat	Do eat	Serving Size	Number of Servings Per Week
I. Animal and vegetable protein foods				
Chicken				
Beef, hamburger, veal				
Liver, kidney, tongue, etc.				
Lamb, goat				
Cold cuts, hot dogs				
Pork, ham, sausage				
Bacon				
Fish				
Kidney beans, pinto beans, lentils				
Soybeans				
Tofu				
Eggs				
Nuts or seeds				
Peanut butter				
II. Milk and milk products				
Milk, fluid: Type: _____				
Milk, dry				
Milk, evaporated				
Condensed milk				
Cottage cheese				
Cheese (all kinds except cottage)				
Yogurt				
Pudding and custard flan				
Milkshake				
Sherbert				
Ice cream				
Ice milk				

(continued)

Table 13.4 *(continued)*

Food	Don't eat	Do eat	Serving Size	Servings Per Week
III. Grain Products				
Whole grain bread				
White bread				
Rolls, biscuits, muffins				
Crackers, pretzels				
Pancakes, waffles				
Cereals: Brand: _____				
White rice				
Brown rice				
Noodles, macaroni, grits, hominy				
Tortillas (flour)				
Tortillas (corn)				
Bulgar				
Popcorn				
Wheat germ				
IV. Vitamin-C-rich fruits and vegetables				
Tomato, tomato sauce, or tomato juice				
Orange or orange juice				
Tangerine				
Grapefruit or grapefruit juice				
Papaya, mango				
Strawberries, cantaloupe				
White potato, yautia, yams, plantain, yucca				
Turnip				
Peppers (green, red, chili)				
V. Leafy green vegetables				
Dark green or red lettuce				
Asparagus				
Swiss chard				
Bok choy				
Cabbage				
Broccoli				
Brussel sprouts				
Scallions				

(continued)

Table 13.4 *(continued)*

Food	Don't eat	Do eat	Serving Size	Number of Servings Per Week
Spinach				
Greens (beet, collard, kale, turnip, mustard)				
VI. Other fruits and vegetables				
Carrots				
Artichoke				
Corn				
Sweet potato or yam				
Zucchini				
Summer squash				
Winter squash				
Green peas				
Green and yellow beans				
Beets				
Cucumbers or celery				
Peach				
Apricot				
Apple				
Banana				
Pineapple				
Cherries				
VII. Snacks, sweets, and beverages				
Potato chips				
French fries				
Cakes, pies, cookies				
Sweet rolls, doughnuts				
Candy				
Sugar or honey				
Carbonated beverages (sodas)				
Coffee: Type: _____				
Tea: Type: _____				
Cocoa				
Wine, beer, cocktails				
Fruit drink				
VIII. Other foods not listed that you regularly eat				
_____				
_____				

Modified from California Dept. of Health, 1975.

Table 13.5 Food Diary

Name: _____ Date: _____

Please write down everything you eat for 3 days before your next appointment.

To do this:

1. Write down everything you eat or drink in the order in which it was eaten. Use brand names.
2. Include meals and snacks as well as gum and candy.
3. Write down the amount you eat. Use standard measuring cups and spoons. Record meat portions as ounces.
4. Write down items added to food (sugar on cereal, butter on bread, salad dressing to salad, etc.).
5. Write down the time you eat.
6. Write down how you prepared it (baked, fried, broiled, etc.).
7. Include a list of any vitamin and/or mineral supplements you take. Write down the name of the supplement, the amount of vitamins or minerals it contains, and the amount taken.

Examples:

Day 1: Time	Food and Preparation	Amount
12:30 PM	Peanut butter sandwich	1 tablespoon peanut butter 2 slices bread, whole wheat
	Milk, 2%	6 ounces

Make a separate sheet for each day.

Modified from California Dept. of Health, 1975.

Table 13.6 Food and Activity Record

Date _____ Name _____

Time	Food (quantity-type)	Activity and Length of Time	Where/ with whom	Mood*	How hungry
Examples					
9:00 AM	Hershey's chocolate candy bar (1 large)	15 min. in hall	School friend	Tired	Very
3:00 PM	Potato chips ½ medium bag	30 min. watching TV	Home, alone	Bored	A little
5:30 PM	Cola (regular) 1 can	Thirsty	Work, another store clerk	"Down"	Thirsty
7:00 PM	Cookies (3 small chocolate chip)	Late for dinner	Work, alone	Upset	Very

*Anxious, bored, content, depressed, "down," angry, tired, happy, relaxed, "up," celebrating, other

Modified from J. Endres & R. Rockwell (1985). *Food, Nutrition, and the Young Child*. Columbus, OH: Merrill Publishing Co.

Biochemical and Clinical Assessment: Fitness and Laboratory Tests

The biochemical and clinical assessment of an athlete through fitness and laboratory tests is an essential component to a complete nutrition assessment. Some settings, such as sports medicine clinics or fitness centers, allow partial or full access to these types of tests. Other settings, such as schools or athletic facilities, may not be equipped for the collection of such complete data. In these settings the information in the athlete's medical records, such as blood tests, diagnoses, or histories, can assist in the development of a comprehensive nutrition care plan. The importance of medical data can be determined by the counselor or medical practitioner, depending on the age, sex, and health status of the athlete. A list of suggested physical fitness, laboratory, and clinical tests can be found in table 13.7.

Psychosocial Influences

The psychological and social influences on an athlete can be positive and negative. In either case, these influences affect the eating habits and overall lifestyle of an athlete (see table 13.8). Sports medicine professionals need to be aware of the relevant issues affecting dietary intake, even though a complete psychological assessment is outside the scope of practice of most individuals acting as nutrition counselors. During the nutrition assessment and counseling, many psychological issues may be uncovered. Since most nutrition counselors are not qualified to accurately assess and treat these issues, referrals to qualified professionals are recommended to evaluate and care for potential problems.

Table 13.7 Physical Fitness and Laboratory Tests

Test/assessment	Relevant information
Fitness assessment	Heart rate
	Blood pressure
	Aerobic capacity
	Strength
	Flexibility
	Percent body fat
Blood tests	Cholesterol (total, HDL, LDL)
	Triglycerides
	Glucose
	Iron status (hemoglobin/hematocrit, serum iron[a], ferritin[b])
	Plasma electrolytes
Medical assessment	Current health status
	Medical history
	Cardiovascular risk status
	Orthopedic problems
	Recent and past injuries
	Gynecological problems

Note. Appropriateness of some of these tests will depend on the athlete's age and sex. In many practice settings some of this information will not be available.

[a]Serum iron can be evaluated in women; [b]Ferritin can be evaluated if anemia is suspected.

From Storlie, J. Nutrition Assessment of Athletes: A model for intergrating nutrition and physical performance indicators. *International Journal of Sport Nutrition* 1991, 1, 192-204.

Table 13.8   Psychosocial Influences

Dimension	Factors to consider
Social influences	Forms of support
Family members	Sources of conflict/friction
Friends	Vicarious interests
Teammates	Expectations/pressures
Coaches	Role modeling
Celebrities	
Self-concept	Body image
	Self-efficacy
	Self-confidence
	Fears of failure, fears of competition
	Locus of control
Competitive goals and commitment	Realistic aspirations (athletic talent, self-discipline)
	Priority/importance
	Competitive anxieties
Attitudes and philosophy toward life	Balanced vs. imbalanced approach
	Aspirations (career, school, other areas)
	Tendency to be driven or single-minded
	Need for power and control
	Stress patterns/life satisfaction

From Storlie, J. Nutrition Assessment of Athletes: A model for intergrating nutrition and physical performance indicators. *International Journal of Sport Nutrition* 1991, 1, 192-204.

Storlie (1991, p. 199) has described several scenarios in which psychosocial influences commonly affect an athlete's health and physical performance:

Parents may have a vicarious interest in a child's athletic performance borne out of their own past failures. This could pressure a young athlete into experiencing competitive anxieties, obsessions with exercise, and even eating disorders. On the other hand, parents can be supportive and encourage their children's participation in sports. A healthy mentoring relationship with a coach can motivate an athlete's performance, but some coaches badger athletes to the point of rebellion. Family members, friends, peers, coaches, and celebrities are all role models; athletes learn both good and bad practices from these people.

Athletes who are prone to pathogenic weight behaviors appear to be particularly vulnerable to disturbances in body image, fear of failure, and a high need for control and perfection. Major incongruencies between athletic aspirations and abilities, body image and ideal weight, or perceptions of self versus others' perceptions are indicators of potential psychological problems. When exercise and competition become all-consuming, work, school, and other activities are affected and the athlete's lifestyle can become narrow and unbalanced.

NUTRITION COUNSELING STRATEGIES

Nutrition counseling, like screening and assessment, is usually led by the athletic trainer or sports physician. However, the intervention is usually the most successful when a team approach that includes all the sports medicine professionals is used. The athletic trainer or sports physician may take the lead role, conducting the counseling sessions and giving direction to the other sports medicine professionals. The coach and physical therapist are usually involved on a more daily basis, observing the athlete and answering questions or referring the athlete back to the athletic trainer or physician for more specific information.

Eating behaviors are determined by

- biological factors,
- psychological factors, and
- sociocultural factors (Michéner, 1989).

Gut hormones, thermoregulatory mechanisms, and blood glucose levels are biological factors affected by exercise that influences eating behaviors. Depending on these biological changes, an athlete's brain receives messages from the body that it needs to eat or drink. But these natural biological urges can be overcome. Psychological factors are often more powerful in influencing eating behaviors than biological factors. Psychological factors are many and varied and include emotional conflict, self-image, and attitudes toward nutrition. For example, an athlete may be emotionally torn between an internal noncompetitive spirit and an external motivation to compete to make his or her parents proud. This conflict can cause psychological instability that will ultimately affect eating behaviors, the most classic of which is either loss of appetite or overeating.

Sociocultural factors also play a strong role in determining eating patterns and behaviors. Peer influence, time constraints, and lack of accurate information, among other factors, play a significant part in forming the eating behaviors of individuals. The dietary choices of athletes who travel on the road together are clearly influenced by the eating establishments made available to them and the foods that coaches and other teammates select. Nutritional misinformation and the lack of practical and accurate nutritional information are notorious sociocultural factors that influence the eating patterns of athletes. In fact, Madison Avenue may have a greater influence on the eating patterns of many athletes than bona fide sources of nutritional information.

The Nutrition Care Plan

The nutrition care plan is the guide to the nutritional intervention. It includes the recommendations and plan for change, how the plans will be implemented, and the follow-up plan. The general categories of recommendations and plans are obtaining more information, the treatment strategy, and education. The plan is built on the data collected in the assessment, the lifestyle needs of the athlete, the goals of the athlete, and the optimal nutritional recommendations (even though the final negotiations may reach only satisfactory nutritional intake levels). To achieve a successful outcome, the athlete must be an active participant in the development of the plan and must agree to the strategies and goals stated in the plan.

Developing a practical nutrition care plan requires assessing the athlete's present nutritional status and requirements, taking into consideration biological, psychological, and sociocultural determinants of eating behaviors. Most athletes need a normal, well-balanced diet. The design of the diet itself can be based on the U.S. Dietary Guidelines (see figure 13.1) and the athlete's calorie requirements, as previously discussed. In specific situations, however, the demands of training and competition may result in increased physiological demands, which, if not met by diet, may negatively influence performance (table 13.9). To appropriately address these circumstances, a specialist with a sophisticated knowledge and understanding of sports nutrition is required, and such a referral should be made to ensure the health and performance of the athlete.

Table 13.9 Physiological Demands of Exercise and Possible Nutrient Needs

Physiological demand	Possible nutrient needs
Aerobic energy production for endurance exercise	Increased calories Increased carbohydrates Increased protein Increased B-complex vitamins Increased water and electrolytes

Prolonged anaerobic workout[a]
  Hockey
  Soccer
  Downhill skiing
	Increased carbohydrates
	Increased B-complex vitamins
	Increased water

Musculoskeletal stress	Increased protein Increased carbohydrates[b] Adequate calories[c] Increased vitamin C Increased iron and zinc Increased vitamins B_6 and B_{12}[d] Increased calcium[e]

Thermoregulatory stress
  Endurance sports
  Environmental conditions
  Long or frequent air travel
	Increased water
	Increased electrolytes

Weight loss
  Wrestling
  Body building
  Gymnastics
  Ballet
	Decreased calories
	Increased nutrient density of foods
	Increased water

Immune system
  Frequent injuries or illness
  Overtraining
  Fatigue[f]
	Increased protein
	Increased vitamin C
	Increased water and electrolytes
	Increased iron and zinc
	Increased B-complex vitamins

[a]While anaerobic sports do not typically deplete carbohydrate stores, intermittent anaerobic workouts that last for several hours could delpete muscle glycogen through anaerobic glycolysis; [b]Carbohydrates will spare protein; [c]Caloric requirements must be adequate to spare protein and promote proper healing, but could decrease due to inactivity during injury rehabilitation; [d]Associated with protein metabolism; [e]In bone injuries; [f]Due to the hectic schedules that some athletes must keep to handle long workouts, travel, jobs, and/or school schedules, they may not get enough sleep and relaxation.

From Storlie, J. Nutrition Assessment of Athletes: A model for intergrating nutrition and physical performance indicators. *International Journal of Sport Nutrition* 1991, 1, 192-204.

Counseling Strategies for Lifestyle Change

It should be clear that dietary change is really lifestyle change. Altering eating behaviors often requires changing other life habits beyond diet. For instance, an athlete who lacked an appetite after most training sessions and never ate much until the next day learns that eating good carbohydrate sources immediately after training assists with the replenishment of spent glycogen in the muscles, thereby improving endurance for the next day's training session. This athlete has decided to make one dietary change—to consume a good source of carbohydrates shortly after each training session. This singular dietary change might involve the following lifestyle changes:

- Changes in shopping habits to have an appropriate food on hand after training
- Knowledge acquisition about good food sources of carbohydrates
- Time management skills, as the athlete never had to stop to eat after training before
- Some experimentation and emotional considerations, as the athlete will have to find foods that are satisfying and convince his or her body that even though there is no hunger it needs to eat (Laquatra & Danish, 1988)

Obstacles block the path of many changes, but lifestyle changes seem to be the most difficult to achieve. Athletes are motivated to improve their performance. If they understand that these diet and lifestyle changes will assist their performance, they generally put forth a good effort.

It is crucial for sports medicine professionals to recognize that food is more than just a mode of transportation for nutrients into the body. Food is a very intimate and emotional component of our lives. It is at the center of many religious and cultural celebrations and is often linked to significant family memories, both good and bad. Food has been used for reward and punishment and may represent a powerful emotional concept to some individuals (Kleiner, 1993).

Sports medicine professionals must recognize that although athletes may cognitively understand the benefits of changing their eating behaviors, they cannot do so until they overcome the emotional barriers to that change. Instead of the professional designing a strategy for diet and behavioral change, the athlete must be involved in the process to set his or her own goals for gradual change. This helps to secure the athlete's commitment and ensure effective and permanent change (Kleiner, 1993).

Regular follow-up is essential to successful behavioral change. If monitoring the athlete's progress indicates that the athlete appears to be having difficulty in adhering to the jointly established plan for change, the sports medicine professional should consider involving other health professionals, such as social and psychological counselors, registered dietitians, and nurse educators.

The counseling process can be divided into the following 10 strategies (Michener, 1989):

1. Develop a partnership with the athlete.
2. Educate the athlete.
3. Explain behavior–health–performance relationships.
4. Assess barriers to behavioral change.
5. Obtain the athlete's commitment.
6. Encourage the athlete's participation.
7. Use a combination of strategies.
8. Design a behavior modification plan.

9. Monitor progress.
10. Involve other health professionals.

To best describe how these strategies can be applied, the following sections use practical scenarios to explain and demonstrate each counseling strategy.

Develop a Partnership With the Athlete

Since it is essential that the person undergoing counseling trust the counselor, taking the time to get to know the athlete and for him or her to get to know you is essential to a successful counseling outcome.

As the coach of a high school swim team, Tim Wrigley has little time to get to know each athlete individually. But he knows that one way to hear about the personal goals and home lives of his athletes at the beginning of each year is to ask them what they eat. Coach Wrigley knows that even though most of his athletes are at a healthy weight, they still need to eat a healthy diet to promote growth, health, and athletic performance. He begins the process by talking to the team in a group setting about a healthy diet. Sometimes he invites a registered dietitian to talk to the team as well. Each team member is given the job of recording his diet for three days, including what, when, where, and why foods were eaten. Then each team member meets individually with the coach to discuss his diet diary.

During this meeting the coach and the athlete discuss each other's goals: the athlete's personal goals and the coach's goals for the team. Together they determine how the athlete can best contribute to the team. With these goals in mind, the athlete's diet is discussed and compared with a healthy dietary pattern. This evaluation process leads to dietary goal setting for the athlete.

This process has allowed the coach and the athlete to develop a partnership, with recognition of each other's goals and desire to change.

Educate the Athlete

Accurate information is a powerful tool in behavior modification. Bright, motivated athletes looking for information often succumb to false or misleading nutritional information. By giving them accurate information and not berating them for following poor advice, they often will change their behaviors quite easily.

Janet began running cross-country for her high school team this season. It is her first experience at long-distance running. She had always competed at short-distance events before. When she started training, she was doing fairly well, but as the season wore on, her performance seemed to diminish, especially toward the latter half of her runs. Sometimes she felt so weak that she would have to stop and walk for awhile.

The team athletic trainer noticed that Janet didn't stop for fluid breaks very often. Since the weather had gotten warmer, she wondered whether Janet wasn't well hydrated enough to perform at peak levels. When the athletic trainer asked Janet how often she replenished her fluids, Janet replied that it was too hard to run with water in her stomach, so she skipped most of her fluid stops.

The athletic trainer realized that Janet's performance was probably suffering because of dehydration but that the only way to get Janet to change her behavior was to educate her about the importance of fluids and exercise. Then they could begin to talk about how Janet could get used to having fluid in her stomach while she was running without discomfort.

She gave Janet educational materials that she had about fluids and exercise. She also suggested that Janet talk with other successful athletes who had discovered their own strategies for comfortably replacing fluids during running. Without the initial education Janet would probably have been resistant to discussing how to go about including fluids during training and competition. Now she was willing to experiment and was motivated to get used to replenishing her fluids during exercise.

Explain Behavior–Health–Performance Relationships

Like the previous strategy, another powerful technique is giving the athlete more information about how his or her health ultimately affects athletic performance. Again, never berate an athlete for following incorrect or unscientific information. Instead, educate the athlete about the positive influences of behavior based on accurate information.

Malcolm is a bodybuilder. Since Malcolm used to be out of shape, he really likes the way his body looks since he began training, especially how flat his stomach is. Malcolm is very serious about his diet and sticks to his dietary regime religiously. Malcolm generally feels great, but lately his bowels have been irregular enough that he has begun to feel rather constipated. Being very meticulous, Malcolm went to see his family physician.

After examining Malcolm, his physician asked him about his training and diet program. It soon became evident that Malcolm had very little fiber in his diet: no fruits, few vegetables, and only refined breads, cereals, and pastas. This was probably the cause of his constipation. When the physician asked why Malcolm had eliminated so much fiber from his diet, Malcolm responded that he didn't want his stomach distended from the gas that he usually got from eating high-fiber foods.

Malcolm's physician explained that by eliminating these foods in his diet, he had removed many important vitamins and minerals essential to health and physical performance. In addition, without fresh fruits, vegetables, and whole grains, fiber was lacking in his diet, leading to his problem with constipation. Even though Malcolm felt that he looked better when he avoided gas-forming foods, the constipation was inhibiting his training and ultimately his body-shaping goals.

Together Malcolm and his physician worked out a plan to include enough fibrous foods in his diet to eliminate his constipation problem. Then they both agreed that there would be no harm if Malcolm eliminated the most gas-producing foods just a few days before a competition so that there would not be any distention in his abdomen from gas.

Assess Barriers to Behavioral Change

Just as one cannot drive a car through a brick wall, athletes cannot make behavioral changes with barriers in the way, be they real or imagined. Barriers to behavioral change must be discussed at the outset of counseling so that they can be dealt with in a way that either allows the athlete to eliminate them or work around them.

Cynthia is a member of a semiprofessional volleyball team. During the off-season and preseason she tries to eat well. She lives in an apartment with two roommates, and they each do their own shopping and cooking, giving Cynthia pretty good control over the food that she eats. When volleyball season begins in earnest and the team goes on the road, Cynthia begins to have a hard time making healthy food choices. When the team is traveling for a week at a time, Cynthia feels that her performance diminishes by the end of the week because she isn't eating as well as she would have been at home. She finally goes to see the team's athletic trainer to ask for help.

After they discuss her problem, the athletic trainer asks Cynthia what her biggest roadblocks are to eating well while traveling. Cynthia explains that to save time and money she usually eats breakfast at a fast-food restaurant. When the team eats together, she feels that her choices are limited because of the food available on the menu. And often she finds that if she gets hungry during the day she eats out of vending machines.

Listening to Cynthia's description gave the athletic trainer the opportunity to assess the problems and address the barriers that were keeping her from changing her behavior. Even though Cynthia thought that she had no healthy food choices, she really did. She just had to learn what those choices were.

The athletic trainer suggested that for breakfast, Cynthia choose cereal with low-fat milk and orange juice, selections that are available at most fast-food restaurants that serve breakfast. When eating at a restaurant, she could order all side dishes, such as vegetables, salad, baked potato, cottage cheese, and fruit, if there was no healthy alternative on the menu. The athletic trainer also told her that she could ask to have something broiled rather than fried and have sandwiches served without spreads and dressings to try to lower their fat content. Another important suggestion was that Cynthia pack her own snack foods, such as pretzels, low-fat granola bars, fruit, and juices, to avoid succumbing to vending machines when she needed some extra energy.

This information was exactly what Cynthia needed. What appeared to be insurmountable barriers fell by the wayside once Cynthia had the information she needed to make healthy food choices.

Obtain the Athlete's Commitment

The athlete must want to change and must concur with the method of achieving change. Without a commitment from the athlete, it is unlikely that any positive changes will occur. Without such commitment, to the athlete behavioral change will appear to be someone else's responsibility (e.g. the nutrition counselor, the coach, the athletic trainer) rather than the athlete's own responsibility.

Steve, a competitive cyclist, walked into the registered dietitian's office with a grocery bag full of the dietary supplements that he'd been taking for the last year. He was there to have his diet evaluated and to see whether he could improve his athletic performance. After describing his diet, he showed the dietitian what supplements he used. She asked him how and why he took each supplement. Steve explained that most of the supplements were recommended by a friend who was an Olympic contender and who had sold Steve the supplements.

After analyzing Steve's diet, the dietitian showed him the strong points and weak points of his diet. Basically, he was eating great. His diet wasn't lacking any of the components found in the supplements that he was taking. But Steve was still sure that at least some of those supplements were making a difference.

After the dietitian explained that there may be a few nutrients that are needed in extra amounts by athletes performing high-energy exercise, she and Steve negotiated the supplements that he would continue to take and those he was willing to give up. They decided that as long as his performance did not diminish, he would stay away from the supplements that he had given up, and they agreed to discuss whether he felt the need to continue on any supplements at a future meeting. In a way, Steve was partially relieved because he was spending over $50 a month on the bagful of pills and powders. Obtaining Steve's commitment to this strategy was critical to a positive outcome. If Steve didn't really believe that this was his own decision, his performance could possibly diminish from emotional or psychological reactions, rather than physiological ones, to withdrawing from the supplements.

Encourage the Athlete's Participation

By having some control of the process, the athlete becomes involved and committed to the goal. Participating in the design of their own nutrition plan places athletes in a role of responsibility for the outcome of the plan. Most athletes do not want to fail.

Teri is a 14-year-old gymnast who is beginning to become concerned about her body weight. Dr. Wright, the team physician, is aware of the potential for the development of eating disorders in female gymnasts. Dr. Wright has learned some techniques for giving the young girls healthy tools that will help them understand and control their diets and hopefully decrease their risk of eating disorders.

Dr. Wright has set up a meeting with Teri and her coach to discuss Teri's diet and body weight. After evaluating her body weight and body fat, Teri, Dr. Wright, and her coach agreed that Teri could safely lose about six pounds (three kilograms). This would keep her competitive yet maintain her health and growth. Next they looked at Teri's diet and discovered that she could cut back on some calories in order to assist with weight loss. Most of Teri's extra calories were coming from fat.

Dr. Wright enlisted Teri's participation in her own diet planning by teaching Teri about fat and then showing her how to determine the number of fat grams and calories that she was eating each day. Teri discovered that by eating lots of fried foods and snacks such as chips, cookies, and candy, she had been eating 30 to 40 extra grams of fat every day. The extra fat grams meant extra calories that she didn't need. By just decreasing her fat grams, Teri could lose weight at a healthy rate of one-half to one pound (one-quarter to one-half kilogram) per week.

Teri's job was to make sure that she ate a healthy, balanced diet and to count her fat grams every day. Thus she learned how to make healthy food choices and to control her fat and calorie intake. Teri would now have these practical dietary tools to use throughout her life and lose her unwanted pounds at the same time.

Use a Combination of Strategies

Not all strategies work for every athlete, but at least one of the strategies should work for any athlete who really wants to change. Sometimes the appropriate strategy is not obvious, so trying a variety or combination of strategies might prove to be successful when a singular approach did not work. As long as an athlete is still interested, keep trying.

Derrick has enjoyed cross-country skiing and target shooting since he was a child. He recently met a coach who trains athletes for the biathlon event. Derrick thought that he'd give it a try. His skiing was excellent, but his precision with a rifle was slightly off. With practice Derrick improved and was able to win some events, but he still wasn't as accurate as his coach thought that he could be. At this point they began discussing Derrick's lifestyle. It soon became clear that Derrick really enjoyed drinking coffee. When the coach explained that the caffeine in coffee might decrease his shooting precision, Derrick refused to believe that coffee affected him at all. And he continued to drink his usual three to five cups a day.

The coach's next strategy was to educate Derrick. He brought him research studies and professional articles written about the effects that caffeine can have on precision rifle shooting. He also brought articles about the dehydrating effects of caffeine, an undesirable effect for a cross-country skier. He even had testimonials from other biathletes about how their performances had improved since eliminating caffeine from their diets. None of this information seemed to make an impression on Derrick.

Next the coach asked Derrick why his coffee was so important to him and why it was such a big deal to even switch to decaffeinated coffee, if not quit altogether. Derrick replied that his dad had always labored hard outside and was always a big coffee drinker. To the end of his days, his dad had said that the only reason he could work so hard for so long was because he drank coffee. It was the coffee that kept him going. If not for the coffee that Derrick's mom had made his dad every day, he never would have been able to accomplish what he had in his life. Derrick was sure that his dad was right, so he was afraid to give up drinking coffee, thinking that he would fail rather than improve his performance.

Once the coach learned this information, he challenged Derrick to a test. Derrick would slowly eliminate caffeine from his diet. If his caffeine-free performance was not better than his performance on caffeine, he could go back to drinking coffee. Derrick agreed. Together they mapped a set of goals for Derrick to achieve: a timeline for slowly eliminating the caffeine from his diet, then the point when he would begin the test.

Derrick stuck to his coffee-elimination goals and took the test. His performance was significantly better compared with his performance on caffeine. Derrick had shown himself that he could overcome his fear of eliminating coffee from his diet and proved to himself that it made a difference in his performance.

Design a Behavior Modification Plan

Most athletes like to know where they are going and how they are going to get there. A behavior modification plan allows the athlete to design a set of small, short-term goals, as well as larger, long-term goals. This plan allows for the achievement of frequent successes, supporting further positive change. When failures occur, they do not seem so overwhelming, and since the plan is clearly laid out, it is easy to get back to it and continue toward the goal.

Mark plays high school football in the fall and wrestles in the winter. He needs to bulk up for football and get lean for wrestling. Each year Mark stuffs himself to gain weight before football and then starves himself and sweats to lose weight for wrestling. After doing this for two years in a row, Mark's mother intervened and suggested that he see a registered dietitian to help him design a healthier strategy to manage his body weight.

With the dietitian, Mark designed a long-term weight control strategy that included several short-term goals. Instead of trying to gain and lose weight in very short amounts of time, Mark set several short-term goals for his body weight over periods of several months. He also decided that he wouldn't try to have such a dramatic weight change between wrestling and football. He stated, in fact, that he probably performed better in the heavier wrestling weight class. He also planned to add strength training to his training routine so that he would gain muscle before football and maintain muscle before wrestling. Thus the management of his body weight wouldn't be as difficult and certainly not as unhealthy. Mark's specific plans looked like this:

Long-term goals:

- *Maintain a more stable body weight year round.*
- *Eat a high-carbohydrate, low-fat, moderate-protein diet that meets my energy needs.*
- *Combine training workouts with strength training.*

Short-term goals:

- *May—Begin to increase strength training and calories to gain about one pound (one-half kilogram) per week (weight gain may not show for two to three weeks).*
- *July—Evaluate weight-gain progress. Adjust calories and training to maintain or continue to gain body weight.*
- *August—Same as July.*
- *Late August—Begin football season. Adjust calories and training to maintain weight.*
- *Late November—Increase aerobic training and decrease calories to lose one to two pounds (one half to one kilogram) of body weight per week (depending on weight-loss needs) until wrestling season begins.*

Monitor Progress

As a health professional, it is important for you to monitor the athletes that you have counseled to make sure that there have been no misunderstandings between you and your client in the delivery of information and in the planning and execution of their nutrition goals. In addition, it is reassuring to the athlete for you to check up on them periodically. Monitoring progress is a helpful tool for reinforcing the goals that have been set for behavioral change, answering any questions that have arisen, and dealing with any new barriers or situations that might occur during the process.

Ted plays professional football. At the beginning of training camp in the summer, he felt that he wasn't eating quite right and that if he lost some weight, he could improve his performance. Ted and his athletic trainer set up a meeting to talk about diet and weight loss. A plan was set up for Ted to follow, and he felt that he could stick to it.

Once the regular playing season began, Ted believed that he was following his diet, but he began to gain weight. His athletic trainer noticed Ted's weight gain and asked Ted how his diet and weight-loss plan were going. They both realized that even though it was now the regular playing season, Ted wasn't getting as hard a workout on a daily basis as he had been during training camp, so he needed to eat fewer calories to maintain his weight loss. After adjusting Ted's diet plan, his athletic trainer recommended that they meet again every few weeks just to check on Ted's progress and make sure that nothing else had changed to interfere with their weight-loss strategy. At the end of the season, they would evaluate how his body weight had changed and probably would need to readjust his diet plan again to compensate for his off-season activity level.

Involve Other Health Professionals

Frequently, an athlete has a problem that can be taken care of only by a nutrition professional. An athlete may also encounter a problem that requires other health care expertise, such as a physician or a psychologist. It is imperative that sports medicine professionals understand their own practice limitations and involve other health professionals when necessary to provide adequate care for the athletes whom they counsel.

Dave is a diver on his college swim team. He has always watched his weight because he knows that it makes a difference in his performance. He recently went to see the team physician because he's had several colds back to back, making it hard for him to train.

During his examination the physician asked Dave to get on the scale. He had lost 15 pounds (7 kilograms) since last season, placing him in the underweight category for his height. When the physician asked Dave about his diet, Dave was rather reluctant to talk about how much he was eating.

At this point the physician became concerned that Dave was engaging in some abnormal eating behaviors or possibly had an eating disorder. The physician talked to Dave about the effects of low body weight on health, immune function, and ultimately athletic performance. He told Dave that because he was not an expert with diet but was concerned that Dave's diet might be inadequate, he thought it would be good for Dave to meet with a team of experts with experience in working with athletes, diet, and behavior. Dave agreed to the referral. The group of experts included a registered dietitian, a psychologist, and a physician. The team physician assured Dave that he would be in close contact with this expert team so that Dave's athletic goals were not set aside and he could continue to dive for the team as long as he remained healthy and able.

CASE STUDY

At the end of his senior year of college, Tim was drafted to play professional basketball for the NBA. After graduation Tim weighed 225 pounds (102 kilograms) and was 6 feet 7 inches (2 meters) tall, with a medium frame size. He felt that he was a little overfat, so before basketball training camp, Tim had been trying to lose weight. His two-week precamp diet consisted of the following:

Weekdays:

8:00 A.M.   Six ounces (177 milliliters) orange juice or 8 to 12 ounces (237 to 355 milliliters) of cola drink

1:00 P.M.	*Fast-food chicken sandwich, french fries, lemonade*
8:00 P.M.	*Sometimes just fruit; sometimes a casserole that included noodles or potatoes, meat, and a vegetable*

Only breakfast changed on the weekend.

Weekend breakfast:

10:00 A.M.	*Three eggs, three sausage links, a piece of fruit, six ounces (177 milliliters) orange juice*

Tim drinks beverages only with meals, never between meals, and rarely while he is in practice or playing. He states that he does not drink much during practice or games because his former coach believed strongly that full bellies inhibit performance on the court. Tim does not drink any alcohol.

When training camp began and Tim moved from his family home to his new city with the team, he lived at a hotel until he knew that he would have a permanent position with the team. Soon into training camp, Tim lost his appetite. After the first week of training camp his performance began to diminish. After the second week the coach asked the team physician to take a look at Tim. After stepping on the scale, Tim and the physician learned that Tim had lost 13 pounds (6 kilograms) since the beginning of training camp two weeks before. He now weighed 203 pounds (92 kilograms).

QUESTIONS FOR ANALYSIS

1. Tim is suffering from several problems. What is the most likely and serious health concern?

2. What are Tim's other health concerns?

3. What would be your first counseling strategy in this case?

4. What barriers does Tim have to behavioral change?

5. Design a care plan of strategies for Tim that will support his efforts to win a spot on the NBA team in the next few weeks while helping him maintain his health now and in the future.

SUMMARY

The relationship between diet and exercise is clear: what, where, and how an athlete eats affects health and physical performance now and in the future. Athletes obtain nutritional information from many sources. Unfortunately, many of those sources are either incorrect or unscrupulous, and athletes suffer the consequences of nutritional misinformation.

Dietary practices are affected by physiological and psychosocial influences. Changing dietary behaviors is a complex issue and often requires lifestyle changes. Sports medicine professionals must be aware of their athletes' nutritional health. By offering appropriate education and experience, sports medicine professionals can counsel athletes regarding dietary requirements, eating behaviors, and food choices. At the least, they must be able to spot a problem and refer the athlete to an appropriate health care practitioner.

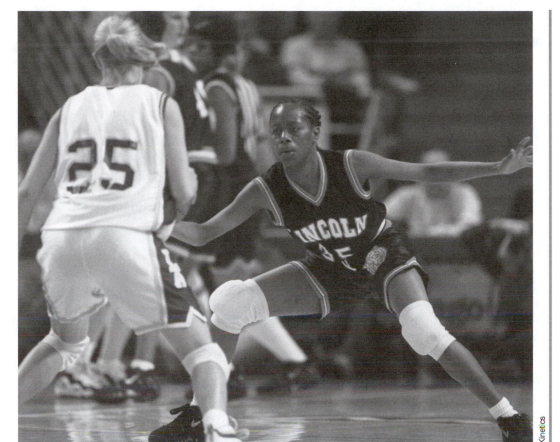

chapter 14

Counseling for the Management of Stress and Anxiety

Vikki Krane, PhD, *Bowling Green State University*
Christy Greenleaf, MS, *University of North Carolina at Greensboro*

CHAPTER OBJECTIVES

Identify the stages of the stress process

Explain the relationship between stress and injury

Differentiate between stress and anxiety theories and apply them to injury and rehabilitation

Implement strategies to reduce stress and anxiety in injured athletes

stress—An imbalance between the perceived demands of a situation and an individual's perceived abilities to meet those demands.

anxiety—The emotional or cognitive dimension of physiological arousal.

Stress and **anxiety** are very common in athletic environments. Stress may result from sport-specific concerns such as performing up to one's ability, improving on one's last performance, not performing well, fear of failure, feelings of inadequacy, and losing (Gould, Horn, & Spreeman, 1983; Scanlan & Passer, 1978). Fear of becoming injured or aggravating an injury can lead to stress and anxiety. Athletes also experience stress and anxiety related to nonsport situations, such as keeping up with school work, family problems, relationship issues, financial concerns, and life direction concerns (Gould, Jackson, & Finch, 1993; Scanlan, Stein, & Ravizza, 1991). Often these concerns follow athletes into the sport environment and affect their performance. Additionally, stress and anxiety may increase athletes' possibility of becoming injured and can affect how they cope with injury and rehabilitation when an injury occurs. Because of the prevalence of stress and anxiety experienced by athletes, it is essential to understand how it may affect athletes and its role in athletic injury and rehabilitation.

Gould and Krane (1992) emphasized the need to differentiate among stress-related terminology. Specific to the focus of this chapter is the distinction between stress and anxiety. Stress occurs when there is an imbalance between perceived environmental demands and perceived response capability, when failure to meet the demand has important consequences (McGrath, 1970). Anxiety, on the other hand, is the cognitive dimension of physiological arousal (Gould & Krane, 1992). Thus stress is a person's interpretation of the environmental demands, and anxiety is the cognitive reaction to perceived inability to cope with those demands. For example, a swimmer who recently returned to competition after rehabilitating a shoulder injury is preparing for a regional swim meet. She questions her ability to achieve her goal of qualifying for the state meet because she is not sure of her endurance and the strength of her shoulder. This swimmer is experiencing stress. The regional swim meet is important to her because it is her last chance to qualify for the state meet, yet the swimmer doubts her ability (i.e., she perceives an imbalance between her ability and the demands of the environment). The swimmer may also experience anxiety in reaction to this stress. During warm-ups at the meet, she may notice that her muscles feel tense, her stomach feels funny, and she is having a hard time concentrating. Consequently, stress is the response to her appraisal of the situation, and anxiety is her cognitive reaction to the stressful situation.

Although often the terms *stress* and *anxiety* are used interchangeably, the distinction between them is important for theoretical and practical reasons. Stress and anxiety can influence injured athletes differently, and each can be addressed through different intervention strategies. Accordingly, the purpose of this chapter is to provide (1) theoretical frameworks for understanding the relationships among stress, anxiety, and athletic performance and (2) practical applications or interventions based on these theoretical frameworks to decrease the negative impact of stress and anxiety on injured athletes.

A CONCEPTUAL FRAMEWORK OF STRESS

McGrath (1970) described stress as a process during which an individual interprets environmental demands as threatening or nonthreatening. Based on that interpretation, psychological reactions (e.g., fear) or physiological reactions (e.g., increased heart rate or perspiration) occur, which then affect behavior. This process perspective of stress emphasizes the environmental influences inherent in stress and differentiates it from anxiety, which can be considered a cognitive manifestation of stress (Gould & Krane, 1992). It is important to note that stress involves one's perception of a situation, while anxiety refers to a cognitive appraisal of one's self (i.e., expectations, body sensations).

Palmer and Dryden (1995) developed a **multimodal-transactional model of stress** as the foundation to their approach to stress counseling and stress management. As they stated: "This model provides a simple but realistic explanation of the complicated nature of stress as it addresses the inter-relationship between the internal and external worlds of individuals" (p. 4). Consistent with a process view of stress, this model emphasizes the importance of individuals' reactions to a situation and their perceived abilities to cope with the situation.

The multimodal-transactional model of stress is described as a five-stage process, as depicted in figure 14.1 (Palmer & Dryden, 1995). In stage 1, an individual perceives pressure from an external source (e.g., a meeting with coach or teammates, a strength test). "Stage 2 reflects the individual's perception of the pressure or demand and her appraisal of her ability to deal with it" (Palmer & Dryden, 1995, p. 4). In stage 3, psychophysiological responses occur. As table 14.1 illustrates, these responses include affective, behavioral, biological, cognitive, imaginal, interpersonal, and sensory responses. Collectively, these psychophysiological responses are referred to as the **stress response** (Girdano, Everly, & Dusek, 1993; Palmer & Dryden, 1995). The stress response includes attempts by the individual to cope with the situation.

multimodal-transactional model of stress— A model of stress that considers the interrelationship between internal and external factors, an individual's reactions to a situation, and his or her perceived abilities to cope with the situation.

stress response— Psychological and physiological responses that occur when exposed to a stressor.

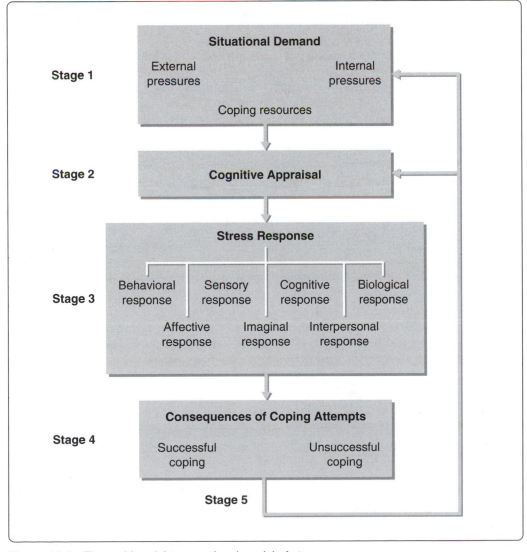

Figure 14.1 The multimodal-transactional model of stress.

From Palmer & Dryden (1995). *Counseling for stress problems.* Thousand Oaks, CA: Sage.

Table 14.1	Psychophysiological Responses to Stress That May Be Experienced by Injured Athletes
Affective	Anxiety; Anger; Guilt; Depression; Shame; Feeling sorry for oneself
Behavioral	Sleep disturbances; Restlessness; Aggressive behavior; Alcohol or drug abuse; Sulking, crying; Poor performance; Absenteeism; Clenched fists
Biological/ physiological	Muscular tension; Increased heart rate; Indigestion; Spasms in stomach; Pain; Headaches
Cognitive	Frustration; Worries; Distortion, exaggeration; Unrealistic performance expectations; Self-defeating statements; Self-handicapping
Imaginal	Images of failure; Images of reinjury; Flashbacks of being injured; Images of helplessness; Images of embarrassment
Interpersonal	Withdrawal; Manipulation; Argumentation
Sensory	Tension; Nausea; Cold sweat; Clammy hands; Pain; Butterflies in stomach

From Palmer & Dryden (1995). *Counseling for stress problems.* Thousand Oaks, CA: Sage.

The consequences of individuals' coping attempts constitute stage 4; they may successfully or unsuccessfully cope with the demands of the situation. The perceived success of coping attempts is important. When athletes perceive coping attempts as unsuccessful, this perpetuates the perception of their inability to cope with the situational demand, resulting in continued stress. However, positively perceived coping attempts eliminate further stress. The more importance placed on successfully meeting the demands of the situation by the individual, the greater the negative reaction to unsuccessful coping attempts.

Finally, stage 5 involves a feedback system in which the individual returns to a state of equilibrium (i.e., coping attempts were successful) or the individual continues to perceive the situation as threatening, and stress is prolonged (i.e., coping attempts were unsuccessful).

For example, an athlete perceives pressure from her coach to return to competition, yet she lacks confidence in her current physical ability to meet the demands of competition. This leads her to view meetings with the coach as threatening and stressful (stage 1). She is worried about meeting with the coach because she feels unable to stand up to the coach (stage 2). Knowing that she will be meeting with the coach later in the day, she is distracted, and her stomach is in knots (stage 3). To minimize the stress she is experiencing, she cancels the meeting so that she does not have to face the coach (stage 4). This alleviates her stress (stage 5) until the next time she is expected to meet with the coach. In this example, stress occurred because the athlete experienced an injury. Stress also may lead to the occurrence of injury.

INJURY AS A SOURCE OF STRESS

An injury, or the fear of injury, can be a source of stress experienced by athletes (Ievleva & Orlick, 1991). Athletes who have been injured most likely will have some negative emotional reaction or mood disturbance (Smith, Scott, & Wiese, 1990). The more serious the injury, the more likely that negative emotional disturbance will occur (A.M. Smith et al., 1990). When injured, athletes commonly experience anger, frustration, depression, and concerns about their future (Leddy, Lambert, & Ogles, 1994; Williams & Roepke, 1993). Injured athletes have to cope with feelings of helplessness, dependency on others, and withdrawal from physical activity and the social environment of their team (Lynch, 1988; McDonald & Hardy, 1990). They may become concerned about their perceived inability to cope with the injury and reha-bilitation process (A.M. Smith et al., 1990). All these feelings and concerns create a stressful situation for injured athletes.

STRESS AS A PRECURSOR TO INJURY

Andersen and Williams (1988) proposed a model of stress and athletic injury that suggests that the stress response may lead to increased injury risk (see figure 2.1 and a preliminary discussion of this model in chapter 2). Their model shows that a potentially stressful athletic situation is appraised by the individual athlete. Per-ceiving the situation as threatening (i.e., stressful) results in physiological responses (e.g., muscle tension) and attentional responses (e.g., lack of concentration, inappro-priate focus of attention), which increase the likelihood of injury. Andersen and Williams's model also proposes three categories of factors that affect the stress re-sponse: personality, history of stressors, and coping resources. Each of these factors may directly affect the stress response. Personality (e.g., anxiety, motivation, hardi-ness) and coping resources (e.g., stress management skills, psychological coping skills, social support) also may indirectly affect the stress response through the effects of the history of stressors. This model also specifies interventions that may lessen the impact of the stress response; these are discussed later in the chapter.

> *The model is predicated on the assumption that the two basic mechanisms behind the stress–injury relationship are increases in general muscle ten-sion and deficits in attention during stress. It is hypothesized that indi-viduals with a lot of stress in their lives who have personality traits that tend to exacerbate the stress response and few coping resources will, in a stressful situation, be more likely to appraise the situation as stressful, ex-hibit greater muscle tension and attentional changes, and thus be at greater risk of injury compared to individuals who have the opposite profile. (Andersen & Williams, 1988, p. 298)*

Much research exists that supports Andersen and Williams's (1988) stress and injury model. Specifically, there has been considerable focus on the relationship be-tween stress and the incidence of injury (Williams & Roepke, 1993). Typically, life stress is measured as the number of major changes or disruptions (e.g., death of a loved one, moving to a new home, changing schools) that an individual has experi-enced recently. These changes, however, may be interpreted by an individual as posi-tive or negative.

Although several studies have failed to support the stress–injury relationship (Passer & Seese, 1983; Williams, Haggert, Tonyman, & Wadsworth, 1986; Williams, Tonyman, & Wadsworth, 1986), negative life stress generally has been associated with the incidence of injury (e.g., Hardy & Riehl, 1988; Passer & Seese, 1983; Petrie, 1993b). For example, stress has been found to be associated with the frequency of injury in high school football players (Coddington & Troxel, 1980; Thompson & Mor-ris, 1994), alpine skiers (May, Veach, Reed, & Griffey, 1985), physical education ma-jors (Lysens, Auweele, & Ostyn, 1986), noncontact sport participants (baseball, soft-ball, tennis, and track; Hardy & Riehl, 1988), and gymnasts (Kerr & Minden, 1988; Petrie, 1992). Research also has shown that as the number of stressful life events increased, so did the number and severity of injuries (Hanson, McCullagh, & Tonyman, 1992; Kerr & Minden, 1988).

Additionally, studies have considered the role of factors theorized to moderate the stress–injury relationship (i.e., personality factors and coping resources). Studies examining the role of coping resources have supported that athletes with high stress and few coping resources are more likely to become injured than athletes with low coping resources alone (Hanson et al., 1992; Petrie, 1993a; Smith, Smoll, & Ptacek, 1990). High levels of social support seem to buffer the effects of stress and reduce the likelihood of injury in high-stress athletes (Petrie, 1993b; Williams & Roepke, 1993). Psychological skills also appear to affect the stress–injury relationship. R.E. Smith and colleagues (1990) found that athletes with low social support and few psychological skills were most likely to show a strong association between stress and injury. Athletes who have high levels of stress and low social support, psychological skills, and coping resources appear to be at highest risk of injury (R.E. Smith et al., 1990; Williams & Roepke, 1993).

Overall, studies have supported the Andersen and Williams (1988) model of stress and injury, suggesting that high levels of stress may increase the risk of sport injury. Generally, life events considered as negative are most likely to be associated with injury, especially if the athlete has few coping resources.

MULTIDIMENSIONAL ANXIETY THEORY

cognitive anxiety—Negative thoughts, concerns about performance, disrupted attention, and inability to concentrate.

Most current research on competitive anxiety is grounded in the multidimensional anxiety theory (Martens, Burton, Vealey, Bump, & Smith, 1990). This theory is based on the premise that anxiety consists of two subcomponents that have different antecedents and different relationships with performance. **Cognitive anxiety** includes a person's negative thoughts, concerns about performance, disrupted attention, and inability to concentrate (Davidson & Schwartz, 1976; Martens et al., 1990). **Somatic anxiety** is a person's perceptions, or cognitive awareness, of physiological reactivity, which may include excessive sweating, shakiness, increased heart rate, or butterflies in the stomach (Davidson & Schwartz, 1976; Martens et al., 1990).

Cognitive anxiety is proposed to result from evaluative cues and negative feedback. For some athletes the mere thought of a competitive (i.e., evaluative) situation may invoke cognitive anxiety. Heightened cognitive anxiety has been found to be associated with the following variables (Alexander & Krane, 1996; Caruso, Dzewaltowski, Gill, & McElroy, 1990; Jones, Swain, & Cale, 1990; Krane, Williams, & Feltz, 1992):

somatic anxiety— Perceptions of physiological aspects of arousal, such as excessive sweating, shakiness, increased heart rate, or butterflies in the stomach.

- Previous poor performance
- Negative individual or team performance expectations
- Lack of perceived readiness for competition
- Negative attitude toward previous performance
- Negative verbal feedback

Because of the intrusive nature of cognitive anxiety, it has been theorized to negatively affect performance (Martens et al., 1990). As an individual's cognitive anxiety increases, attentional focus turns to worries and self-doubts. This focus away from important performance cues increases the likelihood of committing an error (Bird & Horn, 1990). This negative relationship between cognitive anxiety and athletic performance has been supported consistently (e.g., Burton, 1988; Krane, 1990).

Unlike cognitive anxiety, somatic anxiety is not the result of concerns about evaluation. Rather, Martens et al. (1990) proposed somatic anxiety to be a classically conditioned response to the competitive environment. Athletes often respond to competitive situations with heightened physiological activity (e.g., increased heart rate). This reaction is repeated frequently, to the point that the association between competition and heightened reactivity becomes automatic. It has been suggested that this response is common and not necessarily detrimental to performance (Jones, Swain, & Hardy, 1993). Generally, increases in somatic anxiety enhance performance up to an optimal level, when best performances are experienced. However, further increases in somatic anxiety result in a decline in performance (Burton, 1988; Krane, Joyce, & Rafeld, 1994).

Jones and his colleagues (1993) suggested the importance of considering how athletes interpret their cognitive and somatic anxiety. Perhaps the mere presence of cognitive or somatic anxiety may not be detrimental to performance. Instead, whether an individual considers her or his anxiety as helpful or harmful directly affects performance. This has been referred to as the **direction of anxiety**, or athletes' interpretations of anxiety symptoms (Jones et al., 1993). For example, one athlete may interpret butterflies in the stomach (i.e., somatic anxiety) as feeling "psyched up," or excited and ready for competition. Those same feelings may be interpreted by another athlete as being "psyched out," or not ready for the event. Research has supported that the first athlete will not be adversely affected by somatic anxiety, yet the second athlete likely will be impeded by somatic anxiety. For example, gymnasts who interpreted their cognitive anxiety as facilitative performed better than gymnasts who interpreted their cognitive anxiety as debilitative (Jones, Swain, & Hardy, 1993). Additionally, more-elite swimmers interpreted their cognitive and somatic anxiety as facilitative, whereas less-elite swimmers interpreted anxiety as debilitative (Jones, Hanton, & Swain, 1994).

direction of anxiety—How an athlete interprets anxiety (i.e., as helpful or harmful to performance).

MULTIDIMENSIONAL ANXIETY AND ATHLETIC INJURY

Both cognitive and somatic anxiety are experienced by injured athletes. Fear, which may be considered a component of cognitive anxiety, is a common reaction to an injury (Faris, 1985; Williams, Rotella, & Heyman, 1998). Tension, or somatic anxiety, also is commonly experienced after becoming injured (A.M. Smith et al., 1990; Weiss & Troxel, 1986). Injured athletes may experience increases in cognitive or somatic anxiety upon diagnosis and during injury evaluation or rehabilitation sessions. They may worry about increased pain or be concerned about the reactions of their teammates or coaches. Quackenbush and Crossman (1994) found that negative thoughts tended to be greatest immediately after injury and then dissipated over time. Also, it is likely that athletes will experience anxiety as they prepare to return to competition after rehabilitating an injury. At this time athletes may be concerned about reinjury, their skill level, and their status on the team, as well as other common competitive concerns.

It is important that cognitive and somatic anxiety resulting from an injury be addressed. Negative thoughts may interfere with concentration on rehabilitation exercises, and cognitive and somatic anxiety may lead to physiological reactions (e.g., muscle tension) that will increase athletes' pain (Lynch, 1988; A.M. Smith et al., 1990). Additionally, gymnasts who had high cognitive anxiety experienced a greater number of injuries than gymnasts with low cognitive anxiety (Kolt & Kirby, 1994), so cognitive anxiety also may be an antecedent of injury.

In summary, research has supported the multidimensional nature of competitive anxiety. When considered negative by athletes, cognitive and somatic anxiety negatively affect performance. Cognitive and somatic anxiety can result from an injury or can increase the possibility of the incidence of an injury.

THE INTERRELATIONSHIP AMONG STRESS, ANXIETY, AND INJURY

Although the multimodal-transactional model of stress and the multidimensional anxiety theory have been addressed independently so far, stress and anxiety are closely interwoven. Stress may be manifested though increased cognitive and somatic anxiety, and research has supported that situational variables affect cognitive and somatic anxiety (Caruso et al., 1990; Krane et al., 1994). An injured athlete, for example, may associate the training room with pain. Thus treatment sessions are perceived as stressful. In response to the perceived stress, this athlete has negative thoughts (e.g., I hate treatment, I can't do this) and increased muscular tension, which leads to increased pain. In this situation stress and anxiety have become entwined.

The combination of anxiety and stress also may lead to increased incidence of injury. Supporting this notion, Petrie (1993a) found that high trait anxiety and high life stress were associated with a high number days of practice or competition missed due to injury. Perhaps, as Bandura (1995) suggested, negative self-evaluation and cognitive anxiety are exhibited through erratic thinking and reduced employment of strategic thinking. Such cognitions most likely interfere with performance and potentially increase the risk of injury. In fact, injured gymnasts reported feeling that a lack of concentration or thinking of other things led to their injury (Kerr & Minden, 1988).

The interaction between stress and anxiety is important when considering intervention strategies. Most likely, strategies to reduce stress will reduce anxiety, and vice versa. However, it is important to target interventions at the primary symptoms that the athlete is experiencing (Maynard & Cotton, 1993; Maynard, Hemmings, & Warwick-Evans, 1995; Maynard, Smith, & Warwick-Evans, 1995). Thus, effective stress management strategies target symptoms that reflect external or environmental sources of stress, and anxiety management strategies target internal thoughts or feelings.

EFFECTIVENESS OF STRESS AND ANXIETY MANAGEMENT INTERVENTIONS

stress management— Techniques to reduce the negative impact of stress by reducing the perceived demands of a situation or increasing one's ability to cope with those demands.

Although few studies have specifically examined the impact of **stress management** or **anxiety management** interventions on the rehabilitation or reduction of injury, there is support for their effectiveness in sport environments in general (Greenspan & Feltz, 1989). Stress management programs have been effective in lowering athletes' stress levels (Mace & Carroll, 1985), decreasing negative thoughts, and increasing performance (Crocker, Alderman, & Smith, 1988). Additionally, Kerr and Leith (1993) found that athletes who participated in a stress management program showed better performance, better mental rehearsal and attentional skills, and less cognitive interference than athletes who did not receive this training. Similarly, an educational program focused on reducing dysfunctional thought processes significantly decreased the cognitive anxiety levels of gymnasts (Elko & Ostrow, 1991) and was effective in increasing pain tolerance (Pen & Fisher, 1994).

anxiety management— Techniques to reduce the negative impact of anxiety by reducing negative thoughts or the physical aspects of anxiety.

In a series of studies (Maynard & Cotton, 1993; Maynard, Hemmings, & Warwick-Evans, 1995; Maynard, Smith, & Warwick-Evans, 1995), athletes who were taught applied relaxation or positive thought control (aimed at developing a positive mental attitude) showed reductions in cognitive and somatic anxiety and an increase in self-confidence. Athletes were placed into these programs based on their anxiety symptoms; highly cognitively anxious athletes received positive thought control training while highly somatically anxious athletes received applied relaxation training. Results showed that

- applied relaxation effectively reduced somatic anxiety and, to a lesser extent, cognitive anxiety;

- positive thought control effectively reduced cognitive anxiety and, to a lesser extent, somatic anxiety; and
- athletes who participated in these programs showed an increase in a facilitative interpretation of cognitive and somatic anxiety.

These studies show the importance of considering the symptoms experienced by the athletes when developing an intervention strategy. Overall, although injury prevention or treatment were not the focus of these intervention studies, they support the effectiveness of these interventions.

The positive effects of stress or anxiety management on injury reduction have been supported in two studies. Swimmers who participated in a progressive relaxation program had a 52 percent reduction of injury, and football players in the program had a 33 percent reduction in severe injury (Davis, 1991). DeWitt (1980) also observed a decline in injuries when examining the effectiveness of cognitive and biofeedback training. Although injury was not the primary focus of the study, the participants (college football and basketball players) reported a decrease in minor injuries and stated that they felt more relaxed, in control over tension, and generally looser during games.

Thus it appears that stress and anxiety management aid in minimizing the risk of injury and are important when considering injury prevention as well as treatment (Ievleva & Orlick, 1991). As Andersen and Williams (1988) proposed, physiological and attentional aspects of the stress response may lead to injury; thus interventions aimed at reducing the physiological or attentional aspects of the stress response and anxiety may prevent injury.

Benefits of Stress and Anxiety Management Interventions

- Reduced stress
- Reduced cognitive anxiety
- Reduced somatic anxiety
- Reduced pain
- Reduced incidence of injury
- Increased adherence to rehabilitation
- Possibly enhanced physical healing
- Assistance in adjustment to being injured
- Improved coping with stress of injury
- Enhanced mental readiness to return to full participation

STRESS MANAGEMENT

Consistent with the multimodal-transactional model of stress, stress management interventions can be approached from two perspectives: (1) reducing the perceived demands of a situation or (2) increasing the ability to cope with the situational demands. The first approach involves making changes in the sports medicine environment to minimize the potential stress experienced by injured athletes. The second approach provides injured athletes with skills and strategies to change their perception of the environment and its accompanying demands.

Developing a Positive Environment

A very effective mechanism to reduce potential stress is to develop a positive and helpful environment in the training room or rehabilitation center. This can be accomplished through providing every athlete with positive feedback, encouragement, and helpful information and instruction. It is important that athletes feel comfortable in the athletic therapy environment. When sports medicine professionals yell at athletes for missing sessions, it only increases the likelihood that athletes will avoid future sessions as well. Rather than telling athletes what they have done incorrectly (e.g., completed a practice drill they were advised not to do), remind them of the reason that their actions were incorrect and instruct them about what they should be doing (e.g., avoid certain movements, only walk through drills). This type of response from sports medicine professionals increases adherence to rehabilitation and minimizes athletes' viewing the training room as a source of stress. Additional suggestions for developing a positive environment include the following:

- Focus on what athletes are able to do, not their limitations.
- Provide a lot of verbal praise as athletes progress in their rehabilitation.
- Be encouraging and supportive when athletes have setbacks during their rehabilitation.
- Avoid punishing athletes when they are unable to complete rehabilitation assignments.
- When athletes act in a manner incongruent with recommendations, rather than punish athletes, instruct them about what they should have done and what to do in the future.

Modeling

modeling—
Demonstrating the necessary behaviors, attitudes, and skills needed to be successful in a particular situation.

Modeling is another strategy to reduce the stress experienced by injured athletes (Flint, 1993). Modeling, or observational learning, involves exposure to someone who demonstrates the necessary behaviors, skills, and strategies to be successful in a particular situation (Bandura, 1995). Modeling is most effective when the model is similar to the observer in physical characteristics (e.g., size, physique), status (e.g., skill level), sex, and other pertinent characteristics (Bandura, 1995).

A common concern of athletes after a serious injury is whether they will be able to make a complete comeback and return to their previous ability level. This concern is exacerbated when injured athletes lack accurate information about their rehabilitation and prognosis. An injured athlete is able to gain important information about effective coping and rehabilitation by learning from another athlete's experiences. By seeing another athlete who has overcome the setback of a similar injury, athletes may regain an optimistic perspective that they too can do so.

Modeling can be implemented in the sports medicine environment in several ways. Informally, models who are progressing successfully in their rehabilitation can be pointed out to recently injured athletes (Flint, 1993). Modeling can be implemented formally by pairing together a recently injured athlete with someone who has successfully recovered from a similar injury. Recovered athletes can share their experiences and give newly injured athletes encouragement. Flint (1993) suggested that models can be used with preoperative athletes so that they can gain valuable information about what to expect and how to cope with the upcoming surgery. Another modeling strategy is the use of videotape. Flint developed a videotape of interviews with athletes who had recently undergone knee surgery. Athletes were interviewed at varying stages of recovery and asked to describe how they felt, problems they faced during recovery, and how they overcame those problems. The videotape also included images of the athlete back in full sport participation. This video was used as a psychological intervention with injured athletes, who responded with increased motivation and a positive attitude during rehabilitation.

In the rehabilitation environment, models can be used to effectively demonstrate successful coping skills, proper form in rehabilitation exercises, use of psychological skills, positive attitude, and strategies for challenging situations (e.g., moving about campus on crutches). Benefits of modeling include

- reduced fear,
- provision of accurate information about an injury,
- increased perceptions of control,
- enhanced expectations of successful recovery,
- decreased anxiety, and
- increased confidence (Flint, 1993).

Providing an Opportunity to Voice Needs and Concerns

Some athletes may feel intimidated or unable to express their needs in athletic therapy environments. When their concerns remain unknown, they can build up, leading to distress and apprehension related to the training room. Thus it is important to empower athletes with the skills and opportunities to voice their fears, concerns, and needs. Sports medicine professionals should provide an avenue for discussion of how athletes are feeling. This should become a regular component of each treatment session. Providing an opportunity for athletes to acknowledge their fears or concerns can be accomplished through the following mechanisms:

- Devote time at the beginning of each treatment session for injured athletes to ask questions, discuss their feelings, or simply voice frustrations.
- Have athletes keep a journal of their concerns, feelings, and frustrations that can be shared with a sports medicine professional or sport psychology consultant.
- Ask athletes about their feelings often, keeping the lines of communication open.
- Be empathic when athletes voice concerns: Show concern, listen intently, and treat all concerns and fears as important.

Once athletes are provided an avenue to voice their feelings, they also should be provided the skills to do so. Some athletes may not be comfortable sharing their feelings. They may feel that the sports medicine professional will not understand what they are going through or that they will appear weak. Thus it may be necessary to teach communication skills and allow athletes to openly express their feelings. Chapter 4 presents more specific information on developing rapport with athletes and improving communication skills.

Behavioral Rehearsal

A common source of stress is uncertainty and fear of the unknown. Through **behavioral rehearsal** (Palmer & Dryden, 1995) injured athletes can "walk through" various situations that may occur and become prepared to cope with varying conditions. For example, a soccer player returning from knee surgery may be concerned about whether she is able to make the cuts needed when dribbling the ball downfield. This action can be rehearsed in the rehabilitation environment before returning to the field: The athlete can work through a progression of actions similar to the cuts she would like to use on the field. She could first walk slowly through the cutting action.

behavioral rehearsal— Becoming prepared to cope with situations by practicing or going through a trial run of situations that may occur.

As the athlete progresses, she can gradually add speed and eventually complete the motion at full speed. This should be accomplished before returning to full participation. In this manner the athlete will feel confident in her abilities before she steps back on the soccer field.

Other situations also can be similarly rehearsed. The sports medicine professional and athlete should list potentially stressful situations and develop strategies to overcome them. Then these strategies should be practiced. For example, a high jumper may feel confident that his strained hamstring is healed and strong, yet he may be concerned about reinjury from slipping on the wet approach when participating in a meet in the rain. One manner to alleviate such concerns is to address them before they occur in a competitive setting. This high jumper could wet the approach during practice (with a hose or bucket of water) and get used to the feeling of jumping on a wet surface. Then, when it happens to rain during competition, he will already know that he is strong and able to jump well on a wet approach, thus decreasing his stress and enhancing his confidence.

Assertiveness Training

A perceived inability to meet the demands of a situation leads to stress. However, communicating such concerns allows athletes to negotiate change. By acknowledging their needs, athletes may learn that they have inaccurate perceptions (e.g., the athlete may expect recovery time to be much shorter than the athletic trainer does). When athletes state their needs, athletic trainers are able to determine when athletes need to learn additional skills (e.g., how to eliminate negative thoughts, how to cope with minor pain). Through assertiveness training, athletes can be empowered to express their thoughts and feelings in a constructive manner; they are given the communication skills necessary to negotiate change and reduce stress.

"Verbal assertiveness is saying what you like or dislike about someone or something without using degradation; it is getting what you want, but not at the expense of someone else's self-esteem" (Girdano et al., 1993, p. 218). Assertiveness includes being able to voice one's needs in a positive manner, complain appropriately, give positive feedback to others, stand up for oneself, and express one's feelings (Girdano et al., 1993; Palmer & Dryden, 1995). Being assertive does not mean being argumentative or aggressive.

Girdano et al. (1993) suggest that assertiveness training be accomplished by working through the following exercises:

1. Greet others: Initiate at least two exchanges or conversations each day.
2. Use complimentary statements: Compliment others whenever it is appropriate.
3. Use "I" statements: Be willing to take a position and let your preferences be known.
4. Ask why: Be willing to ask for additional information.
5. Spontaneously exchange your feelings: Express how you are feeling to others. Begin slowly, then gradually increase the level of self-expression.
6. Disagree: If you truly believe what someone is telling you is wrong, state what you feel is correct.
7. Make eye contact: Maintain eye contact when talking with another person. Begin slowly, maintaining eye contact for a few seconds at a time, then gradually increase the length of your eye contact.

Increasing assertiveness takes time. Athletes should work through these steps one at a time. When they feel comfortable at one level, they should move on to the next. As injured athletes become more comfortable expressing themselves, they will be able to state their feelings and frustrations about their injury and rehabilitation. Only when these feelings are acknowledged can sports medicine professionals assist athletes' adjustment to a situation.

Coping With Frustration

Athletes also may be taught skills that enhance their ability to cope with frustration. When athletes feel frustrated by the constraints of their injury or a perceived lack of progress, they should be encouraged to work through these feelings. Developing an action plan allows them to acknowledge and work through feelings of frustration (Girdano et al., 1993). An action plan can be accomplished by athletes through the following steps:

1. Voice your frustration and state what you would like to happen.
2. State the benefits of reducing your frustration.
3. Develop specific indications of success (e.g., lifting a certain amount of weight, stretching a certain distance).
4. List your resources.
5. Acknowledge potential barriers to achieving your goal.
6. Note ways to overcome the barriers.

For example, a baseball player with a broken wrist is frustrated that he needs help doing many simple tasks (e.g., buttoning his shirt, tying his shoes). He voices his frustrations and develops an action plan with his athletic trainer. First, he wants to be as independent as possible while still in his cast. He will be satisfied with his progress when he is able to use his arm and does not need help getting dressed in the mornings. However, realizing that this will be several weeks away, he lists his resources as his roommate, who has been very helpful, and other friends and teammates. This baseball player also realizes that his biggest obstacle is his own attitude. He gets angry when he needs help, and his foul mood makes it less likely that others will be willing to assist him. His plan is to appreciate the help of others by being polite and thanking them and to remind himself that this is a temporary situation.

ANXIETY MANAGEMENT

As proposed by the multidimensional anxiety theory, cognitive and somatic anxiety may affect athletes differently. Some athletes may be more affected by the cognitive manifestations of anxiety, whereas other athletes may be more affected by the physical, or somatic, aspects of anxiety. It is therefore important to match the type of anxiety management intervention to the situation or symptoms experienced by the athlete. For example, an athlete who is struggling with doubts and worries (i.e., cognitive anxiety) will benefit from cognitively based interventions. Another athlete who is hindered by muscular tension will benefit from physical relaxation techniques.

Cognitive Anxiety Management Interventions

One of the most common manifestations of cognitive anxiety is negative thoughts. Learning to think positively and eliminating negative thoughts is thus an effective mechanism to decrease cognitive anxiety. Although often people are told "think positively" or "do not be negative" (a negative thought in and of itself), rarely are athletes told how to remove negative thoughts and think positively. Thought stoppage and reframing are two techniques that increase positive thinking and reduce negative thoughts.

Thought Stoppage

Thought stoppage is a technique to reduce or eliminate unwanted negative or counterproductive thoughts that may lead to cognitive anxiety (Palmer & Dryden, 1995; Zinsser, Bunker, & Williams, 1998). Thought stoppage can be accomplished in three steps:

1. Identify and acknowledge negative thoughts.
2. As soon as you notice a negative thought, say or think "Stop!"
3. Replace the negative thought with a productive, positive thought.

For thought stoppage to be effective, athletes must become aware of their negative thought patterns. Athletes can accomplish this by keeping a log and writing down their thoughts as they occur (e.g., while icing an injury) or during breaks (e.g., between exercise sets). Once their thoughts are on paper, athletes will be able to notice common negative statements or situations when negative thoughts are common. Athletes then should prepare a list of positive thoughts that can be used to replace their negative thoughts (see table 14.2 for examples). Finally, athletes should practice stopping negative thoughts and replacing them with positive replacement thoughts as often as possible.

As an example of thought stoppage, consider this scenario. An athlete comes to the training room for a rehabilitation session. As she begins her stretching exercises, she complains about her lack of progress and the futility of doing rehabilitation exercises. The athletic trainer reminds her to use thought stoppage and to think positively. The athlete continues her stretching in silence, but as she prepares for strength exercises she begins to say, "I hate doing . . . Stop! . . . I can do this." Here she has interrupted her negative thought and replaced it with a motivating thought. As athletes practice using thought stoppage, they will find that they have fewer and fewer negative thoughts. Instead, they will be focusing on the motivating or positive replacement thoughts.

Reframing

Athletes who take responsibility for their role in the rehabilitation process seem to enhance their rehabilitation and healing (Ievleva & Orlick, 1991). Although no one wants to be injured or to have to go through a long rehabilitation process, it is important to make the best of the situation. This can be accomplished by learning to reframe self-defeating thoughts into self-enhancing thoughts.

Reframing is "the process of creating alternative frames of reference or different ways of looking at the world" (Zinsser et al., 1998, p. 235). It involves transforming negative perceptions or weaknesses into positive attitudes or strengths. For example,

---

Table 14.2 Common Negative Thoughts and Positive Replacement Thoughts

Negative thoughts	Positive replacement thoughts
This hurts too much.	Be tough; hang in there.
I hate rehab.	Rehab will make me stronger.
I can't do this.	Little by little, I can do this.
This is useless.	This will get me back on the court.
I'll never be able to do this.	I'm getting better.
I'm too weak.	Look how far I've come; I'm getting stronger.

an athlete who views the training room as a drudgery can be encouraged to view it as a challenge or as the road to recovery. Another example is an athlete who had a negative attitude about not being able to complete her prescribed exercises. In her mind each repetition of an exercise that was not completed was a sign of weakness. She would envision herself stepping down a ladder each time she could not complete a set. Through reframing she learned to see herself climbing the ladder toward full recovery. Each completed set was a step upward, while an incomplete set left her on the same rung. She thus was able to focus on her steps toward recovery rather than on her perceived failure. This change in focus made a huge difference in her attitude, which became much more positive.

Somatic Anxiety Management Interventions

Consistent with multidimensional anxiety theory, interventions that focus on controlling the physiological manifestations of anxiety decrease somatic anxiety. The most common techniques in this category are those aimed at inducing muscular relaxation. There are many different relaxation techniques that can be used to reduce somatic anxiety. Two methods are described here: deep breathing and progressive relaxation.

Deep Breathing

When athletes experience anxiety, often their breathing patterns change. An anxious person breathes rapidly and shallowly, whereas a relaxed person breathes deeply and easily (Girdano et al., 1993). Deep breathing facilitates a relaxed feeling, strengthens the cardiovascular system, and increases the oxygen in the blood, which carries energy to the muscles and waste products away from the muscles (Girdano et al., 1993; Williams & Harris, 1998). Thus proper breathing leads to a relaxed mental state and may facilitate the healing process.

Deep breathing is a simple, three-step process of completely filling the lungs with air and fully exhaling:

1. Inhale deeply through the nose, feeling the stomach expand outward during inhalation (placing a hand on the stomach allows you to feel the stomach expanding).
2. Pause slightly (for about two to three seconds).
3. Exhale slowly, saying "relax" during exhalation.

This deep breathing technique, when practiced regularly, will become associated with a calm and relaxed state. For example, before beginning a stretching routine, an athlete recovering from a pulled muscle can take a few deep breaths. This action will help relax the muscles to minimize discomfort and increase the athlete's mental readiness to begin the rehabilitation session. Deep breathing can be used whenever an individual feels the need to relax.

Progressive Relaxation

Progressive relaxation (Jacobson, 1938) is a form of deep muscle relaxation. It consists of a series of exercises involving tensing and relaxing the major muscle groups in the body.

> The contraction phase teaches an awareness and sensitivity to what muscular tension feels like. The letting go, or relaxation phase, teaches an awareness of what absence of tension feels like and that it can voluntarily be induced by passively releasing the tension in a muscle. (Williams & Harris, 1998, p. 225)

Progressive relaxation entails performing an action that will tense a particular muscle or muscle group, holding that tension for about five seconds, and then relaxing those muscles by releasing the tension. Table 14.3 lists the major muscle groups and directions for tensing and relaxing them. The procedure will take approximately 20 to 30 minutes to complete. As athletes practice progressive relaxation, they will find that they can decrease the time needed to relax by increasing the speed in which they progress through the exercises, eliminating the active tensing portion, or focusing on only the tensest areas in the body.

Table 14.3   Progressive Relaxation Procedure

For each of the following muscle groups, do the tense–relax exercise twice. Hold the tension for about 5 seconds, relax for 10-15 seconds, then move on to the next muscle group.

Muscle group	Instructions	Tension location
Right hand	Clench your hand and feel the tension build. Relax and let hand and fingers hang loosely.	Back of right hand and wrist
Left hand	Clench your hand and feel the tension build. Relax and let hand and fingers hang loosely.	Back of left hand and wrist
Wrists	Bend hand back, hyperextending your wrists. Relax.	Wrists, fingers, lower forearm
Upper arms	Bend elbows toward your shoulders and tense the biceps muscles. Relax.	Biceps muscles
Shoulders	Bring shoulders up toward your ears. Relax, let your shoulders drop down.	Shoulder muscles, lower part of neck
Forehead	Wrinkle your forehead, raise your eyebrows. Relax.	Forehead area
Eyes	Close eyes tightly. Relax.	Eyelids, muscles around eyes
Jaws	Clench your jaws tightly. Relax.	Jaws and cheeks
Tongue	Press your tongue against the roof of your mouth. Relax.	Area around tongue
Mouth	Press your lips together tightly. Relax.	Area around mouth
Neck	Turn your head so that your chin is over your right shoulder. Straighten and relax.	Back and side of neck
Neck	Turn your head so your chin is over your left shoulder. Straighten and relax.	Back and side of neck
Neck and jaws	Bend your head forward, pressing your chin against your chest. Straighten and relax.	Front of neck, muscles around jaw
Chest	Take a deep breath and hold it for 5 seconds. Slowly exhale and relax.	Chest and shoulder area
Abdomen	Tighten your stomach muscles (as if anticipating a punch in the stomach). Relax.	Abdominal area
Back	Arch your back. Relax.	Lower back
Thighs	Stretch your legs out in front of you. Tighten your thigh muscles. Relax.	Top of thighs (quadriceps)

(continued)

Table 14.3	(continued)	
Muscle group	**Instructions**	**Tension location**
Hamstrings	Push your heels down into the floor, tighten your hamstring muscles. Relax.	Back of thighs (hamstrings)
Calves	Point your toes toward your head. Relax.	Back of calves
Calves	Point your toes toward the floor. Relax.	Front of calves
Feet	Curl your toes toward the bottom of your feet. Relax.	Arches and toes

Relax all the muscles of your body. Just let them go limp. Breathe naturally. Let any last traces of tension drain out of your body. Scan your body for any remaining tension and go back and tense–relax those muscles.

INTERVENTION SUMMARY

The stress and anxiety management strategies described in this chapter can be used before the incidence of injury to reduce the likelihood of injury or to help athletes cope with stress and anxiety due to injury. In either situation, stress and anxiety can be managed in manners consistent with the multimodal-transactional stress model and multidimensional anxiety theory. Sports medicine professionals who teach athletes stress and anxiety management strategies can decrease the incidence of injury, enhance adherence to rehabilitation programs, help athletes cope with their injury and debilitation, increase athletes' feelings of self-worth and self-esteem, and provide skills that will benefit athletes in other sport and nonsport situations. All these potential outcomes benefit the athlete within and beyond the sport environment.

CASE STUDY

Beth is a first-year college gymnast. She was actively recruited and was expected to be one of the team's top scorers. Unfortunately, just before the first meet, she sustained a severe ankle sprain. Beth had been putting in many hours of training and practicing, even though she knew that she needed to spend more time on her school work. She was having difficulty balancing her time between academics and gymnastics; Beth was constantly worrying about her grades, and the demands of college courses were much more time-consuming than she had expected. After her ankle injury Beth experienced a range of emotions. At first she felt a bit of relief because she had time to rest and catch up with some school work. However, soon she began to feel isolated from her teammates. She had become good friends with the other gymnasts and now was not able to spend much time with them. Beth also noticed the improvements her teammates were making and began to feel depressed and left behind.

Beth's experiences are quite common. Very often college athletes experience a great deal of stress related to both their sport and school in general. This stress may increase the possibility of an injury occurring. When injured, athletes often experience many different emotions. Sports medicine personnel need to be able to recognize these emotions and provide appropriate strategies for coping with them. Addressing the psychological aspects of an injury is just as important as addressing the physical aspects of the injury. A complete and successful recovery will not occur without a positive environment that both allows athletes to express their feelings and emotions and addresses the physical components of their injury.

Questions for Analysis

1. Based on the models of stress described in this chapter, describe factors that may have led to Beth's injury.

2. What emotions did Beth experience after her injury? What other emotions might she also experience?

3. How should the athletic trainer approach Beth?

4. Which stress and anxiety management strategies might be most helpful for Beth?

5. Describe how a positive sports medicine environment could be attained for Beth.

6. Describe the process of thought stoppage, and give examples of how Beth could use it.

SUMMARY

According to the multimodal-transactional model of stress, stress is the result of athletes' interpretation of situational demands and their ability to meet those demands. This process view of stress focuses on athletes' perceptions of a situation, whereas anxiety is athletes' perceptions of their own thoughts, feelings, and behaviors. Cognitive anxiety consists of athletes' worries; it negatively affects performance. Somatic anxiety, on the other hand, consists of perceptions of physical manifestations of anxiety; it has an inverted-U-shaped ($\cap$) relationship with performance. The most recent research suggests that whether athletes interpret anxiety as helpful or harmful to performance determines how they will be affected by their cognitive or somatic anxiety.

Stress, cognitive anxiety, and somatic anxiety are related to injury. Stress and anxiety can occur in reaction to an injury, or stress and anxiety can increase the likelihood of the occurrence of injury. Because of the bidirectional relationship between stress or anxiety and injury, stress and anxiety management are important areas of focus in the prevention of and rehabilitation from injury (Ievleva & Orlick, 1991).

Stress management techniques taught to healthy athletes may minimize the risk of injury, and interventions after an injury may help the athlete cope more effectively with her or his injury and rehabilitation. Stress management techniques include reducing the perceived demands of a situation through developing a positive environment, modeling, and behavioral rehearsal. Athletes can also be taught to cope with situational demands by providing opportunities to express needs and concerns, assertiveness training, and coping with frustration. Cognitive anxiety can be reduced through thought stoppage and reframing, while somatic anxiety can be reduced through deep breathing and progressive relaxation.

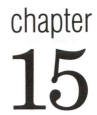

chapter

15

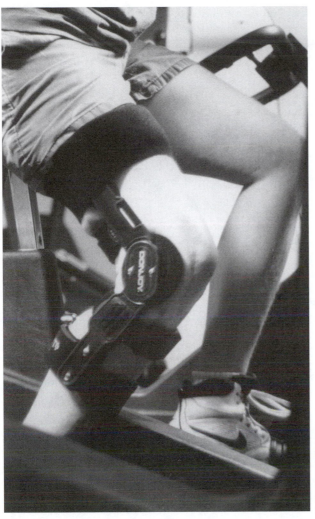

© 1994 Terry Wild Studio

Counseling for Improved Rehabilitation Adherence

A. Craig Fisher, PhD, *Ithaca College, New York*

CHAPTER OBJECTIVES

Understand the cognitive, affective, and behavioral challenges an athlete faces upon injury

Understand the complexity and multidimensional nature of rehabilitation program adherence and the major predisposing factors

Implement competence, control, and commitment strategies to promote rehabilitation adherence

Understand and avoid the major pitfalls to rehabilitation adherence

The purpose of this chapter is to give you an indication of the problems injured athletes and their sports medicine professionals face in achieving satisfactory rehabilitation outcomes. Several potential solutions are offered to address these problems in ways that will enable you to integrate these solutions into your repertoire.

CHALLENGES THAT INJURED ATHLETES FACE

Injured athletes face numerous challenges that affect their subsequent rehabilitation treatment effectiveness. These challenges can be categorized as cognitive, affective, and behavioral (Pedersen, 1986).

Cognitive Challenges

Injured athletes frequently agonize over the question, "Why me?" When they eventually gain control of their thinking, they are next faced with understanding the nature of their injury, the planned rehabilitation regimen, and the prognosis for recovery. Focusing on rehabilitation is difficult with all these competing thoughts.

Affective Challenges

Although there is limited evidence to document the precise nature and magnitude of athletes' emotional responses to injury, it seems clear that the range of emotions is large (Wiese-Bjornstal & Smith, 1993). Many athletes have limited mood disturbances and handle their adverse circumstances well. Others show elevations in depression, anger, anxiety, denial, and hopelessness. In fact, at least five injured athletes treated at the Mayo Clinic Sports Medicine Center (all possessing serious preinjury stress) have attempted suicide.

Injured athletes' emotional responses depend on a number of factors, such as the severity or perception of severity of the injury, time in the season or career, and the significance of anticipated absence from the sport scene. Not surprisingly, the more athletes have invested in their sport, the greater the likelihood of a negative emotional response following injury (Evans & Hardy, 1995). Unless injured athletes gain control of their postinjury disruptive emotional responses, successful rehabilitation is in jeopardy.

Behavioral Challenges

Injured athletes must commit to rehabilitation regimens that are often long and difficult. Some pain is likely, and both athletes and their sports medicine professionals have to be wary and deal with its possible ramifications. Pain can become overwhelming, demand immediate attention, disrupt ongoing plans, and motivate athletes to behavior aimed at stopping the pain as quickly as possible (Melzack, 1980). If injured athletes have less than optimistic thoughts and feelings, it is difficult for them to make the kind of commitment needed to successfully complete their rehabilitation programs.

These challenges cause problems for sports medicine professionals. Commitment is essential to rehabilitation **adherence**, and sports medicine professionals are typically ready to do their part; however, injured athletes are not always capable of delivering their end of the bargain. The sports medicine professional can rely on clinical expertise and rehabilitation protocols, but the key to rehabilitation adherence is the injured athlete's commitment to the program and the ability of the sports medicine professional to enhance that commitment.

adherence—*The degree of commitment an individual makes to a particular goal. Adherence implies compliance with instructions and suggestions to achieve a goal.*

Injury rehabilitation adherence is a motivational issue, not a physiological one. Injured athletes are not always completely ready to begin rehabilitation. Sports medicine professionals can compound the problem by spending more time establishing the validity of their treatment programs and less time enhancing injured athletes' adherence to their programs.

THE NATURE OF PROGRAM ADHERENCE

Approximately 40 to 65 percent of patients or clients drop out of a variety of medical regimens (Ice, 1985). Physical therapists report that 64 percent of their patients comply with their prescribed short-term exercise programs, whereas only 23 percent adhere to their long-term programs (Sluijs, Kok, & van der Zee, 1993). Perhaps these statistics seem inflated for your particular circumstances, but even one injured athlete who does not adhere to your prescribed rehabilitation exercises creates a problem for you.

Solutions to the problem of adherence are as complex as the problem itself. Meichenbaum and Turk (1987) claim that there are more than 200 variables that affect adherence. This is too much information for even the most intelligent among us to digest, and the sheer number of variables might cause us to throw our hands in the air.

When faced with such a complex, multidimensional equation, it is common to look for a way to consolidate or simplify. Injured athletes' commitment to their rehabilitation programs can be understood best by considering characteristics germane to the issue of adherence, the conduciveness of sports medicine settings, and the nature of sports medicine professional–injured athlete interactions. Treatment adherence is therefore a function of the qualities that injured athletes possess and the conditions surrounding their rehabilitation (Fisher, 1990).

Athlete's Characteristics

Investigations (e.g., Fisher, Domm, & Wuest, 1988) have shown the importance of self-efficacy and pain tolerance in enhancing rehabilitation adherence. Optimistic beliefs about both the effectiveness of the treatment program and one's capacity to endure the treatment are a powerful predictor of rehabilitation adherence. Conversely, pessimistic beliefs usually reduce rehabilitation adherence. Adherence is a motivational issue, and persistence is the key to motivation. Optimists tend to stick with their tasks until completion; pessimists tend to give up and fail (Seligman, 1990).

Rehabilitation Setting

Adherence to rehabilitation can be enhanced by removing as many environmental barriers and lifestyle disruptions as possible. Athletic training rooms, for example, are often crowded and noisy, especially during prepractice times. The sports medicine professional's attention and availability for counseling and supervision are strained during these busy times. Injured athletes are more motivated to pursue their rehabilitation workouts in less socially evaluative situations and under conditions that allow more personal attention from sports medicine professionals.

Time availability can be just as problematic. We all know only too well how convenient the excuse "not having enough time" is to explain why somebody "can't" do something. A wise sports medicine professional will fit the rehabilitation schedule around the athlete's other commitments rather than attempt to fit the athlete to a predetermined and perhaps inconvenient schedule.

Sports Medicine Professional–Athlete Interactions

Rehabilitation adherence can be enhanced by the sports medicine professional's attitudes and actions. It might be argued that treatment adherence is the responsibility of athletes, but this logic removes responsibility from the very individuals who can offer strategies to enhance rehabilitation adherence—sports medicine professionals. Moreover, sports medicine professionals can motivate rehabilitating athletes only if they have positive expectations about athletes' completion of the rehabilitation program (Wilder, 1994).

COUNSELING STRATEGIES TO PROMOTE REHABILITATION ADHERENCE

Not much information is available about the effectiveness of rehabilitation counseling with injured athletes (Wiese-Bjornstal & Smith, 1993). By using what is known, however, it is possible to develop some specific suggestions and strategies based on sound principles.

multitreatment—Combining one treatment approach with one or more other treatments and using them simultaneously.

Rehabilitation adherence is complex and multidimensional. Combination strategies and **multitreatment** approaches to counseling injured athletes are essential. The fields of counseling and clinical psychology offer many strategies that sports medicine professionals might find useful to help them enhance their athletes' rehabilitation efforts. But what is needed is some type of organizing system to facilitate reasoned choices. Elsewhere, I have proposed that self-confidence is the key to rehabilitation adherence (Fisher, 1990). Self-confidence is a multifaceted construct comprising three major components: (1) *competence,* the feeling and understanding that a particular task can be completed in a successful manner; (2) *control,* the ability or at least the perceived ability to control the significant aspects of a particular task; and (3) *commitment,* the willingness or capability to persevere at a particular task until completion. There is a reciprocal relationship among all three component parts (see figure 15.1). Heightened competence leads to an increased sense of control, caused by a willingness to deal with adversity and a positive belief that difficult situations can be overcome. Taking greater control over adverse conditions (e.g., pain) leads to enhanced competence. Increased positive beliefs lead to increased commitment because people tend to stick to tasks that they feel they can handle. Enhanced competence results when one commits to a task. When one exercises control over the difficult aspects of a task, it loses some of its negative complexion and commitment is more likely. When people make up their minds to commit to task completion, that goal orientation is often strong enough to wash away some of the day-to-day difficul-

Figure 15.1

The model of self-confidence showing the three main components and the reciprocal interactions among these components.

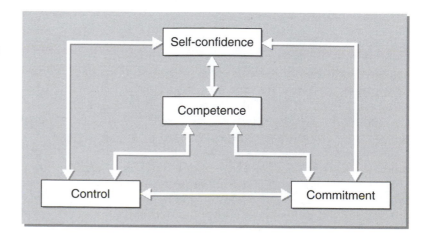

ties that might predispose less-motivated athletes to rehabilitation dropout. Self-confidence is increased when each of the components is elevated; when overall self-confidence is raised, so are the component parts. Self-confident athletes have a greater sense of perceived competence, a greater sense of personal control, and behave in a more committed manner.

Any counseling strategy that promotes one or more of these components increases the likelihood of enhancing injured athletes' rehabilitation adherence. Remember, though, that injured athletes bring their unique constellation of differences to the rehabilitation setting.

Competence Strategies

Injured athletes need to feel that they can achieve their prescribed treatment goals in spite of bouts of uncertainty and other negative emotions. Educating them about their injuries and rehabilitation, along with encouraging positive beliefs and expectations, helps enhance athletes' competence.

Education

In this section I explain the significance of working with injured athletes who are knowledgeable about their condition and its rehabilitation—the reasons why education is important. The questions that beginning sports medicine professionals most often pose are, What should be communicated? and How much information should be offered? The timing of the information raises the question of when to address particular aspects of the rehabilitation. Some guidelines for communicating with injured athletes to enhance their feelings of competence conclude this section on education.

Educating athletes about their rehabilitation is a necessary first step in the process. Knowledge about the rehabilitation regimen, especially the likelihood of pain and the effort needed to rehabilitate fully, may lead to increased pain tolerance, which increases athletes' feelings that they can and will commit to the treatment program. With more information comes reduced uncertainty, and greater certainty leads to a greater sense of knowing what to expect. Sports medicine professionals should not assume that other health care professionals (e.g., orthopedic surgeons, team physicians, health center nurses) have given injured athletes all the information they desire, but instead should offer to fill in any gaps as needed or at least test their injured athletes' knowledge base. Increased knowledge and insight do not automatically guarantee an increase in rehabilitation commitment, but failure to offer the needed and expected information may lead to uncertainty and confusion—conditions that undermine injured athletes' competence and predispose them for reduced treatment adherence (Meichenbaum & Turk, 1987).

Injured athletes need to understand their bodies' normal responses to injury, the concomitant reduction in functional capacity, the treatment rationale, and the objective criteria to be met before successful completion of the rehabilitation program. In addition to the usual rehabilitation treatment details that all sports medicine professionals typically share with their injured athletes (e.g., type of exercises, frequency, intensity, duration), you should consider discussing briefly the nature of human motivation. Mention the tendency for most of us to continue to do the things we like and to avoid the things we do not like. Even if we are determined to stick to tasks, we sometimes lose our motivation for short periods of time. Explain that these lapses in motivation are common, but unless they become a pattern, we can still achieve our goals. It is highly unlikely that injured athletes will be totally committed to all aspects of their rehabilitation every day.

Adherence to rehabilitation programs needs to be seen as continuous, ongoing, and incremental—not all or none. There will be times when injured athletes are really motivated to make the needed commitment to achieve a certain result in the shortest time possible. Full recovery—regardless of the time frame—is still the ultimate goal, however. Athletes need to be taught to recognize that rehabilitation is a sequential and developmental process that will not be obliterated by the odd day off. Failure to grasp this reality may undermine sports medicine professionals' best efforts.

How much should be explained? Clearly, some information is necessary, but how much is crucial? I suggest that you ask injured athletes some of the following questions and let their responses tell you how much they need to know:

- Do you understand the nature of your injury, particularly its severity?

- Do you understand generally what needs to be done to return your knee to its normal function?

- Do you understand the scope of your rehabilitation program, particularly the reasons for any specific exercise?

- Do you understand why the rehabilitation program is designed to last two or three months?

- Do you understand that progress will be slow at first, followed by moderate advances in mobility, then slow toward the end of the program?

- Are you clear about the criteria we'll use to adjust your workouts and the progressions we'll use to judge your progress?

The types of verbal and nonverbal responses (e.g., hesitant/certain, clear/quizzical) allow sports medicine professionals to prompt injured athletes for specific details regarding the questions asked. It would be very surprising if these questions failed to generate some dialogue between the sports medicine professional and the injured athlete. My suggestion, then, is to create the teachable moment and satisfy athletes with the amount of information they need to know, when they need to know it.

The following communication principles are designed to improve adherence to therapeutic regimens (L.W. Green, 1979; Meichenbaum & Turk, 1987).

Brevity

Be selective and simple; avoid medical jargon. This is no place to impress anybody with your knowledge of anatomy, physiology, or rehabilitation protocols. Give athletes only as much information as they need to become a full partner in their rehabilitation (Becker, 1979).

Organization

Categorize your topics and stay on task. For example, focus on particular aspects of the injury, focus on details of the treatment program, or focus on motivation, persuasion, and confidence. It is poor educational practice to address parts of several topics at the same time. Recall the best teachers you have had; chances are they delivered their content in nicely organized modules.

Primacy

Make your key points early in the discussion because your injured athletes will tend to remember the earlier information.

Repetition

Repeat important points to reinforce them. Supplement your information and cautions with written material where possible (e.g., published articles, case studies). Repetition is the essence of learning.

Specificity

Avoid being vague; be specific, concrete, and clear. For example, set particular standards for a particular workout rather than request athletes to do their best.

Other Educational Considerations

Despite your best efforts to comply with the preceding principles, you sometimes have to make adjustments to meet the circumstances. For example, certain questions do not permit discrete and definitive replies. When the injured athlete asks, "How long am I going to be out?" the most appropriate response might be, "How hard are you prepared to work at your rehab?"

Two important messages are delivered with this brief reply. First, it lets the athlete know that you view rehabilitation as a partnership—one that both athlete and sports medicine professional share. Injured athletes must understand their place in the partnership and accept the major responsibility for their rehabilitation outcomes. Second, it is evident from what we know about the complexities of rehabilitation that a discrete response is not always truthful or even possible. Rehabilitation outcomes are too variable to guarantee specific completion dates. But if the athlete persists and presses you for an answer, your best response is to offer a time range, with minimums and maximums derived from your knowledge of the type of injury that the athlete suffered. For example, "If you attend all your rehab sessions, work hard on all your exercises, handle the physical and psychological demands of your rehabilitation, and are a fast healer, then you could be back in 10 days. However, if you don't work at your rehabilitation as you should and you heal slowly, then you might not return to the team for three weeks. Much of this depends on you."

It is important to conclude this section on educational strategies on a positive note. The message that injured athletes need to extract from the sports medicine professional's discussions and interactions with them is one of hope and recovery rather than one of despair and deficit. Therefore, consider the following overarching principle as the prime prerequisite to all the other communication guidelines previously described. The principle of *optimism* should rule, and all disseminated information should leave injured athletes with a sense that they can accomplish their rehabilitation tasks rather than leaving them with lingering doubts and reservations. An example of how this principle governs discussions concerning injuries is discussing and paying more attention to the details of the rehabilitation (hope for the future) than to the specifics of the injury (despair from the past). Because a positive approach on the part of both injured athletes and sports medicine professionals is so important, the next section deals with this in more detail.

Positive Beliefs and Expectations

Injured athletes must enter into their rehabilitation with a positive attitude. There are many roadblocks to recovery, and they will need all the optimism they can muster to sustain their needed perseverance and coping. Injured athletes need to believe that their rehabilitation, if pursued with vigor, will result in successful outcomes. Most important, injured athletes must feel competent in completing their rehabilitation in the prescribed manner.

Bandura's (1977) theory of **self-efficacy** suggests several counseling principles and strategies that can be useful in athletic rehabilitation. This theory, which deals with positive beliefs and expectations, is useful in predicting successful behavior implementation in areas where making the correct behavior choices is difficult (Lewthwaite, 1990). Clearly, injury rehabilitation presents a certain degree of difficulty because of the aversive nature of injury.

There are four main methods for instilling optimism in injured athletes: personal accomplishments, vicarious experiences, verbal persuasion, and emotional arousal

self-efficacy—An individual's feeling of personal effectiveness, in either a global or specific sense.

(Bandura, 1977). Success tends to beget success, and even little accomplishments can motivate injured athletes to better adhere to their rehabilitation.

Sports medicine professionals should structure their rehabilitation environments and interactions with injured athletes to enhance positive beliefs and expectations (Lewthwaite, 1990). The following suggestions take into account the different methods for developing and maintaining a positive approach to rehabilitation.

Personalize the Program

Tailor the rehabilitation regimen, at least in part, to the individual athlete's unique characteristics and circumstances. Some key characteristics to consider are the athlete's effort orientation, frustration tolerance, pain tolerance, and optimism or pessimism. Complex regimens tend to lead to greater nonadherence, especially if they are not tailored to athletes' daily routine or situations (Sluijs et al., 1993).

Minimize Pain

Design your exercise protocols to keep negative sensations (e.g., fatigue, soreness, pain) at a minimum or tolerable.

Increase Gradually

Start athletes' rehabilitation slowly, and gradually build the intensity. You want athletes to be successful in order to enhance their feelings of competence. Early disappointment or lack of expected progress may lead to reduced competence, which in turn may lead to lower adherence. Build success early, and that will normally be enough to inoculate injured athletes against the frustrations they may face later.

Provide Warnings

When it is not possible for athletes to avoid negative sensations, educate them about what to expect. Uncertainty leads to heightened anxiety, and elevated anxiety might be enough to predispose them to reduced commitment. Describe the feeling that the athlete is likely to experience, for example, "Don't be surprised if you feel a little tenderness on the inside of your knee" or "You might feel some tightness in your shoulder as you rotate it, but that's good because you need to stretch it out."

Use Your Experience

If previously injured athletes have shared with you any of their successful strategies for dealing with their rehabilitation, pass these on to your current athletes. For example, the athlete riding the bicycle ergometer might think about traveling toward a particular destination.

Offer Reassurance

Athletes' perceptions about the severity and uniqueness of their injuries can be allayed by reminding them, "I've seen knee injuries much worse than yours, and all those athletes' rehabilitations were successful." Perhaps some of those athletes are still around and might also offer some psychological support.

Monitor Progress

ceiling effects—The fact that further change comes more slowly after most of the advancement has been made.

Athletes need sports medicine professionals to monitor their progress. Progress can be viewed in two ways. First, you can point out the incremental improvement made by the rehabilitating athlete. Second, you should reinforce athletes for working hard at their rehabilitation because it is the process that will eventually lead to the anticipated product. Athletes need to understand that every trial of each exercise gets them just a little closer to recovery. In most injuries neural, vascular, and muscular damage must be corrected before much substantial overt progress can be noticed.

What about the plateaus, or **ceiling effects**, that athletes on long-term rehabilitation regimens routinely face? It is important that athletes recognize that plateaus exist only in overt performance. As long as the athlete is positively stressing the injured area, there is bound to be some advancement, whether noticeable or not. Plateaus are simply periods of necessary neural consolidation and integration, which are necessary before "breakthroughs" can occur.

There is a parallel to be drawn between learning a sport skill and rehabilitation progress. Skill, strength, endurance, and range-of-motion gains are realized in smaller and smaller increments at advanced stages. This is the law of diminishing returns. Injured athletes cannot expect the same rate of progress later in their rehabilitation as they achieved earlier. Unless this reality is accepted, athletes are bound to become frustrated with their lack of progress, and this may negatively affect their beliefs and expectations.

Be Realistic

It is not only athletes who must come to grips with the ceiling effects previously mentioned; so too must sports medicine professionals. Repeated girth measurements of the quadriceps are not going to be very reinforcing unless adequate time between assessment periods is allowed. Rehabilitation takes time. Both athletes and sports medicine professionals need to acknowledge and accept this fact. Expecting results too fast is bound to produce discouragement, and this is counterproductive to the kinds of commitment athletes need to make to their rehabilitation. Sports medicine professionals need to be careful not to exacerbate athletes' frustration by overdoing progress assessments.

Two questions will help you assess your athlete's level of optimism:

1. Do you believe that your rehabilitation regimen will work?
2. Do you feel confident that you can commit yourself to your prescribed treatment?

Most injured athletes can predict with a fair amount of accuracy the likelihood of their rehabilitation adherence, and anything less than an enthusiastic positive reply should give you cause for concern. This concern should give rise to its remediation before rehabilitation begins.

Believing that you have the competence to adhere is not the same as adhering (Caplan, Robinson, French, Caldwell, & Shinn, 1976). Beliefs need to be turned into actions, and this demands that sports medicine professionals use all their knowledge and all their clinical and counseling skills to enhance the likelihood of rehabilitation adherence. Sports medicine professionals can assist rehabilitating athletes in controlling some of the factors that lead to reduced adherence.

Control Strategies

Athletes must exercise control over all aspects of their rehabilitation. If that control is not exerted, then thoughts, feelings, and actions will control personal outcomes. The previous section explained how important positive beliefs and expectations are to rehabilitation adherence, but positive beliefs are going to be effective only as long as injured athletes can maintain them. There are plenty of negative circumstances to pull competence and control away from rehabilitating athletes.

Coping With Negative Thoughts and Feelings

At the beginning of this chapter, some attention was directed at the affective challenges injured athletes are likely to face. If rehabilitation is going to have any chance of success, athletes must eventually come to grips with the negative emotions caused by their injuries. Sports medicine professionals can assist in this task by facilitating the open expression of athletes' emotional responses (Pedersen, 1986). Injured athletes should be encouraged to talk about their injuries and their reactions to them.

When emotional reactions are brought out into the open, they can be dealt with and discharged. Consider how much better this is than holding the negative emotions in or attempting to deny their existence. Rehabilitation, especially long term, provides enough challenges to injured athletes without adding negative affect to the equation.

You understand how important it is for athletes to listen to what you tell them. Athletic trainers claim it is one of the most important factors leading to the development of coping responses (Fisher, Mullins, & Frye, 1993; Wiese, Weiss, & Yukelson, 1991). But, surprisingly, athletic trainers do not rate their own capacity to listen to athletes as that significant (Wiese et al., 1991). This is unfortunate, considering how important listening to athletes can be. The essence of effective communication is that both parties listen to what the other has to say.

Although it is doubtful that sports medicine professionals intend to prevent athletes from dealing with their emotional responses to injury, it can happen innocently enough. Consider the following statements that lead athletes to believe that it is inappropriate for them to express their feelings (Caplan et al., 1976); pay attention to the countering statements that encourage athletes to channel their feelings into positive outcomes:

Stifle feelings	**Channel feelings**
You shouldn't be so upset.	It's natural to be upset, but you must turn this energy into motivation to rehabilitate your injury.
There's nothing to worry about.	Of course you're worried about your injury and your future playing status. Use that worry creatively to motivate you.
You know, injury is just a part of sport.	Undoubtedly, you always knew that you might get injured. That's unfortunate, but you need to spend more of your focus on our present rehabilitation plans.
Do you think you're the only athlete who's ever blown out a knee?	Sometimes bad things happen to good people. Knee injuries are a real problem in this sport, but in almost all cases athletes return to perform at their preinjury level.

The most difficult athlete attitude you will face is learned helplessness. This severe feeling of pessimism is typified by a "give-up" attitude, created because the injured athlete does not believe that anything can be done to alter the negative circumstances (e.g., "It's hopeless. Nothing I try works."). Athletes with learned helplessness use less effective strategies after failure, withdraw their effort, express frustration with their progress, and consistently blame themselves for their circumstances (Sluijs et al., 1993).

Most injured athletes handle the reality of their injuries quite well, but those who show any signs of learned helplessness can likely benefit from attempts at changing their thinking or, in Seligman's (1990) terms, their **explanatory style**. Athletes can think their situations are hopeless because they adopt one or more of the following fallacies, when instead they could adopt the respective counter-thinking.

explanatory style—Reasons people give to explain why things happen to them.

Fallacy of permanence

I'll never return to the form I once had.   There's every reason to believe you'll be as good as new once we've rehabilitated your knee. This is just a temporary setback.

Fallacy of pervasiveness

I'll always be thinking about my injury, wondering when it's going to happen again.

Your knee and surrounding ligaments will be as strong, maybe even stronger, when your rehabilitation is complete.

Fallacy of personalization

Why does everything bad have to happen to me?

Injuries are random, and everyone feels bad when they're injured. Let's make the best of it and return to play better than before. Others have done it.

Most injury treatment programs are going to end up as rehabilitation successes. Injuries are not permanent; they are temporary. It is only because the injury just occurred that it colors the athlete's perceptions so dramatically. In time, especially with some initial progress, injured athletes will realize that thoughts and feelings about their injured condition are not generalizable to other situations. Injuries are unfortunate, but athletes for the most part are blameless in causing them. There are many reasons why injuries happen, but the point to emphasize is that athletes do not have to deal with their injuries by themselves. Sports medicine professionals are there every step of the way to educate, motivate, and assist injured athletes in their rehabilitation efforts.

Coping With Pain

Pain is a component of many injury rehabilitation programs, and this fact is problematic for rehabilitation adherence. For most people in most situations, pain is a signal to stop the activity that is causing the pain. Injured athletes, on the other hand, sometimes need to work through particular aspects of their pain sensations if their rehabilitation efforts are to be maximized. Pain management is one of the keys to successful injury rehabilitation (Pen, Fisher, Sforzo, & McManis, 1995).

What does the sports medicine professional need to know about pain? Can anything be done about how injured athletes react to potentially painful exercise prescriptions? Pain has both physiological and psychological properties; it hurts, but the magnitude of the sensation depends on the injured athlete's perception and labeling (Pen & Fisher, 1994). Everybody has heard the stories of athletes performing in championship games after they incurred serious injuries. Pain tolerance depends on injured athletes' capacities to handle pain and the importance they place on their rehabilitation. Athletes who believe in the efficacy of their treatment programs and believe in their ability to adhere to these programs are better able to cope with their pain. These positive beliefs and attitudes lead to increased resourcefulness and persistence in applying coping strategies, enhanced mobilization of cognitive resources to direct attention away from pain sensation, and even reduced distressing anticipation of pain (Williams & Kinney, 1991). Cognitive strategies work to alleviate pain because there is such a strong mental component to pain.

At the very least, sports medicine professionals should assist injured athletes in understanding the nature of pain they might encounter. As long as pain is an unknown, there is bound to be uncertainty and anxiety associated with rehabilitation. Neither of these states promotes rehabilitation adherence. If it is likely that the athlete will have to face some pain, the sports medicine professional needs to help the athlete distinguish the "good pain" from the "bad pain."

Following are some brief strategies that can be employed to assist athletes with the pain associated with rehabilitation. These interventions can assist athletes' coping with the broad range of emotional disruption brought on by athletic injuries.

Relaxation

Thoughts and feelings can be controlled if athletes decide what their focus will be, rather than letting their thoughts and feelings have the upper hand. Negative thoughts and emotions can be disrupted if athletes are reminded to focus on a word or phrase, sound, prayer, or body sensation.

Calming Imagery

There seems to be something inherently pleasurable and restful about being at the beach, at the ocean, or near a lake. Teaching athletes to imagine themselves in such a setting can help decrease their sensation of pain. More information about the application of imagery to injury rehabilitation can be found in L.B. Green (1992) and Ievleva and Orlick (1993).

Association

Emotions and pain tend to be pervasive sensations in the sense they can flood all aspects of an athlete's existence. By focusing directly on the specific locus of pain, it may be possible to "frame" the pain. There are various suggestions that athletes can be given to deal with pain: "Focus on your pain, and feel cool running water splash over the joint." "Place a black frame around the pain, and make the frame get smaller and smaller." "On a 10-point scale, how high would you rate the pain? Can you reduce the magnitude of the pain?"

Dissociation

If the injured athlete's attention can be directed away from the pain, the pain sensations may become more manageable. Some of the points made earlier about relaxation are applicable here. For example, focusing on breathing with the purpose of slowing it down tends to direct attention away from other sensations and thoughts. Other distractions that might prove useful are listening to music, watching videos, or imagining doing other activities that demand the deployment of attention.

pain threshold—An individual's degree of sensitivity to painful cues.

There is some indication that dissociation works better for pain management than does relaxation or general calming imagery (Beers & Karoly, 1979), although this does not negate the potential benefits of the latter two interventions. Also, it has been found that dissociation strategies are more effective than association strategies in increasing **pain threshold**. Increased attention to internal cues, without the learned capacity to cope, results in a greater focus on the problem, not on a solution. Dissociation may be more helpful in preparing athletes to cope with pain before its onset, but it may not be as successful as association in dealing with the sudden impact of pain and its aftermath. Just having a strategy, be it associative or dissociative, that can be directed at painful or disruptive sensations can provide injured athletes with the confidence that they can handle their rehabilitation.

Thought Stoppage

Negative thoughts can be interrupted and stopped. Failure to do so tends to result in ever-increasing pessimistic rhetoric in the minds of injured athletes. In a worst-case scenario the negative internal dialogue or self-talk sends the pessimistic thinker into a downward spiral, resulting in reduced motivation to pursue the task of rehabilitation. These are the steps to teaching athletes to control their thinking:

Step 1. Ask athletes to recognize their negative self-talk. If the content is "It's really going to hurt" or "I don't think I can do it," these statements will harm rehabilitation adherence. Convince athletes that these are not attacking statements; they are defensive and self-defeating.

Step 2. When athletes hear their expected negative phrases, have them shout "Stop!" under their breath, forcefully but not audibly to others. Alternatively, a sharp slap to the thigh or the snap of a rubber band worn around the wrist interrupts the thought. Have athletes practice stopping thoughts, and they will realize that it works.

Step 3. An alternative thought has to replace the one just stopped, or the original thought will recur. Here are a couple of suggestions: "I can handle the soreness," "I want to return to play again this season." It is even better if the positive thought can be represented by a cue word or phrase. The entire thought-stopping dialogue would then sound as follows: "Stop! . . . Handle it" or "Stop! . . . Work hard to return."

Commitment Strategies

The bottom line of treatment adherence, which is essentially a motivational issue, is commitment. This section describes three major approaches to increase athletes' persistence, perseverance, and dedication to their rehabilitation programs for sports medicine professionals to consider as they interact with and counsel injured athletes.

Social Support

A positive relationship exists between social support and medically related adherence. This is not that surprising when we consider how significant other people are to our decision making and behavior. To whom do we normally address our problems? Clearly, we turn to those who tend to support us and give us the strength and resolve to stick to our tasks.

The relationship between social support and commitment, although powerful, does not take a direct path. Figure 15.2 illustrates how and why social support mediates injury rehabilitation adherence. When sports medicine professionals encourage injured athletes during their rehabilitation, help them through the tough times, and portray an optimistic outlook about athletes' progress, they increase athletes' belief in themselves. This increased competence leads to greater rehabilitation adherence. Perceived competence and social support appear to be powerful allies. Caplan et al. (1976) reported that high perceived competence leads to enhanced rehabilitation adherence only under conditions of high social support. Apparently the lack of support tends to undermine a person's positive approach to rehabilitation. Feeling competent enough to adhere to a rehabilitation regimen is not the same as actually adhering. Neither does the sense of personal control over negative thoughts and feelings guarantee adherence. Positive thoughts and feelings must get translated into committed behavior. Social support increases this likelihood.

When sports medicine professionals share motivational strategies with injured athletes and encourage them to use these coping strategies, the likely result is greater commitment to rehabilitation. Weiss and Troxel (1986) suggested two supportive strategies that deserve consideration. The first, peer modeling, involves putting an injured athlete currently undergoing rehabilitation in touch with previously injured and successfully rehabilitated athletes, preferably ones who had similar injuries. Success stories can be swapped, and suggestions about how to cope with the difficulties inherent in rehabilitation can be shared. Empathy, honest realism, and optimism are the intended results. For those athletes who seem to be less optimistic and have less coping capacity, an alternative strategy can be employed. Peer support groups, an idea taken from clinical and counseling settings, allows small groups of athletes to feed off each other's resolved difficulties and successes in ways that lead them to the resolution of their own coping problems.

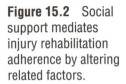

Figure 15.2 Social support mediates injury rehabilitation adherence by altering related factors.

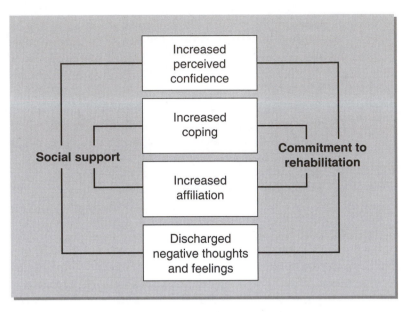

By caring, supporting, and orchestrating a support network, sports medicine professionals can increase injured athletes' sense of belonging, something that suffers because of the distancing that injuries create. Sports medicine professionals are in the best position to encourage coaches and teammates to maintain contact with injured athletes. Team members may need to be counseled about their facilitative role in enhancing teammates' rehabilitation adherence.

Anything that can minimize the physical or psychosocial distance between injured athletes and their sport environments is likely to enhance rehabilitation adherence. Transporting equipment to the practice area for injured athletes' on-site rehabilitation allows them to rehabilitate within their sport context. This makes athletes feel that they are still a part of the team, and this increased affiliation serves as motivation to return to the sport.

When sports medicine professionals listen to their injured athletes, empathize with their expressed concerns about their rehabilitation, and understand and accept what they hear, the effect may prove cathartic. Allowing athletes to discharge their uncertainties and negative thoughts and feelings removes a resistive force that works against rehabilitation adherence. Becker (1979) claimed that rehabilitating individuals tend to be more motivated to adhere to their prescriptions when warmth and empathy are shown and when respect and concern are present. Social support does not mean—nor do injured athletes need—sympathy, pity, or coddling (Caplan et al., 1976). Beware of these well-meaning behaviors because they tend to create an emotional dependency on the sports medicine professional and end up undermining athletes' sense of personal control. This is a caution that all health care professionals must heed. How much support should you provide? The best response is enough support to help athletes commit to their rehabilitation without creating the feeling that the sports medicine professional has to be with them all the time or else their rehabilitation efforts are doomed.

The rehabilitation goals that are set and the means by which they are set may have an important effect on injured athletes' perception of the social support offered by sports medicine professionals. The next section addresses some salient features of goal setting as it relates to injury rehabilitation adherence.

Goal Setting, Goal Attainment, and Incentives

It has been argued that behavioral facilitation (of which goal setting is a major strategy) is severely underestimated and underused in the field of athletic injury rehabilitation (DePalma & DePalma, 1989). That being the case, let's address some key aspects of goal setting and goal attainment that relate to injury rehabilitation adherence.

A brief discussion on why and how goals enhance motivation is in order. Goals direct attention toward some purpose (e.g., return to normal function), and planned outcomes are more likely to be realized when attention is deployed in a particular direction. For example, Ievleva and Orlick (1993) reported that fast healers were more involved in setting goals than were slow healers. Goals also create positive expectations by providing a framework for positive beliefs about goal attainment. Goals provide standards against which progress can be measured. They are the benchmarks needed to adjust the injured athlete's rehabilitation schedule so that the treatment program can be individually tailored.

Rehabilitation goals will not necessarily achieve the desired results unless they adhere to the following principles.

- Goals must be stated specifically.
- Short-term goals are superior to long-term goals.
- Goals must be challenging yet reasonable.
- Target dates for goal attainment must be set.
- Goal progress must be monitored and recorded.
- Goals must not be viewed as permanent and unchangeable.
- Goals must contain both performance and outcome components.

As you consider implementing some of these goal-setting principles, be wary of some of the common pitfalls in goal setting (Gould, 1998):

- Setting too many rehabilitation goals too soon
- Setting rehabilitation goals that are too general
- Failing to recognize the individual differences in the athletes you treat
- Failing to modify unrealistic rehabilitation goals
- Failing to create a supportive yet challenging atmosphere in which rehabilitation goals can be attained

Injured athletes' commitment to their rehabilitation can be enhanced when sports medicine professionals implement goal-setting principles into their prescribed rehabilitation regimens. But merely setting rehabilitation goals and expecting increased motivation is naive. Consider the "expect, record, and inspect (especially if suspect)" strategy (Fisher, Scriber, Matheny, Alderman, & Bitting, 1993). As an athlete completes the expected rehabilitation goal (e.g., three sets of 10 repetitions using 25 pounds, or 11 kilograms, of resistance), the athlete records the achievement on the rehabilitation progress report. Periodically, the sports medicine professional in charge of this athlete's rehabilitation inspects the progress. If the sports medicine professional suspects that the athlete is not achieving the expected results, more positive reinforcement for goals attained, personal attention, and supervision are needed.

Threats Versus Challenges

Fear is a powerful motivator. But there is a danger in using threats and ultimatums. Perhaps the largest drawback is deciding what to do if the threat does not achieve its intended purpose. At best it is a win/lose situation. The sports medicine professional who threatens an athlete with a "do it or else" ultimatum runs the risk of damaging rapport with the athlete, even if the athlete complies (Fisher & Hoisington, 1993). The sports medicine professional wins because today's rehabilitation is completed, but the athlete loses respect for the sports medicine professional. If the athlete does not complete the prescribed rehabilitation workout, it can even end up being a lose/lose situation. Both athlete and sports medicine professional lose because the rehabilitation was not completed as specified, and to further exacerbate the situation the sports medicine professional is compelled to make good on the threat and withhold future services or prevent the athlete from returning to competition.

A threat acts like a two-edged sword. It may work to achieve certain rehabilitation goals, but it may just as readily work against the sports medicine professional wielding the threat. Your experience with ultimatums should tell you that threats work for some of the people some of the time, but the risks are great, and there is an alternative that can achieve the same desired rehabilitation outcomes: Change the threat into a challenge. Instead of dictating a particular outcome, such as "90-degree knee flexion by the end of week or else," ask "Can you get to 90-degree knee flexion by the end of the week? I believe you can." The adversarial component of the threat can be removed by personalizing the demand and by providing support for the outcome.

As long as there are no mitigating circumstances (i.e., physical or psychological reasons), use threats, if you must, as your last resort when all other motivational strategies have failed. They might work, and at the point when an athlete shows little interest in adhering to the prescribed rehabilitation, you have little to lose. Maybe the threat will motivate the athlete to pursue the treatment program with enough diligence that a successful rehabilitation will ensue.

THE OUTLOOK—PESSIMISTIC OR OPTIMISTIC?

When we consider the apparent inevitability of treatment dropout or low adherence, the outlook for successful rehabilitation seems dim. If Ley (1986, p. 183) is accurate in his assertion that "there is enough evidence of professional noncompliance for it to seem likely that even if clinicians were aware of these techniques [the ones described in this chapter, for instance], they would not necessarily use them," then this makes the outlook even more pessimistic.

Sports medicine professionals can fall into a common trap if they are not careful. There is a definite parallel between how negative beliefs and feelings play themselves out in athletes' and sports medicine professionals' approaches to rehabilitation. When injured athletes have low expectations of success and adopt a pessimistic outlook, they tend not to commit to their treatment initially, fail to cope with the inherent frustrations and difficulties, and do not persist with their prescribed programs. When sports medicine professionals adopt similar fatalistic attitudes, they tend to ignore a number of suggested rehabilitation guidelines: They fail to explain the nature of the injury and the proposed treatment program adequately, they fail to support and motivate athletes to adhere, they fail to request athletes' participation in the rehabilitation, and they fail to monitor progress and reinforce athletes' rehabilitation successes.

Adherence to rehabilitation is tough enough without sports medicine professionals exacerbating the situation, consciously or not. Working with unmotivated athletes can be demoralizing, but sports medicine professionals must be mindful of their calling and be quick to recognize when their approach to rehabilitation is in neither their athletes' nor their own best interests. If you ever hear yourself emitting any of the following statements, take heed because your fatalism is showing:

- It's up to them whether or not they listen to me; after all, it's their life, not mine.
- They don't pay me enough to put up with . . . .
- Look, I'm not a shrink, I'm an athletic trainer.

- All this rehabilitation adherence stuff sounds good in theory, but it doesn't work in practice; there's just no time for this adherence stuff.

I suggest you spend some time disputing this kind of thinking because it can lead to a pessimistic outlook.

Treatment dropout or low commitment to an injury rehabilitation program is not inevitable. Sports medicine professionals need to use the information they derive from their initial meetings with injured athletes, minimize the barriers that might predispose athletes to low motivation, foster the kinds of interaction styles that are perceived by injured athletes as supportive, and counsel athletes on the salient features of the rehabilitation process as described in this chapter. When this behavioral recipe is applied, rehabilitation adherence is enhanced.

CASE STUDY

Bill is a running back in a highly successful college football program. In his freshman year he played with the junior varsity, and this is his third year on the varsity roster. One of the hallmarks of this team is its depth of players. Underclassmen typically wait their turn to get playing time. It has almost become expected that players' patience will be rewarded by great personal performances once they have earned their opportunity.

Bill is just such an individual. By most estimates, he would have been a starter elsewhere, but he worked hard waiting for his chance, like so many before him. In the first game of the year of his final season, Bill has earned a starting running back position. And, as has often happened before, Bill's first touch of the ball as a starter goes for 50 yards, down to the opponent's 3-yard line. Bill, his teammates, and those around the team are happy for Bill. On the next play Bill's number is called to score the touchdown that he helped set up. He takes the handoff, runs into the intended hole, and is met by a linebacker's helmet on his right knee. He hears a popping sound as he falls to the ground, clutching his leg.

The athletic trainers rush onto the field, evaluate the injury, and conclude that Bill has incurred some serious knee damage. Bill has to be carried off the field. In fact, Bill has torn the anterior cruciate ligament in his right knee, and his football career is over. He waited three years to get a starting position, and it was over in two plays. Now he's facing reconstructive surgery, followed shortly thereafter by a long-term rehabilitation program. In an instant Bill has gone from "the thrill of victory to the agony of defeat."

Questions for Analysis

1. What may prevent Bill from adhering to his upcoming rehabilitation following knee surgery?

2. At the onset of his rehabilitation, how can Bill's sports medicine professional maximize his chances for a quality rehabilitation?

3. As Bill's rehabilitation progresses, what can be done to enhance his motivation to adhere?

4. Construct a goal-setting scenario that you would present to Bill if you were his sports medicine professional.

5. Which rehabilitation principles will Bill's sports medicine professional undoubtedly have to deliver several times throughout the rehabilitation?

6. What plans might the sports medicine professional implement if Bill becomes depressed with his rehabilitation progress and begins to question his motivation to continue?

SUMMARY

Injured athletes face several challenges that tend to increase the difficulty of rehabilitation. They must commit themselves to their prescribed rehabilitation regimens if they are to achieve successful outcomes, but high commitment to the task is difficult when they are upset about their injuries. Injured athletes are not always in the best frame of mind at the time rehabilitation needs to begin.

Not every athlete who begins a rehabilitation program commits enough effort and successfully deals with the inherent difficulties associated with injury rehabilitation. Treatment dropout sometimes reaches 40 to 65 percent in a number of medically related domains. Adherence to athletic injury treatment programs is substantially better than in some other fields, but it is less than 100 percent.

Treatment program adherence is a complex issue; there are as many as 200 variables involved. These variables can be categorized into three major factors: athletes' personality characteristics, rehabilitation setting characteristics, and sports medicine professional–athlete interactions.

Self-confidence is an umbrella concept comprising competence, control, and commitment. Treatment adherence is enhanced when injured athletes feel that their prescribed rehabilitation exercises will achieve their intended outcome and that they will be able to successfully deal with the difficulties that arise. Adherence is enhanced when injured athletes sense that they can control the thoughts, emotions, and actions that otherwise may alter their focus and intentions. Adherence is enhanced when injured athletes find ways to commit themselves to their treatment programs. The bulk of the chapter describes counseling strategies that foster competence, control, and commitment.

Sports medicine professionals must maintain an optimistic outlook on their injured athletes' rehabilitation. Athletes do not always behave in a committed fashion, and it is up to the sports medicine professional to model and facilitate the degree of optimism necessary for athletes to achieve their rehabilitation goals. Sports medicine professionals must accept this professional responsibility and be as committed as they can be to the successful progress of athletes' rehabilitation programs.

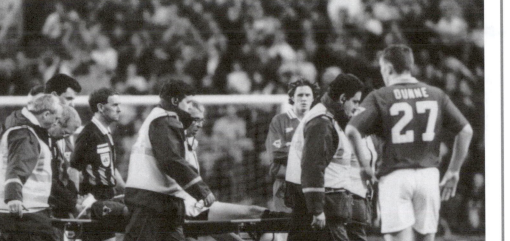

© Action Images

Counseling Athletes With Catastrophic Injury and Illness

Michael J. Asken, PhD, *Pinnacle Health System, Polyclinic Medical Center*

CHAPTER OBJECTIVES

Define catastrophic injury and illness

Summarize the typical and normal psychological response to such events

Understand adjustment problems associated with catastrophic injury and illness

Appreciate the role of counseling in helping the athlete cope with such events

Identify the components of a therapeutic relationship

Describe ways to promote coping and support for the athlete

A bolt from the blue! Unimaginable! Totally unexpected! Devastating! These are all terms attached to catastrophic events, injuries, and illnesses.

First it was a big booboo in a delicate area, a big laugh from John Kruk on a slow day in Clearwater, Florida. Now, two days after a cancerous testicle was removed from the Phil's first baseman, the laughter is gone, replaced by concern over the All-Star's future in uniform and out. (Donellon & Hagen, 1994)

Catastrophic illness and events are much more common than once thought. Table 16.1 lists the percentages of people reporting ever having experienced a specific traumatic event in their lives. According to Norris (1992), the percentage of the total population that ever experiences a traumatic event may be as high as 69 percent.

Athletes, however, are often seen as different from the general population in terms of psychological strength, makeup, and response (Heyman, 1987; Horvat, French, & Henschen, 1986; Morgan & Pollock, 1977). It often seems that the greatest challenges to athletes are on the field and in competition. Unfortunately, it is becoming clear that this is not the case. Catastrophic events, injuries, or illnesses confront athletes at all levels, just as they do the general population. Although the prevalence of traumatic and catastrophic events for athletes is not clear, other than for performance-related injury (Heil, 1993), the occurrence of such an event always stands out, as the aforementioned newspaper report on John Kruk demonstrates.

Whether catastrophe occurs as a result of competition, physical illness, injury outside of sport, or a traumatic event, athletes are not excepted from such tragedies. John Kruk's cancer, Magic Johnson's HIV infection, the paralyzing injuries of Dennis Byrd and Darryl Stingley, the failing of Micky Mantle's liver and his development of lung cancer, the sudden death of Reggie Lewis, the assault on Monica Seles, the murder of Michael Jordan's father, the death of Dan Jansen's sister from leukemia before his Olympic competition, the car crash that Lenny Dykstra and Darren Daulton survived, and the car crash that Pelle Lindbergh did not survive all attest to the potential catastrophes that athletes and their families can face.

This chapter addresses catastrophic injury and illness in athletes. **Catastrophic injury or illness** is defined rather broadly to include injury or illness of an extreme or traumatic nature that is characterized by the devastating impact it has on the

catastrophic injury or illness—An injury or illness of an extreme or traumatic nature, which is characterized by the devastating impact it makes on an individual's life and the adaptation required to recover from it.

Table 16.1 Percentage of People Reporting Ever Having Experienced a Specific Traumatic Event	
Tragic death	30.2
Robbery	24.9
Motor vehicle crash	23.4
Other hazard	15.2
Physical assault	15.0
Other disaster	13.3
Fire	11.0
Combat	9.2
Sexual assault	4.4

From Norris (1992). Epidemiology of trauma: Frequency and impact of different potentially traumatic events on different demographic groups. *Journal of Consulting and Clinical Psychology, 60*(3), 409-418.

athlete's life and the adaptation required to recover from it. Such injuries or illnesses are associated not only with significant challenges to medical and physical treatment and recovery, but also with psychological reactions and adaptation. Weiss and Troxel (1986) have noted that for the athlete almost any injury has the potential to elicit strong and devastating emotions; thus sports medicine professionals must constantly be on the alert to extreme reactions. Comments from Wiese and Weiss (1987, p. 318) about sport injuries in general are even more emphatic in the context of catastrophic injury or illness. They observe that it is "critical to the ultimate goal of recovery and return to competition that athletes are indeed rehabilitated both physically and psychologically."

The description of Monica Seles's return to competition from the knife attack she sustained illustrates this concept: "Her body came back first. It was the easiest part to rebuild" (Price, 1995, p. 24). Psychological intervention in catastrophic situations can be a significant challenge and underscores the need for the material in this chapter about the implementation of appropriate principles of care in the rehabilitation of such catastrophically injured athletes.

ATHLETES' RESPONSE TO CATASTROPHIC INJURY AND ILLNESS

The reaction of athletes to catastrophic injury and illness can be very complex. The response shares many of the same features as reactions to sport injury in general (see chapter 2 for a discussion of response to sport injury). But what is described as the typical impact of injury on the athlete must be amplified severalfold to approach the degree of impact of a catastrophic event. Impact, intensity, and need for intervention are all increased in catastrophic injury or illness.

The difficulty that injury presents for the athlete in terms of restricted activity and uncertainty about the future (Weiss & Troxel, 1986) is put into perspective in the catastrophic situation by Wortman and Silver (1987, p. 189):

In fact, the major coping task faced by individuals who encounter such events is to reconcile themselves to a situation that cannot be changed and over which they have little, if any, control.

It is not surprising then that myriad psychological reactions have been described in relation to catastrophic events. This section discusses four of the most common reactive responses: stages of reaction to catastrophic events, with a special emphasis on the critical nature of the injury or illness immediately after injury or after diagnosis; depression as a response to injury; the potential for post-traumatic stress symptoms when trauma is involved; and the social impact on the athlete, family, and others.

Stages of Reactions to Catastrophic Injury and Illness

The most popular description of psychological response to injury, whether catastrophic or not, is a stage model (Suinn, 1967). These stages may resemble those first described by Kubler-Ross (1969) in the area of death and dying; indeed, athletic injury has been likened to a **grieving process** (Pedersen, 1986).

The stages have been variously described in different models and writings but generally involve the following reactions:

- Shock
- Denial

grieving process—The process involved when dealing with a loss of someone or something of value to the individual.

- Anger and bargaining
- Depression
- Acceptance and adaptation

Initially, there is a period of psychological shock when the individual is confused and disorganized about what has happened. There is a decline in the individual's functioning and ability to respond to the situation.

A period of denial is typically seen as following this stage. Denial is the repudiation or minimization of the implications of the catastrophic situation. Denial may operate with different foci. First, there may be denial of the actual injury or illness, its severity, or its permanence. Just as prevalent, but often overlooked by sports medicine and rehabilitation professionals, is the denial of the emotional response to the catastrophic event. This aspect is often overlooked or disregarded because an athlete or individual engaged in denial may actually seem more positive, be less emotional, and be easier to work with than one who is demonstrating reactions to the situation. While some denial may actually be helpful in terms of coping, adjustment, and the rehabilitative process, excessive or inappropriate denial can inhibit the adaptation process and the rehabilitation program.

With the dissolution of denial, an emotionally turbulent period characterized by questioning, anger, and bargaining emerges. "Why me?" "What did I do to deserve this?" and "What can I do to undo this?" are typical questions and themes at this time.

This period of emotional turmoil gives way to a period of depression as the athlete or individual realizes the reality of the injury, its impact, and requirements of the recovery and rehabilitation process.

The final stage is one of working through toward acceptance, adaptation, or resolution. This is characterized by engaging in those activities, both physical and psychological, that allow maximal return to function.

This process is remarkably similar to that described by Ogilvie (1987) as the stages and reactions that athletes experience when confronted with career termination. He describes stages of denial, projection ("not me"), resentment, anger, hostility, and depression. Certainly where catastrophic injury or illness cannot be resolved, the issue of career termination emerges as well.

Despite the popularity of these paradigms, recent work has concluded that there is little empirical evidence to support them either for athletes (Brewer, 1994) or for the population in general (Wortman & Silver, 1987). Brewer (1994) suggested that cognitive appraisal models (much like those used to describe responses to stress in general) may be more appropriate. Such models propose that reactions are highly influenced by the individual's perception of the catastrophe.

While these often-described stages may or may not be universal or present in any specific or distinct order, they have relevance in clinical settings and for practitioners as a backdrop of likely issues and responses that may be encountered. Many of these themes are poignantly captured in a letter written to Ogilvie (1987, pp. 218-219) by a young female athlete whose career was ultimately terminated by knee injuries:

Now my dream really was gone for good, and I felt so lost. It has almost been a year now, and my feelings are still the same. I feel as if I am being punished for something I know nothing about. I feel real confused a lot of the time along with being scared, depressed, and lonely. I had so much going for me. I lost everything and nothing was gained by it. My knees are so dead now that I cannot enjoy most activities I want to do. I can't even play pickup ball. I could have lived with bad knees if I would have reached my goal or fulfilled my dream, but to come up so empty handed. Sometimes

I feel so angry that I just get real upset and cry. I want to be alone a lot now. I even have a hard time talking about it without getting upset. It can be compared to a death in your family. I lost something that was a major factor in my life. . . .

I have briefly told you my story. There is so much more. Your article showed me that you understand all the hurt and disappointment I'm going through. I don't know how to overcome all I've been through. I now have an "I'll-take-care-of-myself" attitude outwardly, but inwardly I'm screaming for help. If anyone could die from a broken heart, I would be dead. I would appreciate any help or advice you could give me.

The stages typically described also make the important point (i.e., the stage of shock) that the immediate postinjury or postdiagnosis period is likely to be one of **crisis**. The defining characteristic of a crisis is that it overwhelms an individual's abilities and resources to cope with the presenting situation.

It is important for sports medicine professionals who become involved with athletes immediately after injury or diagnosis to understand the characteristics of a crisis situation. Such a period begins with a time of psychological disorganization when emotions and behavioral functioning are disrupted. Individuals often have a feeling of reduced confidence and competence, if not outright feelings of hopelessness.

Individuals may appear dysfunctional or inadequate. They often feel alone and isolated and may perpetuate this by shunning offers of support. There is typically a sense of urgency to resolve the situation and to "make it go away." This may result in a frantic search for information and advice, which may end up being confusing and contradictory, given the manner in which it is sought and processed.

At a time of crisis the individual often perceives things to be worse than they are. Multiple somatic discomforts or complaints may be present. On the positive side, individuals in crisis want to trust their care providers and are amenable to help when the proper attributes of the therapeutic relationship are put into place. These attributes are discussed later in the section on managing the athlete with a catastrophic injury or illness.

crisis—A situation that overwhelms an individual's usual resources and abilities to cope.

Depression

Depression, or the effort to combat it, is perhaps the major reactive response to a catastrophic situation. Given the disruption of lifestyle, pain and discomfort, and the uncertainty of the future, this is hardly surprising. Athletes may not always perceive or express their depression in more typical ways such as crying or feelings of hopelessness. However, anger, frustration, or changes in motivation or work ethic that are unusual for a given athlete may suggest the presence of underlying depression in this context.

Clinical experience suggests that depression may also present as anxiety. Individuals may complain of feeling edgy, not at ease, uncomfortable, stressed, or nervous. Because depression is an infrequent or unusual emotion for the athlete, its emergence (or potential expression) often makes the athlete uncomfortable or anxious, and it is perceived as an anxiety state rather than depression. This is important to recognize so that the depression is effectively treated and intervention is not misdirected to the complaint of anxiety.

While beyond the scope of this paper to present in any detail, the availability of effective treatments for depression should be recognized by sports medicine professionals. One example is that of cognitive behavior therapy which posits that depression is related to the negative perceptions that an individual holds about a situation and that changing these perceptions by modifying the person's cognitive self-statements or negative "self-talk" can reduce depression. Since research has demonstrated that pain, negative self-thoughts and pessimistic outlook are related (Gil, Williams, Keefe & Beecham, 1990) and that changing negative cognitions improves ratings of discomfort and pain (Blinchik-Rybstein, 1979), this can be an important treatment approach. Another example is the value of antidepressant medication, which can be effective not only in treating mood but also helpful with other symptoms such as pain and sleep disturbance, as well (King & Strain, 1994; Charney, Miller, Licinio, & Salomon, 1995).

Impact of Depression

Awareness and management of depression are essential for efficient progress in the rehabilitation program. Depression affects the athlete's comfort level, motivation, and overall function. Depression recently has also been shown to affect outcomes in medical and rehabilitative situations such as morbidity and mortality in heart disease (Carney, Freedland, Rich, & Jaffe, 1995), return to work and activity after stroke (Feibel & Springer, 1982), and outcome in pain treatment (Kleinke, 1991).

Work with injured athletes demonstrates that depression is a significant factor. Price (1995) in his description of Monica Seles' rehabilitation notes that years after the knife attack she could not watch highlights of any Grand Slam event without crying "because I should be there."

Profile of Mood States (POMS)—
A widely used psychological measure of personality, especially that of athletes; individual scales include tension, anger, depression, vigor, fatigue, and confusion.

Research shows that the most seriously injured athletes show more depression, anger, and tension and less vigor on the **Profile of Mood States** (POMS) than less-injured athletes or college students in the normative samples. Research also shows that football players exhibit decreases in self-concept postinjury compared with preinjury and that college athletes who were more invested in professional careers at the time of their career-ending injuries had lower postcollege self-esteem and life satisfaction than those who were not so deeply invested in professional careers (Brewer, 1994; Wiese, Weiss, & Yukelson, 1991). Brewer (1991) suggested that a strong and exclusive identification with the athletic role is more likely to be associated with depressed mood after injury. However, Brewer (1994) further suggested that high physical self-esteem may help buffer the negative effects of athletic injury.

Suicide

One aspect of depression deserves special mention. Hopefully rare, when present, suicidal thought and ideation need swift and expert evaluation and intervention. Although data on the frequency of suicidal thought among athletes is difficult to obtain, it should be recognized that suicide is the third leading cause of death among individuals ages 15 to 24, and it is the fifth leading cause of death among individuals ages 25 to 64 (Cooper-Patrick, Crum, & Ford, 1994).

Especially where future participation in sport may be highly questionable, as is the case in catastrophic injury and illness, the possibility of suicidal thought should be considered. Depression, aggressive behavior, substance abuse, hopelessness, and perception of few reasons for living have all been associated with suicidal ideation. Despite this, sports medicine professionals are often uncomfortable in approaching this topic with the athlete.

Several reasons may account for this reluctance. Practitioners may feel uncomfortable asking questions about suicidal thought in the medical and rehabilitation context because that situation is not perceived to be a mental health interview. They may feel embarrassed or worry that such questions will be embarrassing to the athlete. Hesitation may come from discomfort because of a lack of experience or training in this area or discomfort about how to respond if the athlete answers affirmatively to questions about suicidal thought. Lack of time is sometimes offered as another reason why this area is avoided, although this is likely to be a rationalization to cover uneasiness. Finally, there is often a concern among non–mental health specialists (which is unsupported by clinical practice) that asking about suicidal ideation will suggest or institute such ideas.

The foregoing avoidance is unfortunate because sensitivity to and evaluation of suicidal potential can be critical when dealing with certain athletes facing catastrophic situations. It is accepted that, although individuals who harbor suicidal ideation often do not volunteer these thoughts, they do acknowledge them if asked and if the issues are explored (Cooper-Patrick et al., 1994).

To help address some of the concerns and discomfort in assessing suicidal ideation in medical situations, Cooper-Patrick et al. (1994) have developed the Suicidal Ideation Screening Questionnaire (SISQ). The SISQ is presented in table 16.2. It comprises four questions representing symptoms that the authors report to be most highly correlated with suicidal ideation. It is designed to be used with individuals who do not meet the criteria for a psychiatric disorder. It is also designed to reduce intrusiveness and embarrassment in assessing these concerns.

The authors suggest that a positive response to even one of the questions is evidence of the need for further evaluation of suicidal ideation. Where suicidal thought is an issue, it is imperative that it not be overlooked or minimized. The sports medicine professional needs to take action, including providing for the athlete's immediate safety and referral to a clinical sport psychologist or other competent mental health professional.

Post-Traumatic Stress

In the situation of catastrophic injury or illness, especially where the onset is traumatic in nature, it is important to consider the presence of post-traumatic stress symptoms, if not an actual post-traumatic stress disorder.

Post-traumatic stress is a concept that emerged from work with soldiers who experienced traumatic events during war time (e.g., shell shock). Recently it has become clear, however, that post-traumatic stress is not limited to war experiences and can occur in many other instances, including natural disasters, motor vehicle accidents, industrial accidents, physical assaults, and physical injury and illness.

The concept continues to evolve, but the most current definition of post-traumatic stress disorder can be found in the fourth edition of the *Diagnostic and Statistical Manual of the American Psychiatric Association* (DSM-IV; APA, 1994), which contains the accepted guidelines for all psychiatric diagnoses. The essence of post-traumatic stress is that it occurs when a person experiences an event that would be distressing to almost anyone and involves the occurrence or threat of bodily injury or death to oneself or significant others.

post-traumatic stress—A typical constellation of symptoms that emerge after a person encounters a traumatic or catastrophic event.

Table 16.2 Questions Used to Screen for Suicidal Ideation

1. Have you ever had a period of two weeks or more when you had trouble falling asleep, woke up too early, or slept too much?

2. Have you ever had two weeks or more during which you felt sad, blue, or depressed or when you lost interest and pleasure in things that you usually care about or enjoy?

3. Has there ever been a period of two weeks or more when you felt worthless, sinful, or guilty?

4. Has there ever been a period of time when you felt that life was hopeless?

Symptoms of Post-Traumatic Stress

There are a specific set of symptoms that define a post-traumatic stress disorder. The major features are discussed here, but the reader is referred to the DSM-IV for a full discussion of the topic. It is very normal for individuals to experience some or many of these symptoms for a limited time after being involved in a traumatic event. Post-traumatic stress symptoms become a post-traumatic stress disorder when they last longer than one month. Symptoms can also occur after an extended time period and are then referred to as a delayed post-traumatic stress disorder.

A primary symptom of post-traumatic stress disorder is the recurrence of intrusive images, pictures, or memories of a traumatic event. These images and memories seem to come on their own and are different from simply remembering what happened. They are distressing when they occur, and the individual often fights to suppress their occurrence.

These types of intrusive memories occur when the individual is awake, but nightmares are also a form of intrusive images. The nightmares may be a reflection of the actual traumatic event, or they may be symbolically related dreams of a violent or distressing nature. Flashbacks are a more extreme form of intrusive memories. Clinical experience suggests that they are more common in war-related post-traumatic stress disorders and less common in civilian accidents, except for very severe traumatic experiences, such as repeated assaults.

Another important aspect of post-traumatic stress disorders is a tendency to avoid situations or activities that remind the individual of the traumatic event. The individual may have discomfort in discussing the event, as this elicits intrusive thoughts or representative emotions. The individual may tend to avoid the location where the event occurred. Victims of motor vehicle accidents have been known to drive miles out of their way rather than taking a more direct route to their destination to avoid going by the site of the accident. Another form of this manifestation is avoiding reading articles or listening to news reports or shows that remind the individual of the event. It may also be highly uncomfortable for individuals to hear others discussing their event or similar ones.

A final group of symptoms of post-traumatic disorder involve psychological and somatic symptoms. Sleep disturbance is common with or without nightmares. Decreased appetite, low energy, and multiple minor somatic complaints (e.g., minor aches and pains) can occur. A typical expression is an increased sensitivity or jumpiness, such as being easily startled when the phone or doorbell rings.

Frequency of Post-Traumatic Stress

Although clinical experience suggests that post-traumatic stress symptoms and post-traumatic stress disorder may be underrecognized in accidents or injury situations, research now suggests that post-traumatic stress is not that uncommon. Norris (1992) reports that 24 percent of the total population may have experienced post-traumatic stress symptoms. Those experiencing chronic post-traumatic stress—defined as symptoms lasting at least three years—are around 3.4 percent of the total population (Norris, 1992). Resnick et al. (1993) reported that the overall lifetime prevalence of post-traumatic stress disorder in women may be 12.3 percent, with 4.6 percent reporting having experienced it in the six months before their study.

The prevalence of post-traumatic stress symptoms or post-traumatic stress disorder in the athletic population is difficult to determine. However, May and Sieb (1987) report a European study that compared rates of post-traumatic stress symptoms in individuals injured in skiing accidents versus individuals injured in industrial accidents. Rates of post-traumatic stress symptoms were nearly identical, with post-traumatic stress symptoms reported in 12 of 27 workers and 11 of 21 skiers. Vernacchia, Reardon, & Templeton (1997) describe the use of critical incident debriefing techniques to intervene with a team after the sudden death of one of its members.

Anecdotal Evidence of Post-Traumatic Stress

If you read accounts or look at the comments of athletes who have been traumatically injured, you can often see evidence of post-traumatic stress symptoms. For example, Kennedy (1994) described the events surrounding Chris Parker, who was characterized as the best running back in Division I AA football at Marshall University. Parker lost control of his sports car on the Nitro St. Albans Bridge, killing his girlfriend and her two sisters. Memories and survivor guilt, which is another common symptom in such situations, is reflected in his comments: "I think about the accident every day and wonder how I survived." (p. 12)

> *"I have come to recognize the total significance of that bridge. I see it as the crossroads of my life." (p. 11)*

Even more poignant are the comments from Monica Seles in the *Sports Illustrated* article by Price (1995) in which he described her ordeal as she struggled to return to competition. Price described the presence of intrusive thoughts through nightmares:

> *Sometimes her dreams were vivid replays of the attack. She would see Parche's glaring face, lunging down with the knife once and trying again. She'd wake shivering after vague visions of a tennis court and a crowd, and the crowd shouting in fear. She couldn't get the sound of her own voice, howling as the knife came down, out of her mind. "My scream is what stayed with me a long time," Seles says. (p. 24)*

The recurring nature of intrusive thoughts are found in Monica Seles' comments in the same report:

> *It was eating me alive. I would go out on the court, I could be playing great tennis, and it would all start coming back. I'd say I can't do this. I pretty much moved to daylight sleeping times. I couldn't sleep at night. I saw shadows in every corner. (p. 24)*

The impact of the intrusive thoughts and fears in her life was found in further comments:

> *All these fears came back, and it just went into this tailspin, spinning and spinning and the ball was getting bigger and bigger so that I couldn't sleep at all. I would be up all night in my room, just sitting. In the dark or light, I didn't feel comfortable leaving the house. Total depression. I was just reliving the moment. And the knife . . . .(p. 25)*

The change in psychological functioning is depicted as well:

> *For two years and three months, that [the joy and ecstasy of competing and winning] was gone along with her champion's will. During that time Seles became something else, became someone who went to sleep, fearing sleep because he would find her there, too, behind the high white walls of her Sarasota home, behind the locked door. (p. 24)*

The length of the struggle with the symptoms of post-traumatic stress and the adaptation and lingering effects are also represented:

> *Even now it isn't easy for Seles to look in the mirror and see the half-inch scar stitched just a centimeter from her spine. . . . [I]t took seven months to begin piecing together her life. (p. 28)*

Awareness of the potential for post-traumatic stress symptoms in catastrophic injury and illness is essential for sports medicine professionals for several reasons. First, post-traumatic stress symptoms, if not addressed, can solidify into a post-traumatic stress disorder. Post-traumatic stress symptoms and the disorder are distressing conditions that can be a disabling in themselves. Further, without this awareness, the symptoms of post-traumatic stress can be misdiagnosed by sports medicine professionals. Difficulties with avoidance can be misperceived as a lack of will or poor motivation. Multiple somatic complaints can be seen as being hypochondriacal or "wimpy." This does a great disservice to the athlete, denying treatment that is needed and severely hampering the rehabilitation process.

Social Aspects of Catastrophic Injury and Illness

Catastrophic injury or illness does not occur in a vacuum. The emotional effects of such incidents affect not only the athletes but those around them. Families go through the catastrophic situation with the athlete and can experience many of the same reactive responses previously described. The deficits of dysfunctional families can be exaggerated, and even greater dysfunction can occur. Families are not likely to be knowledgeable about either the physical or psychological aspects of catastrophic injury or illness and need education and guidance.

Teammates or friends may be also affected. While injury may not be foreign to sport, catastrophic injury and illness are a different matter. Teammates may also be confused and perplexed about such situations. Some of this is reflected in a comment from Philadelphia Phillies's catcher Darren Daulton in reaction to John Kruk's diagnosis of cancer:

> From what I heard before, I didn't expect to hear the word cancer. And when you hear that, there's always some concern. It certainly puts baseball secondary. (Donellon & Hagen, p. D1)

The impact of catastrophe on teammates, fellow athletes, and significant others needs to be considered and addressed.

PSYCHOLOGICAL MANAGEMENT OF ATHLETES WITH CATASTROPHIC INJURY AND ILLNESS

Just as the basic issues of psychological reactions to all sports injuries are also applicable to catastrophic injury or illness, so it is with the psychological management of the athlete with catastrophic injury or illness. The basic principles of good psychological intervention with athletes and individuals in general apply to athletes with catastrophic injury or illness. Also necessary, however, is an awareness of specialized techniques to manage the unique issues of catastrophic injury or illness, such as crisis situations or post-traumatic stress disorder. This section emphasizes issues in counseling the athlete with catastrophic injury or illness.

counseling—
Advice, guidance, or support given to help an individual make decisions or cope with challenges.

Counseling is defined as advice, guidance, and support and is differentiated from psychotherapy or more structured psychological interventions. Such approaches require specific training, expertise, and typically referral to clinical sport psychologists or other trained mental health specialists familiar with the athletic population.

Counseling is a very appropriate role for primary care physicians, physical therapists, and athletic trainers. These sports medicine and health care professionals are likely to have a unique relationship and unique contact with the athlete, which places them in a situation to be highly effective counselors. And effective counseling can do much to prevent or minimize more severe reactions in catastrophic situations, including the development of full-blown post-traumatic stress disorder (Mitchell & Bray, 1990).

Catastrophic injury or illness is very intense and requires greater ability and experience with counseling skills. Therefore a basic consideration for providing care to athletes in these situations is the degree to which sports medicine professionals feel that they can become involved with counseling or whether they should become involved at all. Shook (personal communication, 1986) has delineated several factors that sports medicine professionals can use to evaluate themselves when they consider the nature of their involvement in counseling an athlete in a catastrophic situation.

First, you should complete an honest appraisal of your own coping style and ability to handle emotionally charged situations. You should consider your level of previous experience in managing such complex situations, and if your experience is limited, the availability of expert guidance and professional support needs to be considered. Second, the demands on professional time (e.g., other patient responsibilities) and personal time (e.g., family responsibilities or concurrent personal stresses) are factors that affect your availability to the athlete. Finally, the nature of other staff members' support for and attitudes toward the sports medicine professional as an individual are important to help deal with personal reactions to crisis in the athlete.

The observant sports medicine professional will note that there are often subtle contradictions in advice about counseling athletes in catastrophic situations. For example, one general principle of athletic counseling is that athletes are independent and therefore should be treated as such by allowing their input into their planning and care, but this principle is sometimes at odds with the crisis counseling principle of individuals needing guidance and direction. Therefore considerable clinical acuity, flexibility, and decision making are required to produce a successful approach to the athlete.

A final overall consideration, even when the sports medicine professional feels comfortable in a counseling role, is when to refer the athlete for more specific interventions. May and Sieb's (1987) suggested indications for referral including the following:

1. A presenting problem that requires intervention beyond the skill of the sports medicine professional

2. Aspects of the athlete's personality that require support or intervention beyond that of general counseling

3. A clinical situation that does not seem to be improving

4. A situation that seems to be worsening

5. Discomfort, reactions, or personal bias on the part of the sports medicine professional that compromises objective treatment of the athlete

See chapter 8 for more detailed recommendations concerning the referral process.

Creating a Therapeutic Counseling Relationship

A fundamental principle of establishing a therapeutic relationship with the athlete in a catastrophic injury or illness situation is found in the comments of Wiese and colleagues (1991). They indicate that psychological rehabilitation programs, like physical rehabilitation programs, need to be individualized. Despite whatever general guidelines are given in treating athletes in specific situations, the athlete must be addressed as a unique individual. A "cookbook" or "one size fits all" approach will not work in this counseling context.

Enhancing Communication

Wiese and colleagues' (1991) survey of athletic trainers revealed that of 12 techniques rated for their effectiveness in facilitating an athlete's ability to cope with injury rehabilitation, the interpersonal aspect and communication quality specifically were rated as primary. Although the establishment of therapeutic rapport and therapeutic communication is a very complex topic, Pedersen (1986) has suggested six guidelines to facilitate an effective relationship, as presented in table 16.3. He suggested that it is important to "be aware," to recognize that emotional reactions to injury and even grief are to be expected as a part of processing the injury or illness. It is also important to "be there." He stresses the need to be available and to be helpful but cautions against doing too much for the athletes and trying to solve problems for them rather than giving them the means to do so for themselves. "Be sensitive" means allowing the expression of emotion and avoiding a tendency to squelch or minimize expression of concerns by athletes. To "be human" represents taking a nonjudgmental view of the emotions or concerns expressed by athletes to allow therapeutic coping to develop. "Be ready" emphasizes the ability and desire to be available and to be available more than once. Finally, "be patient" suggests that repetition will be needed, by the athlete in expressing concerns and by the sports medicine professional in giving guidance. The adaptation process takes time.

Also essential to the establishment of rapport in the therapeutic relationship are the types of responses the sports medicine professional makes in interactions with the athlete. Bernstein, Bernstein, and Dana (1974) describe five typical types of responses that are applicable to counseling the athlete with catastrophic injury or illness: probing, reassuring, evaluative, hostile, and understanding. They note that four of these, although having a potentially positive role, are more likely to create difficulties in establishing a therapeutic relationship.

probing response—A form of counseling interaction that attempts to elicit information through questions.

The **probing response** is essentially asking questions. This is perhaps the most frequent type of response given by sports medicine professionals, and it stems from the training of primary care physicians, athletic trainers, and physical therapists in taking a history or attempting to find out what's wrong. Although a probing response is essential for diagnosis and treatment and potentially helpful in developing a productive relationship, there are some important cautions in probing an athlete's emotional status.

Within a counseling context *excessive* or *misplaced* questions can inhibit the therapeutic process. Excessive questioning can make the athlete become a passive participant in the interaction and imply that he or she should speak only when spoken to or answer only when asked. An overemphasis on questioning may lead to the sports medicine professional's missing spontaneous cues from the athlete about his or her status that are not tapped directly by the questions. Broad or open-ended questions can help prevent unintended negative effects from probing. The simple and general "How's it going?" or "Tell me a little about . . ." allows the athlete to participate, decide on the initial direction of the interaction, and express issues personally seen as important.

reassuring response—A form of counseling interaction that attempts to restore a sense of wellness, confidence, or self-worth.

Another common response from sports medicine professionals in counseling situations, especially those of a catastrophic nature, is the **reassuring response**. Reas-

Table 16.3	Guidelines to Promote a Therapeutic Relationship With Injured Athletes	
Be aware.	Be sensitive.	Be ready.
Be there.	Be human.	Be patient.

suring responses are an attempt to restore sense of wellness, confidence, or worthiness in the athlete. There is a role for reassurance, especially in crisis situations, but problems occur when the care provider's need to reassure is so great that he or she makes unobtainable promises (i.e., invalid reassurances).

A form of false or invalid reassurance is global reassurance: comments that are so general as to be meaningless (e.g., "It'll be okay," "Don't worry—be happy!"). It must be recognized that excessive reassurance serves to minimize the expression of emotional distress. Wortman and Silver (1987) note that in catastrophic injury or illness attempts to "cheer the person up" can be seen as unhelpful and distressing. Encouraging the brighter side or suggesting things are not as bad as they seem minimizes the situation and suggests that negative feelings are inappropriate. Excessive reassurance often represents the sports medicine professional's discomfort with emotional expression and is used to shut down this expression of emotion by the athlete by suggesting that everything will be okay.

The reassurance essential for the athlete to hear is that the sports medicine professional is interested in the athlete as a person and willing to "go the distance" in providing treatment. A verbal contract offering the best care that the sports medicine professional can provide and reassuring the athlete that he or she will not be abandoned at this critical time is what needs to be communicated. A pledge of teamwork and the sports medicine professional's personal best is the type of reassurance that the athlete needs, rather than global promises that may or may not be valid.

The **evaluative response** is one that makes a value judgment about the appropriateness of the athlete's feelings and implies how the athlete should feel. Evaluative responses are problematic because it is not the sports medicine professional's place to judge the appropriateness of the athlete's feelings. It is important to remember the uniqueness of each athlete and his or her responses to the situation. It is also problematic because, by passing judgment on what is expressed, the sports medicine professional fails to recognize what is important to the athlete. It is likely to reduce the athlete's comfort in sharing further feelings and issues with the sports medicine professional.

The **hostile response** is one that is meant to humiliate, punish, or antagonize the athlete. While there may be a role for disagreeing with the athlete or even a role for strong advice, there is no therapeutic function to hostile reactions. Nonetheless, especially in catastrophic situations with prolonged rehabilitation and therapy, such responses can emerge from mutual frustrations. A hostile response to the athlete's anger simply creates a cycle of hostility and counter-hostility, which can destroy the therapeutic alliance. It is better to ascertain the source of the athlete's hostility and to recognize that anger may be justified.

Bernstein and colleagues (1974) feel that the **understanding response** is the most therapeutic and the one that provides the greatest openness and potential for therapeutic change. The understanding response is really a reflective response that summarizes or restates what the athlete has expressed. It attempts to show empathy or understanding of the athlete's perceptions and to communicate this acceptance to him or her. It is an invitation to be more open.

Promoting Coping

An important goal in counseling the athlete with catastrophic injury or illness is to promote **coping**. Coping is the cognitive and behavioral effort to manage specific internal and external demands that an individual sees as stressful and exceeding his or her usual resources and management approaches (Stone & Porter, 1995). Individuals generally have preferred or usual ways that they deal with stresses and challenges. These responses can range from a pragmatic problem-solving approach, to the use of humor, to avoiding the situation. Coping responses, however, may also

evaluative response—A form of counseling interaction that makes a value judgment about the appropriateness of another's feelings or how they should feel.

hostile response—A form of counseling interaction that is meant to humiliate, punish, or antagonize the other person.

understanding response—A form of counseling interaction that attempts to cause an individual to be more open by summarizing, restating, or reflecting what was said.

coping—The cognitive and behavioral effort to manage specific internal and external demands that an individual sees as stressful and exceeding usual resources and means of management.

be situation specific: An individual may use different responses in different situations.

While much has been written about coping, two categories are predominant: emotionally (or affectively) focused and problem (or practically) focused coping (Smith, Scott, & Wiese, 1990; Stone & Porter, 1995). Emotionally focused coping tries to reduce the negative emotional impact of the event or the stress. Problem-focused coping seeks to resolve the problem by removing or reducing the stress or threat. It is important to recognize which style is predominant for the athlete. This awareness can help in reinforcing the strengths of the athlete's style in coping and avoid creating more distress by emphasizing approaches that contradict his or her typical style. Stone and Porter (1995) note that coping style and its understanding have profound effects on health care, affecting prevention, intervention, compliance, communication, symptom perception, care seeking, and emotional responses.

There are several ways that the sports medicine professional can help promote positive coping by the athlete. First, as described, it is important to recognize the athlete's coping style and devise intervention approaches that complement it. Emphasizing any indicators of progress is important because these are often overlooked in the athlete's typical focus only on ultimate (and long-term) goals and success. It is also important to point out evidence of past or present strengths in coping with challenges (good decisions, actions taken, etc.) because an athlete in crisis may not feel effective or capable. Finally, assessing, coordinating, and monitoring sources of social support promote successful coping, as discussed in the next section.

Maximizing Support

Coping is enhanced by the presence of social support when a catastrophic injury or illness occurs. Social support means to have, and to feel as though one has, others to rely on or seek help from when needed. While some reservations have recently been raised about the reported universal benefits of social support (Smith, Fernengel, Holcroft, Gerald, & Marien, 1994), a variety of research studies generally reached the conclusion that the presence of social support facilitates coping and even outcome in medical situations. Berkman (1995) reports that social isolation and social support are related to survival in heart attack patients. There are also reports that show that social support is related to decreased postoperative pain and earlier discharge in individuals undergoing open-heart surgery and is also related to decreased recurrence of heart attacks (King, Reis, Porter, & Norsen, 1993; Reifman, 1995). Wortman and Silver (1987) noted that in bereavement or physical disability the lack of social support may hinder the recovery process.

Support comes in many different forms. Connell, Davis, Gallant, and Sharpe (1994) describe six forms important to health-related situations. These are summarized in table 16.4. Attachment is the sense of an emotional bond with others. Social integration is a sense of belonging to a group with similar activities and beliefs. Guidance refers to the availability of someone to talk with regarding matters of substance or important decisions. Reliable alliance refers to having people to count on in an emergency. Reassurance of worth is the sense that your competence and skills are recog-

Table 16.4 Forms of Social Support

Attachment	Reliable alliance
Social integration	Reassurance of worth
Guidance	Provision of assistance

nized and valued. The opportunity to provide assistance is the sense that there are people who depend on you for help, so you feel needed.

Athletes, when faced with catastrophic injury or illness, for various reasons may not accept support that is offered. Pride or fear of expressing emotions in front of others may cause athletes to try to put some distance between themselves and their support network. Conversely, those who are usually supportive may be confused and uncomfortable in a situation of catastrophic injury and illness. Rather than say the wrong thing, they may consciously or unconsciously withdraw from the athlete. The counseling role of the sports medicine professional is to appreciate the importance of support and to facilitate the support that is needed while preventing misguided emotional withdrawal by either the athlete or the support network.

It is not clear how support exerts influence on emotional and health outcomes. Berkman (1995) suggests three possible mechanisms. First, friends and supporters may be conditioned stimuli or reminders of positive function and feelings of safety and competence. Second, the interaction of social systems that influences each member of the system may positively influence the athlete through the strength of others and the social network. Third, effects may come from social learning, in which behavior and positive belief in successful outcome are learned from others in the social support network. Social support may also promote positive health outcomes by buffering stress, which can be deleterious. Social support may help stave off loneliness and depression.

Finally, it should be remembered that not all significant others are effective in providing social support. Certainly, effective social support presupposes a functional social unit. Beyond this, certain individuals may be better at providing certain types of support. It is suggested that coaches and teammates may not be the best sources of emotional support and that others need to fill this role (Rosenfeld, Richmond, & Hardy, 1989). The challenge to the sports medicine professional is to successfully orchestrate a supportive foundation for the athlete facing catastrophic injury or illness. Chapter 7 provides a number of practical suggestions for providing an effective support system.

Self-Help Materials as an Adjunct to Counseling

One approach that has been used to foster independence in and from the counseling situation and to provide therapeutic variety and reinforcement is the use of self-help books and materials. Self-help books provide an opportunity for independent action, stimulate thinking about dealing with issues, and reinforce advice given by health professionals. Topics in self-help books include managing depression, anger, pain, and much more.

Pantalon, Lubetkin, and Fishman (1995) review the role of self-help books in clinical treatment and make some suggestions for their use that are applicable to the situation of athletic injury. These authors suggest that it is more effective to prescribe self-help books to read than to leave the choice up to the athlete. This provides structure and models a high regard for the material. The authors further suggest that books be purchased by the athlete and not be provided free of charge. This allows the athlete to keep the material and make notes in it as needed. It is also more of an investment (not just financially) in therapy and the self-help book. Finally, they suggest that specific homework assignments be given rather than simply advice to read the book. It is helpful to give an overview, review chapters, emphasize points, and in general customize the self-help book for the athlete.

Santrock, Minnett, and Campbell (1994) rate the usefulness of 1000 self-help books. These ratings are based on a survey of American Psychological Association (APA) clinical and counseling psychologists. It is of course desirable that the sports medicine professional read any material before recommending it to the athlete.

Family Intervention

As has been noted, families react emotionally to catastrophic injury and illness and can be important factors in rehabilitation and recovery. While formal family therapy may be needed at times for special situations or dysfunctional families, the following guidelines can help address some typical concerns.

It is useful to encourage family members to keep communication open and not withdraw from interaction. They should continue to work on expressing emotion. They should have permission to discuss any topic, including disfigurement, permanent disability, and similar topics.

Further, all involved need to understand what the typical reactions to catastrophic injury and illness are and that such responses are normal. Ongoing information about the state of therapy and rehabilitation can help correct or prevent misperceptions and misunderstandings at various points during rehabilitation. Information should be brief, understandable, and given with the opportunity to ask questions.

The sports medicine professional should provide guidance to help the family avoid being overprotective or reinforcing the athlete's dependency. Involving the family in all phases of rehabilitation and including them at conferences, where feasible, can be helpful. All these suggestions, of course, presuppose permission from the athlete to waive confidentiality with family members. Chapter 7 provides additional information on a systems approach to social support, including the role of the family.

Sport Competition for Athletes With Disabilities

When catastrophic injury or illness is permanent, all the preceding considerations become considerably more complex. Even in this situation, however, it must be remembered that sport competition remains a possibility. There appears to be no physical condition or no sporting activity that is not amenable to creative adaptation (Chawla, 1994; Goodling & Asken, 1987; Hoffer, 1995). Sport competition for athletes with physical disabilities is now a well-developed endeavor at all levels, including national and international competition. Further, disabled sport competition can have positive effects not only on function but on adjustment as well (Asken, 1991). When an athlete cannot make a "U-turn" to preinjury competition, disabled sports competition allows the athlete to come full circle and remain active and competitive.

CASE STUDY

Marcus, a versatile 17-year-old male athlete from the eastern United States, had a dream of playing college football. He had played running back in high school and had helped his team win the state tournament in his junior year. Marcus was named All-Conference and had attracted the attention of several scouts who began calling and writing.

When football season was over, his friends and parents persuaded him to go out for varsity hockey, a sport he was good at and enjoyed but not one he intended to pursue. During the middle of the season Marcus sustained a complicated fracture of the right leg involving the tibial plateau. He also avulsed a ligament. Despite being casted, the fracture did not heal properly, and the ligament could not be repaired before the fracture was healed.

Marcus was not able to go out for football during his senior year. He sat on the sidelines in an immobilizer, trying to recover from the ligament repair surgery, bitter as he saw a potential college career slip away. With encouragement from the sports medicine team, he worked diligently on his rehabilitation and on all aspects of football. He practiced imagery, watched tapes of himself and others, maintained a positive attitude, and prepared himself to try out for a junior college team, a major disappointment compared with the Division I teams that had expressed interest in him.

In the fall Marcus attended the tryouts for the junior college football team. A few days later, however, his mother called the sports counselor to say that Marcus had been in his room lying in bed for three days since learning that he had been cut from the junior college team. She didn't know what to do. (Case study from A.M. Smith, personal communication, October 15, 1996)

QUESTIONS FOR ANALYSIS

1. Why might the injury that Marcus sustained be considered a catastrophic injury, based on the definition provided in the chapter?

2. How would you characterize Marcus's emotional responses to the injury?

3. What do you sense is Marcus's current emotional state?

4. What steps would you take if Marcus's mother called you to get a referral?

5. What types of psychological assistance would you recommend for Marcus?

SUMMARY

May and Sieb (1987) note that despite the need, psychological intervention for injured athletes is often overlooked. They suggest these reasons for this oversight: (1) Emotional responses are seen as obvious and normal and therefore are taken for granted, (2) training and treatment in sports medicine are mechanistic and technical and ignore the psychosocial aspects, and (3) athletes are often reluctant to admit their psychological distress.

As identified in this chapter, catastrophic injuries and situations sometimes befall athletes and present psychological as well as physical challenges. Typical reactions and potential problems during the struggle to regain control were described. Issues that affect the athlete but that extend beyond him or her to the team or family were presented. Throughout this chapter suggestions to allow sports medicine professionals to provide effective counseling via an emphasis on communication and support have been provided.

In catastrophic injury and illness the need for counseling is urgent, and the potential for the sports medicine professional to profoundly help the athlete is great. The catastrophically injured or ill athlete needs to have the sports medicine professional in the athlete's emotional corner.

References and Annotated Bibliography

Chapter 1: The Role of the Sports Medicine Professional in Counseling Athletes

American Physical Therapy Association. (1991). Guide for professional conduct. Alexandria, VA: Author.

American Physical Therapy Association. (1992). Evaluative criteria for accreditation of education programs for the preparation of physical therapists. Alexandria, VA: Author.

American Physical Therapy Association. (1995). Criteria for standards of practice for physical therapy. Alexandria, VA: Author.

Bass, J.L., Christoffel, K.K., Widome, M., Boyle, W., Scheidt, P., Stanwick, R., & Roberts, K. (1993). Childhood injury prevention counseling in primary care settings: A critical review of the literature. *Pediatrics, 92,* 544-550.

This review of the literature on childhood injury prevention is useful because it validates the important role of counseling in prevention. Eighteen of the 20 studies reviewed demonstrated that counseling is a factor in injury prevention.

Bass, J.L., Mehta, K.A., Ostrovsky, M., & Halperin, S.F. (1985). Educating parents about injury prevention. *Pediatric Clinics of North America, 32,* 233-243.

This paper summarizes the purposes, methods, and results of the Pediatric Accident Prevention Project (PAPP). Of particular importance was the positive effect of counseling on lowering childhood injury rates among the study population.

Biggs, D.A. (1994). Dictionary of counseling. Westport, CT: Greenwood Press.

Brewer, B.W., Jeffers, K.E., Petipas, A.J., & Van Raalte, J.L. (1994). Perceptions of psychological interventions in the context of sport injury rehabilitation. *The Sport Psychologist, 8,* 176-188.

This paper presents the results of two experiments designed to test the effect of goal setting, imagery, and counseling in sport rehabilitation settings.

Brody, D.S., Miller, S.M., Lerman, C.E., Smith, D.G., Lazaro, C.G., & Blum, M.J. (1989). *The relationship between patients' satisfaction with their physicians and perceptions about interventions they desired and received. Medical Care, 27,* 1027-1035.

Byerly, P.N., Worrell, T., Gahimer, J., & Domholdt, E. (1994). Rehabilitation compliance in an athletic training environment. *Journal of Athletic Training, 29,* 352-355.

This study categorized rehabilitating athletes as adherent or nonadherent with their rehabilitation programs and attempted to correlate their adherence with six variables. The authors conclude that rehabilitation adherence is associated with effective pain control and the presence of emotional support.

Committee on Accreditation of Allied Health Professions. (1992). Essentials and guidelines for an accredited educational program for the athletic trainer. Chicago: Author.

Corsini, R.J. (1994). Encyclopedia of psychology (2nd ed.). New York: Wiley.

Egan, G. (1986). The skilled helper (3rd ed.). Pacific Grove, CA: Brooks/Cole.

This book presents the author's model for integrating the activities of helping professionals. Chapters two through four (Overview of the Helping Model, Attending and Listening, and Empathy and Probing) are of particular value for sports medicine professionals.

Ermler, K.L., & Thomas, C.E. (1990). Interventions for the alienating effect of injury. *Athletic Training, 25,* 269-271.

The authors describe interventions that athletic therapists can use to help injured athletes overcome the effects of powerlessness, anomie, and isolation following injury.

Etzel, E.F., & Ferrante, A.P. (1993). Providing psychological assistance to injured and disabled college student athletes. In D. Pargman (Ed.), *Psychological bases of sport injuries* (pp. 265-283). Morgantown, WV: Fitness Information Technology.

This chapter describes some of the special challenges in counseling college student athletes along with methods athletic therapists and others can use when working with this group.

Fisher, A.C., (1990). Adherence to sports injury rehabilitation programmes. *Sports Medicine, 9,* 151-158.

The author emphasizes the complex nature of rehabilitation adherence and suggests strategies to help strengthen three areas critical to success in this area: competence, control, and commitment.

Fisher, A.C., Mullins, S.A., & Frye, P.A. (1993). Athletic trainers' attitudes and judgments of injured athletes' rehabilitation adherence. *Journal of Athletic Training, 28,* 43-47.

This study examined athletic trainers' perceptions about the factors that were important in enhancing rehabilitation adherence. Eight factors were identified that should help athletic therapists improve their patients' adherence.

Fisher, A.C., Scriber, K.C., Matheny, M.L., Alderman, M.H., & Bitting, L.A. (1993). Enhancing athletic injury rehabilitation adherence. *Journal of Athletic Training, 28,* 312-318.

This paper describes the role of patient education, communication, rapport, social support, personalized treatment, goal setting, progress monitoring, and therapist threats in enhancing adherence to injury rehabilitation programs.

Furney, S.R., & Patton, B. (1985). An examination of health counseling practices of athletic trainers. *Athletic Training, 20,* 294-297.

This study evaluates athletic trainers' health counseling role and perceptions of adequacy for counseling on particular subjects. Athletic trainers feel most competent to counsel athletes on injury prevention and rehabilitation. They feel least competent to counsel in the areas of bereavement, suicide, and child abuse.

Guccione, A.A., & DeMont, M.E. (1987). Interpersonal skills education in entry-level physical therapy programs. *Physical Therapy, 67,* 388-391.

This study attempts to determine the prevalence and characteristics of interpersonal skills education (IPS) in physical therapy schools. The authors found that most physical therapy programs teach IPS, but fewer evaluate their students' mastery of IPS competencies.

Heil, J. (1993). Diagnostic methods and measures. In J. Heil (Ed.), *Psychology of sport injury* (pp. 89-112). Champaign, IL: Human Kinetics.

This chapter describes the process of diagnostic assessment in injury psychology. It describes various tests the sport psychologist can use to assess the psychological state of an injured athlete. Heil emphasizes the value of using input from the sports medicine staff to supplement diagnostic testing.

Heil, J., Bowman, J.J., & Bean, B. (1993). Patient management and the sports medicine team. In J. Heil (Ed.), *Psychology of sport injury* (pp. 237-249). Champaign, IL: Human Kinetics.

Heil, Bowman, and Bean make the case for the sports medicine professional's involvement in the psychological care of the injured athlete. Suggestions for the identification of common psychological problems experienced by injured athletes are provided. The chapter helps supplement the sports medicine professional's counseling experience with psychologically sound techniques.

Henderson, J., & Carroll, W. (1993). The athletic trainer's role in preventing sport injury and rehabilitating injured athletes: A psychological perspective. In D. Pargman (Ed.), *Psychological bases of sport injuries* (pp. 15-31). Morgantown, WV: Fitness Information Technology.

This chapter offers an athletic trainer's perspective to injury and rehabilitation psychology. Several case studies are provided to help the reader apply the theoretical material in a realistic setting.

Henderson, J.G., Pollard, C.A., Jacobi, K.A., & Merkel, W.T. (1992). Help-seeking patterns of community residents with depressive symptoms. *Journal of Affective Disorders, 26,* 157-162.

Hendrickson, T.P., & Rowe, S.J. (1990). The role of sports psychology/psychiatry. In Mellion, W.M. Walsh, & G.L. Shelton, (Eds.), *The team physician's handbook* (pp 95-110). Philadelphia: Hanley & Belfus.

This chapter provides a useful summary of the things team physicians should consider when coordinating the athlete's mental health care.

Holland, J.L., Magoon, T.M., & Spokane, A.R. (1981). Counseling psychology: Career interventions, research, and theory. *Annual Review of Psychology, 32,* 279-305.

This article combines a thorough review of the literature on career counseling with the authors' theory about the origins and patterning of careers. Their concept of counseling seems particularly well-suited for the role of the allied health professional.

Ivey, A.E., & Authier, J. (1978). Microcounseling. Springfield, IL: Charles C. Thomas.

This book describes the microcounseling techniques for interviewing, counseling, and psychological therapy skills.

Janis, I.L. (1983). Short-term counseling. New Haven, CT: Yale University Press.

The primary premise of this book is that a supportive relationship can be developed in just one session between helper and client. This book is appropriate for sports medicine professionals since it defines "helping" quite broadly and emphasizes the importance of the short-term counseling relationship so characteristic in sports medicine.

Kane B. (1982). Trainer in a counseling role. *Athletic Training, 17,* 167-168.

Kane, B. (1984). Trainer counseling to avoid three face-saving maneuvers. *Athletic Training,* 171.

This article describes the steps the athletic trainer can take to intervene with athletes who attempt to "save face" in athletics through accidental injury, intentional injury, and malingering.

Kottler, J.A. (1986). On being a therapist. San Francisco, CA: Jossey-Bass.

Although written primarily for mental health professionals, this book is useful for sports medicine professionals. Of particular value are the sections that highlight the personal hardships that can beset health care professionals who take on a counseling role with their patients.

Makarowski, L.M., & Rickell, J.G. (1993). Ethical and legal issues for sport professionals counseling injured athletes. In D. Pargman (Ed.), *Psychological bases of sport injuries* (p.45-65). Morgantown, WV: Fitness Information Technology.

The authors describe the legal and ethical requirements of counseling injured athletes. The authors describe a process of value-decision making that will help sports medicine professionals maintain a proper counseling relationship with their athletes.

Miller, M.J., & Moore, K.K. (1993). Athletes' and non-athletes' expectations about counseling. *Journal of College Student Development, 34,* 267-270.

The authors conclude that there are no differences between the two groups with regard to their expectations about counseling.

Murray, J. (1992). Prevention and the identification of high risk groups. *International Review of Psychiatry, 4,* 281-286.

This paper is of significant value for sports medicine professionals because it empha-sizes the importance of preventing minor psychological problems through early identifi-cation, referral, and treatment.

National Athletic Trainers Association. (1985). Standards of Professional Practice. Dallas: Author.

National Athletic Trainers Association. (1992). Competencies in Athletic Training. Dallas: Author.

National Athletic Trainers Association. (1993). Essentials and guidelines for development and implementation of NATA accredited graduate athletic training education programs. Dallas: Author.

National Athletic Trainers Association Board of Certification. (1995). Role delineation study (3rd ed.). Philadelphia: F.A. Davis.

Pedersen, P. (1986). The grief response and injury: A special challenge for athletes and athletic trainers. *Athletic Training, 21,* 312-314.

This paper describes the grief response and the role the athletic trainer can play in facili-tating it.

Ramsden, E.L., & Taylor, L.J. (1988). Stress and anxiety in the disabled patient. *Physical Therapy, 68,* 992-996.

The authors describe typical patient reactions to stress and the steps that physical thera-pists can take to ameliorate the problems of anxiety and fear related to the stress of disability.

Ray, R. (1994). Management strategies in athletic training. Champaign, IL: Human Kinetics.

This book describes the basic management functions athletic trainers are expected to carry out in their daily practice. The chapter on legal liability is useful for creating an awareness of the athletic trainer's legal responsibilities in the counseling role.

Ray, R., Hanlon, J., & Van Heest, G. (1989). Facilitating team grieving: A case study. *Athletic Training, 24,* 39-42.

This paper describes an actual case of an athletic trainer–mental health nurse–pastor team and their counseling role with members of a team after the death of a teammate.

Residency Review Committee for Family Practice (1996). *Program requirements for residency eduction in family practice.*

Saunders, C., & Maxwell, M. (1988). The case for counseling in physical therapy. *Physiotherapy, 74,* 592-596.

This paper advocates the use of microcounseling in physical therapy practice. The tech-nique of "reflecting" is examined in particular detail.

Smith, A.M., Scott, S.G., & Wiese, D.M. (1990). The psychological effects of sports injuries. *Sports Medicine, 9,* 352-369.

This review article examines several aspects of athletes' post-injury psychological state. The authors stress the individuality of athlete response to injury which makes careful attention to post-injury signs and symptoms so important.

Stewart, J.T. (1989). Training caregivers. North Vancouver, BC: Para-Professional Training Associates.

Thompson, R.A., & Sherman, R.T. (1993). Helping athletes with eating disorders. Champaign, IL: Human Kinetics.

This is an excellent source of information for sports medicine professionals who wish to improve the understanding and skill in dealing with eating disorders.

Viney, L.L., Clarke, A.M., Bunn, T.A., & Benjamin, Y.N. (1985). The effect of a hospital-based counseling service on the physical recovery of surgical and medical patients. *General Hospital Psychiatry, 7,* 294-301.

Wiese, D.M., & Weiss, M.R. (1987). Psychological rehabilitation and physical injury: Implications for the sports medicine team. *The Sport Psychologist, 1,* 318-330.

This paper focusses on four areas of interest to sports medicine professionals: 1) How do injuries happen?, 2) How do athletes respond to injuries?, 3) How can psychological recovery from injury be facilitated?, and 4) When are athletes psychologically ready to return to competition?

Wiese, D.M., Weiss, M.R., & Yukelson, D.P. (1991). Sport psychology in the training room: A survey of athletic trainers. *The Sport Psychologist, 5,* 15-24.

This study provides evidence of athletic trainer perceptions about the important and effective components of various psychological entities.

Wiese-Bjornstal, D.M., & Smith, A.M. (1993). Counseling strategies for enhanced recovery of injured athletes within a team approach. In D. Pargman (Ed.), *Psychological bases of sport injuries* (p.149-182). Morgantown, WV: Fitness Information Technology.

This chapter provides useful guidance to sports medicine professionals on steps they can take to facilitate a holistic approach to recovery from athletic injury.

Chapter 2: Psychosocial Dimensions of Sport Injury

Andersen, M.B., & Williams, J.M. (1988). A model of stress and athletic injury: Prediction and prevention. *Journal of Sport and Exercise Psychology, 10,* 294-306.

This review paper provides a framework for the prediction and prevention of stress-related sport injuries. A theoretical model of stress and athletic injury is presented, and corresponding research is described.

Andersen, M.B., & Williams, J.M. (1993). Psychological risk factors and injury prevention. In J. Heil (Ed.), *Psychology of sport injury* (pp. 49-57). Champaign, IL: Human Kinetics.

Brewer, B.W. (1993). Self-identity and specific vulnerability to depressed mood. *Journal of Personality, 61,* 343-364.

Brewer, B.W., Linder, D.E., & Phelps, C.M. (1995). Situational correlates of emotional adjustment to athletic injury. *Clinical Journal of Sports Medicine, 5,* 241-245.

Brewer, B.W., Petitpas, A.J., Van Raalte, J.L., Sklar, J.H., & Ditmar, T.D. (1995). Prevalence of psychological distress among patients at a physical therapy clinic specializing in sports medicine. *Sports Medicine, Training, and Rehabilitation, 6,* 139-145.

Brewer, B.W., Van Raalte, J.L., & Linder, D.E. (1991). Role of the sport psychologist in treating injured athletes: A survey of sports medicine providers. *Journal of Applied Sport Psychology, 3,* 183-190.

Brown, M.L. (1995). *Athlete, athletic trainer, and coach perceptions of athletic injury cause and prevention.* Unpublished master's thesis, University of Minnesota, Minneapolis.

Carmen, L., Zerman, J.L., & Blaine, G.B. (1968). The use of Harvard psychiatric service by athletes and nonathletes. *Mental Hygiene, 52,* 134-137.

Chan, C.S., & Grossman, H.Y. (1988). Psychological effects of running loss on consistent runners. *Perceptual and Motor Skills, 66,* 875-883.

Coakley, J.J. (1996). Socialization through sports. In O. Bar-Or (Ed.), *The child and adolescent athlete* (pp. 353-363). Oxford, England: Blackwell Science.

Cromer, B.A., & Tarnowski, K.J. (1989). Noncompliance in adolescents: A review. *Journal of Developmental and Behavioral Pediatrics, 10*(4), 207-215.

Crossman, J., & Jamieson, J. (1985). Differences in perceptions of seriousness and disrupting effects of athletic injury as viewed by athletes and their trainers. *Perceptual and Motor Skills, 61,* 1131-1134.

Crossman, J., Jamieson, J., & Hume, K.M. (1990). Perceptions of athletic injuries by athletes, coaches and medical professionals. *Perceptual and Motor Skills, 71,* 848-850.

Curry, T. (1992). A little pain never hurt anyone: Athletic career socialization and the normalization of sports injuries. *Sociology of Sport Journal, 11,* 273-290.

Daly, J.M., Brewer, B.W., Van Raalte, J.L., Petitpas, A.J., & Sklar, J.H. (1995). Cognitive appraisal, emotional adjustment, and adherence to rehabilitation following knee surgery. *Journal of Sport Rehabilitation, 4,* 22-30.

Duda, J.L., Smart, A.E., & Tappe, M.K. (1989). Predictors of adherence in the rehabilitation of athletic injuries: An application of personal investment theory. *Journal of Sport and Exercise Psychology, 11,* 367-381.

Dugan, D.O. (1987). Death and dying: Emotional, spiritual and ethical support for patients and families. *Journal of Psychosocial Nursing, 25,* 21-29.

Fisher, C.A., Domm, M.A., & Wuest, D.A. (1988). Adherence to sports injury rehabilitation programs. *Physician and Sportsmedicine, 16*(7), 47-51.

Fisher, C. A., Mullins, S.A., & Frye, P.A. (1993). Athletic trainers' attitudes and judgments of injured athletes' rehabilitation adherence. *Journal of Athletic Training, 28,* 43-47.

Fisher, C.A., Scriber, K.C., Matheny, M.L., Alderman, M.H., & Bitting, L.A. (1993). Enhancing athletic injury rehabilitation adherence. *Journal of Athletic Training, 28,* 312-318.

Frey, J.H. (1991). Social risk and the meaning of sport. *Sociology of Sport Journal, 8,* 136-145.

This paper describes the "culture of risk" inherent in sport.

Friedman, I.M., & Litt, I.F. (1986). Promoting adolescents' compliance with therapeutic regimens. *Pediatric Clinics of North America, 33,* 955-973.

Ginsberg, H., & Opper, S. (1979). *Piaget's theory of intellectual development.* Englewood Cliffs, NJ: Prentice Hall.

Gordon, S., Milios, D., & Grove, J.R. (1991). Psychological aspects of the recovery process from sport injury: The perspective of sport physiotherapists. *Australian Journal of Science and Medicine in Sport, 23,* 53-60.

Gould, D., Udry, E., Bridges, D., & Beck, L. (1997a). Coping with season-ending injuries. *Sport Psychologist, 11,* 379-399.

Gould, D., Udry, E., Bridges, D., & Beck, L. (1997b). Stress sources encountered when rehabilitating from season-ending injuries. *Sport Psychologist, 11,* 361-378.

Grove, J.R. (1993). Personality and injury rehabilitation among sport performers. In D. Pargman (Ed.), *Psychological bases of sport injuries* (pp. 99-120). Morgantown, WV: Fitness Information Technology.

Hardy, C.J., & Crace, R.K. (1993). The dimensions of social support when dealing with sport injuries. In D. Pargman (Ed.), *Psychological bases of sport injuries* (pp. 121-144). Morgantown, WV: Fitness Information Technology.

This chapter provides an excellent discussion of how social support can be a facilitative factor in recovery from sport injury.

Heil, J. (1993). *Psychology of sport injury.* Champaign, IL: Human Kinetics.

The content of this book is organized into six parts: psychological perspectives on injury, behavioral risk factors, assessment of injury, treatment of injury, the sports medicine team, and biomedical issues.

Hughes, R.H., & Coakley, J. (1991). Positive deviance among athletes: The implications of overconformity to the sport ethic. *Sociology of Sport Journal, 8,* 307-325.

This paper describes the sport ethic, which involves accepting injury risks and playing through pain as the norm in sport.

Kahanov, L., & Fairchild, P.C. (1994). Discrepancies in perceptions held by injured athletes and athletic trainers during the initial injury evaluation. *Journal of Athletic Training, 29,* 70-75.

Kozar, B., & Lord, R.H. (1988). Overuse injuries in the young athlete: A "growing" problem. In F.L. Smoll, R.A. Magill, & M.J. Ash (Eds.), *Children in sport* (3rd ed., pp. 119-129). Champaign, IL: Human Kinetics.

LaMott, E.E. (1994). *The anterior cruciate ligament injured athlete: The psychological process.* Unpublished doctoral dissertation, University of Minnesota, Minneapolis.

LaMott, E.E., Petlichkoff, L.M., Van Wassenhove, J., Stein, K., Wade, G., & Lewis, K. (1989, September). *Psychological rehabilitation of the injured athlete: An educational approach to injury.* Paper presented at the annual meeting of the Association for the Advancement of Applied Sport Psychology, Seattle, WA.

Lewis, L., & LaMott, E.E. (1992, October). *Psychosocial aspects of the injury response in professional football: An exploratory study.* Paper presented at the annual meeting of the Association for the Advancement of Applied Sport Psychology, Colorado Springs, CO.

Lord, R.H., & Kozar, B. (1989). Pain tolerance in the presence of others: Implications for youth sports. *The Physician and Sportsmedicine, 17* (10), 71-72, 77.

McDonald, S.A., & Hardy, C.J. (1990). Affective response patterns of the injured athlete: An exploratory analysis. *The Sport Psychologist, 4,* 261-274.

Messner, M.A. (1990). Men studying masculinity: Some epistemological questions in sport sociology. *Sociology of Sport Journal, 7,* 136-153.

Messner, M.A. (1992). *Power at play: Sports and the problem of masculinity.* Boston: Beacon Press.

Morrey, M.A. (1997). *A longitudinal examination of emotional response, cognitive coping, and physical recovery among athletes undergoing anterior cruciate ligament reconstructive surgery.* Unpublished doctoral dissertation, University of Minnesota, Minneapolis.

Nixon, H.L. (1993). Accepting the risks of pain and injury in sport: Mediated cultural influences on playing hurt. *Sociology of Sport Journal, 10,* 183-196.

Pearson, L., & Jones, G. (1992). Emotional effects of sports injuries: Implications for physiotherapists. *Physiotherapy, 78,* 762-770.

Rice, P.L. (1992). *Stress and health* (2nd ed.). Pacific Grove, CA: Brooks/Cole.

Rotella, R.J., Ogilvie, B.C., & Perrin, D.H. (1993). The malingering athlete: Psychological considerations. In D. Pargman (Ed.), *Psychological bases of sport injuries* (pp. 85-97). Morgantown, WV: Fitness Information Technology.

Shumaker, S.A., & Brownell, A. (1984). Toward a theory of social support: Closing conceptual gaps. *Journal of Social Issues, 40,* 11-36.

Smith, A.M. (1996). Psychological impact of injuries in athletes. *Sports Medicine, 22,* 391-405.

Smith, A.M., Scott, S.G., O'Fallon, W.M., & Young, M.L. (1990). The emotional responses of athletes to injury. *Mayo Clinic Proceedings, 65,* 38-50.

Smith, A.M., Scott, S.G., & Wiese, D.M. (1990). The psychological effects of sports injuries: Coping. *Sports Medicine, 9,* 352-369.

This review paper summarizes literature on athletes' emotional responses to injury and associated psychological coping strategies.

Smith, A.M., Stuart, M.J., Wiese-Bjornstal, D.M., Milliner, E.K., O'Fallon, W.M., & Crowson, C.S. (1993). Competitive athletes: Preinjury and postinjury mood state and self-esteem. *Mayo Clinic Proceedings, 68,* 939-947.

Smith, R.E., Smoll, F.L., & Ptacek, J.T. (1990). Conjunctive moderator variables in vulnerability and resiliency: Life stress, social support and coping skills, and adolescent sport injuries. *Journal of Personality and Social Psychology, 58,* 360-370.

Strauss, R.H., & Lanese, R.R. (1982). Injuries among wrestlers in school and college tournaments. *Journal of the American Medical Association, 284*(16), 2016-2019.

Thornton, J.S. (1990). Playing in pain: When should an athlete stop? *Physician and Sportsmedicine, 18*(9), 138-142.

Udry, E. (1997). Coping and social support among injured athletes following surgery. *Journal of Sport and Exercise Psychology, 19,* 71-90.

Udry, E., Gould, D., Bridges, D., & Beck, L. (1997). Down but not out: Athlete responses to season-ending injuries. *Journal of Sport and Exercise Psychology, 19,* 229-248.

Weinberg, R.S., & Gould, D. (1995). *Foundations of sport and exercise psychology.* Champaign, IL: Human Kinetics.

Weiner, B. (1985). An attribution theory of achievement motivation and emotion. *Psychological Review, 92,* 548-573.

Wiese, D.M., & Weiss, M.R. (1987). Psychological rehabilitation and physical injury: Implications for the sportsmedicine team. *The Sport Psychologist, 1,* 318-330.

Wiese, D.M., Weiss, M.R., & Yukelson, D.P. (1991). Sport psychology in the training room: A survey of athletic trainers. *The Sport Psychologist, 5,* 15-24.

Wiese-Bjornstal, D.M., & Smith, A.M. (1993). Counseling strategies for enhanced recovery of injured athletes within a team approach. In D. Pargman (Ed.), *Psychological bases of sport injuries* (pp. 149-182). Morgantown, WV: Fitness Information Technology.

Some basic counseling areas and the responsibilities of various members of the sports medicine team are identified in this chapter. The roles of athletic trainers, coaches, teammates, parents, sport psychologists, and physicians are discussed.

Wiese-Bjornstal, D.M., Smith, A.M., & LaMott, E.E. (1995). A model of psychologic response to athletic injury and rehabilitation. *Athletic Training: Sports Health Care Perspectives, 1,* 16-30.

Wiese-Bjornstal, D.M., Smith, A.M., Shaffer, S.M., & Morrey, M.A. (1998). An integrated model of response to sport injury: Psychological and sociological dynamics. *Journal of Applied Sport Psychology, 10* (1), 46-69.

This review paper summarizes current research knowledge on the cognitive and emotional responses of athletes to injury. A sociocultural perspective on the role of playing with pain and injury in North American sport is also provided.

Williams, J.M., & Andersen, M.B. (1998). Psychosocial antecedents of sport injury: Review and critique of the stress and injury model. *Journal of Applied Sport Psychology 10* (1), 5-25.

A review of the literature with specific application to the original predictions of the Andersen and Williams (1988) stress–response model of athletic injury.

Williams, J.M., & Roepke, N. (1993). Psychology of injury and injury rehabilitation. In R.N Singer, M. Murphey, & L. Tennant (Eds.), *Handbook of research on sport psychology* (pp. 815-839). New York: Macmillan.

Young, K., White, P., & McTeer, W. (1994). Body talk: Male athletes reflect on sport, injury, and pain. *Sociology of Sport Journal, 11,* 175-194.

Chapter 3: Psychosocial Intervention Strategies in Sports Medicine

Andersen, M.B., & Williams, J.M. (1993). Psychological risk factors and injury prevention. In J. Heil (Ed.), *Psychology of sport injury* (pp. 49-57). Champaign, IL: Human Kinetics.

This article presents a theoretical model for understanding the relationship between stress and athletic injury. A framework for predicting and preventing stress-related injuries—including cognitive, physiological, attentional, behavioral, interpersonal, and social factors—is discussed.

Bunker, L., Williams, J.M., & Zinsser, N. (1993). Cognitive techniques for improving performance and building confidence. In J.M. Williams (Ed.), *Applied sport psychology* (pp. 225-242). Mountain View, CA: Mayfield.

Danish, S.J., Petitpas, A.J., & Hale, B.D. (1993). Life development interventions for athletes: Life skills through sports. *Counseling Psychologist, 21*(3), 352-385.

> *This article describes sport psychology and a psychoeducational model that counseling psychologists can apply as teachers of life skills for athletes. Specific examples of sport psychology framed within a life-development intervention model are provided.*

Davis, J.O. (1991). Sports injuries and stress management: An opportunity for research. *Sport Psychologist, 5,* 175-182.

Duda, J.L., Smart, A.E., & Tappe, M.K. (1989). Predictors of adherence in the rehabilitation of athletic injuries: An application of personal investment theory. *Journal of Sport and Exercise Psychology, 11,* 367-381.

Fisher, C.A., Domm, M.A., & Wuest, D.A. (1988). Adherence to sports-related rehabilitation programs. *Physician and Sportsmedicine, 16,* 47-52.

Folkman, S., & Lazarus, R.S. (1980). An analysis of coping in a middle-aged community sample. *Journal of Health and Social Behavior, 21,* 219-239.

Granito, V., Hogan, J., & Varnum, L. (1995). The Performance Enhancement Group Program: Integrating sport psychology and rehabilitation. *Journal of Athletic Training, 30*(4), 328-331.

> *This article discusses the implementation of a team approach to athletic injury management. The responsibilities of members of a team composed of sport psychology and athletic training professionals are presented. A program model addressing ways to physically and mentally support the injured athlete throughout rehabilitation is also presented.*

Green, L.B. (1994). The use of imagery in the rehabilitation of injured athletes. In A.A. Sheikh & E.R. Korn (Eds.), *Imagery in sports and physical performance* (pp. 157-174). Amityville, NY: Baywood.

> *This chapter provides an in-depth examination of the application of imagery in athletic injury rehabilitation. Philosophical, historical, and psychological perspectives supporting the use of imagery and specific techniques that can be employed throughout the duration of the injury are provided.*

Hughes, R.H., & Coakley, J. (1991). Positive deviance among athletes: The implications of overconformity to the sport ethic. *Sociology of Sport Journal, 8,* 307-325.

> *This article focuses on developing a definition of positive deviance and on using the definition to scientifically analyze athletes' behavior. The concept of the sport ethic and its influence on the adoption of negative attitudes and behaviors is also discussed.*

Huizenga, R. (1994). *You're okay, it's just a bruise.* New York: St. Martin's Press.

Ievleva, L., & Orlick, T. (1991). Mental links to enhanced healing: An exploratory study. *The Sport Psychologist, 5,* 25-40.

Ievleva, L., & Orlick, T. (1993). Mental paths to enhanced recovery from a sports injury. In D. Pargman (Ed.), *Psychological bases of sport injuries* (pp. 219-245). Morgantown, WV: Fitness Information Technology.

Kerr, G., & Goss, J. (1996). The effects of a stress management program on injuries and stress levels. *Journal of Applied Sport Psychology, 8,* 109-117.

Krane, V., Greenleaf, C.A., & Snow, J. (1997). Reaching for gold and the price of glory: A motivational case study of an elite gymnast. *The Sport Psychologist, 11,* 53-71.

Martens, R. (1987). *Coaches guide to sport psychology.* Champaign, IL: Human Kinetics.

Pargman, D. (Ed.). (1993). *Psychological bases of sport injuries.* Morgantown, WV: Fitness Information Technology.

Petitpas, A., & Danish, S.J. (1995). Caring for injured athletes. In S.M. Murphy (Ed.), *Sport psychology interventions* (pp. 255-281). Champaign, IL: Human Kinetics.

Focused on examining psychological factors that affect athletes with injuries, this chapter emphasizes the psychological rehabilitative process. Specific sections include injury's psychological effects, warning signs of difficult adjustment to injury, typical treatment protocol in psychological strategies, and practical and ethical issues facing sport psychologists in the sports medicine setting.

Rice, P.L. (1992). *Stress and health* (2nd ed.). Pacific Grove, CA: Brooks/Cole.

Richardson, P.A., & Latuda, L.M. (1995). Therapeutic imagery and athletic injuries. *Journal of Athletic Training, 30*(1), 10-12.

Athletic trainers and practicing clinicians are offered basic information about the use of imagery in rehabilitation. This article describes a sample imagery program that incorporates a series of prescribed steps, including the introduction, evaluation, acquisition, and adjunctive use of imagery in a rehabilitation program.

Ryan, J. (1995). *Little girls in pretty boxes: The making and breaking of elite gymnasts and figure skaters.* New York: Doubleday.

Samuels, M., & Samuels, N. (1975). *Seeing with the mind's eye.* New York: Random House; Berkeley: Bookworks.

Shaffer, S.M. (1996). *Grappling with injury: What motivates young athletes to wrestle with pain?* Unpublished doctoral dissertation, University of Minnesota, Minneapolis.

Suinn, R.M. (1987). Behavioral approaches to stress management in sports. In J.R. May & M.J. Asken (Eds.), *Sport psychology* (pp. 59-75). New York: PMA.

Udry, E. (1996). Social support: Exploring its role in the context of athletic injuries. *Journal of Sport Rehabilitation, 5,* 151-163.

Udry, E., Gould, D., Bridges, D., & Tuffey, S. (1997). People helping people? Examining the social ties of athletes coping with burnout and injury stress. *Journal of Sport and Exercise Psychology, 19,* 368-395.

Warner, L., & McNeill, M.E. (1988). Mental imagery and its potential for physical therapy. *Physical Therapy, 68*(4), 516-521.

This article presents existing research to support the useful application of mental imagery in a physical therapy setting. It also presents variables influencing the outcome of mental practice and the advantages and disadvantages of using imagery with physical therapy patients.

Weiss, M.R., & Troxel, R.K. (1986). Psychology of the injured athlete. *Athletic Training, 21,* 104-109, 154.

Wiese-Bjornstal, D.M., & Smith, A.M. (1993). Counseling strategies for enhanced recovery of injured athletes within a team approach. In D. Pargman (Ed.), *Psychological bases of sport injuries* (pp. 149-182). Morgantown, WV: Fitness Information Technology.

Wiese-Bjornstal, D.M., Smith, A.M., & LaMott, E.E. (1995). A model of psychologic response to athletic injury and rehabilitation. *Athletic Training: Sports Health Care Perspectives, 1*(1), 17-30.

Wolpe, J. (1973). *The practice of behavior therapy.* New York: Pergamon Press.

Yukelson, D., & Murphy, S. (1993). Psychological considerations in injury prevention. In P.A.F.H. Renstrom (Ed.), *Sport injuries: Basic principles of prevention and care* (pp. 321-333). Cambridge, MA: Blackwell Scientific.

Chapter 4: Effective Interaction Skills for Sports Medicine Professionals

Cormier, L.S., & Hackney, H. (1993). *The professional counselor: A process guide to helping* (2nd ed.). Boston: Allyn & Bacon.

Davis, C.M. (1990). What is empathy, and can empathy be taught? *Physical Therapy, 70,* 707-715.

The author discusses empathy from both a philosophical and practical perspective as it relates to the work of physical therapists.

Ford, I.W., & Gordon, S. (1993). Social support and athletic injury: The perspective of sport physiotherapists. *Australian Journal of Science and Medicine in Sport, 25*(1), 17-25.

Hardy, C.J., & Crace, R.K. (1993). The dimensions of social support when dealing with sport injuries. In D. Pargman (Ed.), *Psychological bases of sport injuries* (pp. 121-144). Morgantown, WV: Fitness Information Technology.

This chapter provides an excellent discussion of the various dimensions of social support, with specific emphasis on how they relate to the work of sports medicine professionals.

Heil, J. (1993). *Psychology of sport injury.* Champaign, IL: Human Kinetics.

Kahanov, L., & Fairchild, P.C. (1994). Discrepancies in perceptions held by injured athletes and athletic trainers during the initial injury evaluation. *Journal of Athletic Training, 29,* 70-75.

This paper describes the results of a study examining the nature of communication between athletic trainers and athletes during the initial injury examination.

Kottler, J.A., & Brown, R.W. (1996). *Introduction to therapeutic counseling* (3rd ed.). Pacific Grove, CA: Brooks/Cole.

Kottler, J.A., & Kottler, E. (1993). *Teacher as counselor: Developing the helping skills you need.* Newbury Park, CA: Corwin Press.

Martens, R. (1987). *Coaches guide to sport psychology.* Champaign, IL: Human Kinetics.

Communication recommendations for athletic coaches are provided in chapter 4 of this book.

Martin, D.G. (1983). *Counseling and therapy skills.* Prospect Heights, IL: Waveland Press.

Mehrabian, A. (1971). *Silent messages.* Belmont, CA: Wadsworth.

Okun, B.F. (1992). *Effective helping: Interviewing and counseling techniques* (4th ed.). Pacific Grove, CA: Brooks/Cole.

Petitpas, A., & Danish, S.J. (1995). Caring for injured athletes. In S.M. Murphy (Ed.), *Sport psychology interventions* (pp. 255-281). Champaign, IL: Human Kinetics.

Purtilo, R., & Haddad, A. (1996). *Health professional and patient interaction* (5th ed.). Philadelphia: Saunders.

Rosenfeld, L., & Wilder, L. (1990). Communication fundamentals: Active listening. *Sport Psychology Training Bulletin, 1*(5), 1-8.

Schultz, C.L., Wellard, R., & Swerissen, H. (1988). Communication and interpersonal helping skills: An essential component in physiotherapy education? *Australian Journal of Physiotherapy, 34,* 75-80.

This paper describes the rationale for and content of a program on interdisciplinary communication and interpersonal helping skills for physiotherapy students.

Trainers staff. (1993, Fall). Athletic directory/sport psychology. *Trainers, 8,* 1.

Wagstaff, G.F. (1982). A small dose of commonsense—communication, persuasion and physiotherapy. *Physiotherapy, 68,* 327-329.

This very practical article identifies characteristics of the communicator, of the message, and of the audience, with specific recommendations for the work of physiotherapists.

Wiese, D.M., Weiss, M.R., & Yukelson, D.P. (1991). Sport psychology in the training room: A survey of athletic trainers. *The Sport Psychologist, 5,* 15-24.

This paper presents the results of a survey of athletic trainers. In particular, it was noted that athletic trainers recognize the need for strong interpersonal communication skills in working with injured athletes.

Wiese-Bjornstal, D.M., & Smith, A.M. (1993). Counseling strategies for enhanced recovery of injured athletes within a team approach. In D. Pargman (Ed.), *Psychological bases of sport injuries* (pp. 149-182). Morgantown, WV: Fitness Information Technology.

Some basic counseling areas and responsibilities of various members of the sports medicine team are identified in this chapter. Athletic trainers, coaches, teammates, parents, physicians, and physical therapists all have important roles to play in interactions.

Yukelson, D. (1993). Communicating effectively. In J.M. Williams (Ed.), *Applied sport psychology: Personal growth to peak performance* (pp. 122-136). Mountain View, CA: Mayfield.

This chapter provides an overview of effective communication skills for anyone working with athletes. The important role of empathy and active listening skills are described.

Chapter 5: Assessing Athletes Through Individual Interview

Andersen, M.B., & Williams, J.M. (1988). A model of stress and athletic injury: Prediction and prevention. *Journal of Sport and Exercise Psychology, 10,* 294-306.

Anshel, M.H. (1997). *Sport psychology: From theory to practice* (3rd ed.). Scottsdale, AZ: Gorsuch Scarisbruck.

Bianco, T.M., & Orlick, T. (1996). Social support influences on recovery from sports injury. *Journal of Applied Sport Psychology (AAASP Abstracts), 8* (Oct., Suppl. S), 57.

Brewer, B.W. (1993). Self-identity and specific vulnerability to depressed mood. *Journal of Personality, 61,* 343-364.

Grove, J.R. (1993). Personality and injury rehabilitation among sport performers. In D. Pargman (Ed.), *Psychological bases of sports injuries* (pp. 99-120). Morgantown, WV: Fitness Information Technology.

A discussion of the ways in which personality influences the thoughts, feelings, and behaviors of athletes during rehabilitation is presented in this chapter.

Leddy, M.H., Lambert, M.J., & Ogles, B.M. (1994). Psychological consequences of athletic injury among high level competition. *Research Quarterly for Exercise and Sport, 65*(4), 347-354.

McDonald, S.A., & Hardy, C.J. (1990). Affective response patterns of the injured athlete: An exploratory analysis. *The Sport Psychologist, 4,* 261-274.

McNair, D.M., Lorr, M., Droppleman, L.F. (1971). Profile of mood states. San Diego: Educational and Industrial Testing Service.

Morrey, M.A. (1997). *A longitudinal examination of emotional response, cognitive coping, and physical recovery among athletes undergoing anterior cruciate ligament reconstructive surgery.* Unpublished doctoral dissertation, University of Minnesota, Minneapolis.

Myers, D.G. (1990). *Exploring psychology.* New York: Worth.

This general psychology text discusses different theories of learning, development, and personality. It also briefly describes counseling theories.

Rotella, R.J., & Heyman, S.R. (1993). Stress, injury, and the psychological rehabilitation of athletes. In J.M. Williams (Ed.), *Sport psychology: Personal growth to peak performance* (2nd ed., pp. 338-355). Mountain View, CA: Mayfield.

Smith, A.M., & Milliner, E.K. (1995). Injured athletes and the risk of suicide. *Journal of Athletic Training, 29*(9), 337-341.

This paper describes several young athletes who attempted suicide after each sustained a serious athletic injury, required a surgical procedure, and endured a long and difficult rehabilitation. These young athletes had all failed to achieve their preinjury sport competency at the time of their suicide attempts. The emphasis of this paper is that the postinjury depression that may accompany serious athletic injury is not without risk in a vulnerable age group.

Smith, A.M., Scott, S.G., O'Fallon, W., & Young, M.L. (1990). The emotional responses of athletes to injury. *Mayo Clinic Proceedings, 65,* 38-50.

Smith, A.M., Scott, S.G., & Wiese, D.M. (1990). The psychological effects of sports injuries: Coping. *Sports Medicine, 9,* 352-369.

Smith, A.M., Stuart, M.J., Wiese-Bjornstal, D.M., Milliner, E.K., O'Fallon, W.M., & Crowson, C.S. (1993). Competitive athletes: Pre and post injury mood state and self-esteem. *Mayo Clinic Proceedings, 68,* 939-947.

Wiese-Bjornstal, D.M., & Smith, A.M. (1993). Counseling strategies for enhanced recovery of injured athletes within a team approach. In D. Pargman (Ed.), *Psychological bases of sports injuries* (pp. 149-182). Morgantown, WV: Fitness Information Technology.

Wiese-Bjornstal, D.M., Smith, A.M., & LaMott, E.E. (1995). A model of psychological responses to athletic injury and rehabilitation. *Athletic Training: Sports Health Care Perspectives, 1*(1), 16-30.

Williams, J.M., & Roepke, N. (1993). Psychology of injury and injury rehabilitation. In R. Singer & M. Tennant (Eds.), *Handbook of research on sports psychology* (pp. 815-839). New York: Macmillan.

This review chapter outlines key research on personality and psychosocial factors that contribute to injury risk, mechanisms by which these variables might cause injuries, and the psychological aspects of injury rehabilitation.

Chapter 6: Effective Group Health Education Counseling

Anderson, M.K., & Hall, S.J. (1995). *Sports injury management.* Philadelphia: Williams & Wilkins.

This comprehensive sports medicine text provides information on various health-related practices, conditions, and diseases. It is a valuable source of information for undergraduate athletic trainers.

Bull, S.J. (1995). Reflections on a 5-year consultancy program with the England women's cricket team. *The Sport Psychologist, 9,* 148-163.

Carron, A.V. (1982). Cohesiveness in sport groups: Interpretations and considerations. *Journal of Sport Psychology, 4,* 123-128.

Flint, F.A., & Weiss, M.R. (1992). Returning injured athletes to competition, a role and ethical dilemma. *Canadian Journal of Sport Sciences, 17,* 34-40.

Furney, S.R., & Patton, B. (1985). An examination of health counseling practices of athletic trainers. *Athletic Training, 21,* 294-297.

Gill, D.L. (1986). *Psychological dynamics of sport.* Champaign, IL: Human Kinetics.

This book provides an extensive coverage of issues related to sport psychology. The material is presented in a manner conducive for use by coaches, athletes, and sport psychologists.

Hoberman, J.M. (1992). *Mortal engines: The science of performance and the dehumanization of sport.* New York: Free Press.

John Hoberman has written an expose of some of the dehumanizing aspects of sport. This controversial book provides the reader with historical background into health-related issues and practices with athletes.

Lopiano, D.A., & Zotos, C. (1992). Modern athletics: The pressure to perform. In K.D. Brownell, J. Rodin, & J.H. Wilmore (Eds.), *Eating, body weight, and performance in athletes* (pp. 275-292). Philadelphia: Lea & Febiger.

Specific physiological, psychological, and sociological aspects of sport and their impact on athletes are discussed in this book. It provides an in-depth discussion of several topics such as eating disorders and overtraining and could form the foundation for health education counseling programs.

Pate, R.R., McClenaghan, B., & Rotella, R. (1984). *Scientific foundations of coaching.* New York: Saunders.

This book was one of the original texts that attempted to integrate scientific aspects (physiology, biomechanics, and psychology) in a coaching context.

Petruzzello, S.J., Landers, D.M., Linder, D.E., & Robinson, D.R. (1987). Sport psychology service delivery: Implementation within the university community. *Sport Psychologist, 1,* 248-256.

Salmela, J.H. (1989). Long-term intervention with the Canadian men's Olympic gymnastic team. *The Sport Psychologist, 3,* 340-349.

Taylor, J. (1995). A conceptual model for integrating athletes' needs and sport demands in the development of competitive mental preparation strategies. *Sport Psychologist, 9,* 339-357.

Zimmerman, T.S., & Protinsky, H. (1993). Uncommon sports psychology: Consultation using family therapy theory and techniques. *American Journal of Family Therapy, 21,* 161-174.

Zimmerman, T.S., Protinsky, H.O., & Zimmerman, C.S. (1994). Family systems consultation with an athletic team: A case study of themes. *Journal of Applied Sport Psychology, 6,* 101-115.

Chapter 7: Using Family Systems Theory to Counsel the Injured Athlete

Becker, L.A. (1989). Family systems and compliance with medical regimen. In C.N. Ramsey, Jr. (Ed.), *Family systems medicine* (pp. 416-431). New York: Guilford Press.

Brewer, B.W., Jeffers, K.E., Petitpas, A.J., & Van Raalte, J.L. (1994). Perceptions of psychological interventions in the context of sport injury and rehabilitation. *The Sport Psychologist, 8*(2), 176-188.

Cook, A.S., & Dworkin, D.S. (1992). *Helping the bereaved: Therapeutic interventions for children, adolescents, and adults.* New York: Basic Books.

de Schazer, S. (1988). *Clues: Investigating solutions in brief therapy.* New York: Norton.

Fisch, R., Weakland, J., & Segal, L. (1982). *The tactics of change: Doing therapy briefly.* San Francisco: Jossey-Bass.

This book offers background and interventions related to problem cycles.

Grove, J.R., Hanrahan, S.J., & Stewart, R.M. (1990). Attributions for rapid or slow recovery from sports injuries. *Canadian Journal of Sport Sciences, 15*(2), 107-114.

Hardy, L. (1992). Psychological stress, performance, and injury in sport. *British Medical Bulletin, 48*(3), 615-629.

Lanning, W., & Toye, P. (1993). Counseling athletes in higher education. In W.D. Kirk & S.V. Kirk (Eds.), *Student athletes: Shattering the myths and sharing the realities* (pp. 61-70). Virginia: American Counseling Association.

Larivaara, P., Vaisanen, E., & Kiuttu, J. (1994). Family systems medicine: A new field of medicine. *Nordic Journal of Psychiatry, 48*(5), 329-332.

Lynch, G.P. (1988). Athletic injuries and the practicing sport psychologist: Practical guidelines for assisting athletes. *The Sport Psychologist, 2*(2), 161-167.

This article suggests that the emotional component and the role of the mind in athletic injury are often overlooked in the intervention process. It provides practical strategies for the sport psychologist pertaining to the mind–body connection.

Murray, C.I., Sullivan, A.M., Brophy, D.R., & Mailhot, M. (1991). Working with parents of spinal cord injured adolescents: A family systems perspective. *Child & Adolescent Social Work Journal, 3,* 225-238.

Nichols, M.P., & Schwartz, R.C. (1995). *Family therapy: Concepts and methods* (3rd ed.). Boston: Allyn & Bacon.

> *This book describes the latest approaches to family therapy. Two separate chapters on research are included.*

Nideffer, R.M. (1989). Psychological aspects of sports injuries: Issues in prevention and treatment. *International Journal of Sport Psychology, 20*(4), 241-255.

Patterson, J.M. (1991). A family systems perspective for working with youth with disability. *Pediatrician, 18*(2), 129-141.

Petrie, T.A. (1992). Psychological antecedents of athletic injury: The effects of life stress and social support on female collegiate gymnasts. *Behavioral Medicine, 18*(3), 127-138.

Sachs, P.R., & Ellenberg, D.B. (1994). The family system and adaptation to an injured worker. *American Journal of Family Therapy, 22*(3), 263-272.

Thompson, T.L., Hershman, E.B., & Nicholas, J.A. (1990). Rehabilitation of the injured athlete. *Pediatrician, 17*(4), 262-266.

Wiese, D.M., & Weiss, M.R. (1987). Psychological rehabilitation and physical injury: Implications for the sportsmedicine team. *The Sport Psychologist, 1*(4), 318-330.

Wiese, D.M., Weiss, M.R., & Yukelson, D.P. (1991). Sport psychology in the training room: A survey of athletic trainers. *The Sport Psychologist, 5*(1), 15-24.

Zimmerman, T.S. (1993). Systems family therapy with an athlete. *Journal of Family Psychotherapy, 4*(3), 29-37.

> *This paper discusses many issues common in athletic families, including the need to perform and the subsequent anxiety that performance pressure creates.*

Zimmerman, T.S., & Protinsky, H. (1993). Uncommon sports psychology: Consultation using family therapy theory and techniques. *American Journal of Family Therapy, 21*(2), 161-174.

> *This article suggests that the goals of sport system consultants, including conflict resolution and management, symptom removal, and cohesion, are similar to those of family therapists.*

Zimmerman, T.S., Protinsky, H., & Zimmerman, C.S. (1994). Uncommon sports psychology: A qualitative study of systems consultation with athletic teams. *Journal of Applied Sport Psychology, 6,* 101-115.

> *This paper presents the recurrent themes that emerged from a family systems consultation case study with a university women's athletic team.*

Chapter 8: Referral of Injured Athletes for Counseling and Psychotherapy

Andersen, M.B., & Brewer, B.W. (1995). Organizational and psychological consultation in collegiate sports medicine groups. *Journal of American College Health, 44,* 63-69.

Andersen, M.B., Denson, E.L., Brewer, B.W., & Van Raalte, J.L. (1994). Disorders of personality and mood in athletes: Recognition and referral. *Journal of Applied Sport Psychology, 6,* 168-184.

Bobele, M., & Conran, T.J. (1988). Referrals for family therapy: Pitfalls and guidelines. *Elementary School Guidance, 22,* 192-198.

Brewer, B.W. (1994). Review and critique of models of psychological adjustment to athletic injury. *Journal of Applied Sport Psychology, 6,* 87-100.

Brewer, B.W., Jeffers, K.E., Petitpas, A.J., & Van Raalte, J.L. (1994). Perceptions of psychological interventions in the context of sport injury rehabilitation. *The Sport Psychologist, 8,* 176-188.

Brewer, B.W., Linder, D.E., & Phelps, C.M. (1995). Situational correlates of emotional adjustment to athletic injury. *Clinical Journal of Sport Medicine, 5,* 241-245.

Brewer, B.W., Petitpas, A.J., Van Raalte, J.L., Sklar, J.H., & Ditmar, T.D. (1995). Prevalence of psychological distress among patients at a physical therapy clinic specializing in sports medicine. *Sports Medicine, Training and Rehabilitation, 6,* 139-145.

Brewer, B.W., & Petrie, T.A. (1995, Spring). A comparison of injured and uninjured football players on selected psychosocial variables. *Academic Athletic Journal,* pp. 11-18.

Brewer, B.W., Van Raalte, J.L., & Linder, D.E. (1991). Role of the sport psychologist in treating injured athletes: A survey of sports medicine providers. *Journal of Applied Sport Psychology, 3,* 183-190.

Carson, R.C., Butcher, J.N., & Mineka, S. (1996). *Abnormal psychology and modern life* (10th ed.). New York: Harper Collins.

Cerny, F.J., Patton, D.C., Whieldon, T.J., & Roehrig, S. (1992). An organizational model of sports medicine facilities in the United States. *Journal of Orthopaedic and Sports Physical Therapy, 15,* 80-86.

Chan, C.S., & Grossman, H.Y. (1988). Psychological effects of running loss on consistent runners. *Perceptual and Motor Skills, 66,* 875-883.

Daly, J.M., Brewer, B.W., Van Raalte, J.L., Petitpas, A.J., & Sklar, J.H. (1995). Cognitive appraisal, emotional adjustment, and adherence to sport injury rehabilitation following knee surgery. *Journal of Sport Rehabilitation, 4,* 23-30.

Gipson, M., Foster, M., Yaffe, D., O'Carroll, V., Bene, C., & Moore, B. (1989, April). *Opportunities for health psychology in sports medicine services and training.* Paper presented at the Western Psychological Association/Rocky Mountain Psychological Association Joint Annual Convention, Reno, NV.

Heil, J. (1993a). Referral and coordination of care. In J. Heil (Ed.), *Psychology of sport injury* (pp. 251-266). Champaign, IL: Human Kinetics.

This chapter presents considerations in making psychological referrals for injured athletes and integrating service delivery among members of the sports medicine team.

Heil, J. (1993b). Specialized treatment approaches: Problems in rehabilitation. In J. Heil (Ed.), *Psychology of sport injury* (pp. 195-218). Champaign, IL: Human Kinetics.

Henderson, J., & Carroll, W. (1993). The athletic trainer's role in preventing sport injury and rehabilitating injured athletes: A psychological perspective. In D. Pargman (Ed.), *Psychological bases of sport injuries* (pp. 15-31). Morgantown, WV: Fitness Information Technology.

Heyman, S.R. (1993). When to refer athletes for counseling and psychotherapy. In J. Williams (Ed.), *Applied sport psychology: Personal growth to peak performance* (2nd ed., pp. 299-309). Mountain View, CA: Mayfield.

Ievleva, L., & Orlick, T. (1991). Mental links to enhanced healing: An exploratory study. *The Sport Psychologist, 5,* 25-40.

Kane, B. (1982). Trainer in a counseling role. *Athletic Training, 17,* 167-168.

Kane, B. (1984). Trainer counseling to avoid three face-saving maneuvers. *Athletic Training, 19,* 171-174.

Kazdin, A.E. (1979). Nonspecific treatment effects: A methodological evaluation. *Psychological Bulletin, 8,* 729-758.

Larson, G.A., Starkey, C.A., & Zaichowsky, L.D. (1996). The psychological aspects of athletic injuries as perceived by athletic trainers. *The Sport Psychologist, 10,* 37-47.

Leddy, M.H., Lambert, M.J., & Ogles, B.M. (1994). Psychological consequences of athletic injury among high level competitors. *Research Quarterly for Exercise and Sport, 65,* 347-354.

Linder, D.E., Brewer, B.W., Van Raalte, J.L., & DeLange, N. (1991). A negative halo for athletes who consult sport psychologists: Replication and extension. *Journal of Sport and Exercise Psychology, 13,* 133-148.

Linder, D.E., Pillow, D.R., & Reno, R.R. (1989). Shrinking jocks: Derogation of athletes who consult a sport psychologist. *Journal of Sport and Exercise Psychology, 11,* 270-280.

Makarowski, L.M., & Rickell, J.G. (1993). Ethical and legal issues for sport professionals counseling injured athletes. In D. Pargman (Ed.), *Psychological bases of sport injuries* (pp. 45-65). Morgantown, WV: Fitness Information Technology.

Meyer, J.D., Fink, C.M., & Carey, P.F. (1988). Medical views of psychological consultation. *Professional Psychology: Research and Practice, 19,* 356-358.

Misasi, S.P., Davis, C.F., Jr., Morin, G.E., & Stockman, D. (1996). Academic preparation of athletic trainers as counselors. *Journal of Athletic Training, 31,* 39-42.

National Athletic Trainers Association. (1992). *Competencies in athletic training.* Dallas: Author.

This document delineates the standards for entry-level practice in athletic training.

Pearson, L., & Jones, G. (1992). Emotional effects of sports injuries: Implications for physiotherapists. *Physiotherapy, 78,* 762-770.

Petitpas, A., & Danish, S.J. (1995). Caring for injured athletes. In S.M. Murphy (Ed.), *Sport psychology interventions* (pp. 255-281). Champaign, IL: Human Kinetics.

Using case study material to illustrate key points, this chapter explores psychological effects of sport injury and identifies warning signs of a poor adjustment to sport injury. It examines psychological treatments for injured athletes and discusses the role of psychologists in sports medicine.

Smith, A.M., & Milliner, E.K. (1994). Injured athletes and the risk of suicide. *Journal of Athletic Training, 29,* 337-341.

This article describes risk factors for suicide by injured athletes and outlines suicidal risk assessment practices for sports medicine professionals.

Smith, A.M., Stuart, M.J., Wiese-Bjornstal, D.M., Milliner, E.K., O'Fallon, W.M., & Crowson, C.S. (1993). Competitive athletes: Preinjury and postinjury mood state and self-esteem. *Mayo Clinic Proceedings, 68,* 939-947.

Strein, W., & Hershenson, D.B. (1991). Confidentiality in nondyadic counseling situations. *Journal of Counseling and Development, 69,* 312-316.

Van Raalte, J.L., & Andersen, M.B. (1996). Referral processes in sport psychology. In J.L. Van Raalte & B.W. Brewer (Eds.), *Exploring sport and exercise psychology* (pp. 275-284). Washington, DC: American Psychological Association.

Although oriented primarily to psychologists, this chapter presents an overview of referral processes in the sport environment that transcends professional boundaries. Guidelines for appropriate referral practices are provided.

Van Raalte, J.L., Brewer, B.W., Brewer, D.D., & Linder, D.E. (1992). NCAA Division II college football players' perceptions of an athlete who consults a sport psychologist. *Journal of Sport and Exercise Psychology, 14,* 273-282.

Wiese-Bjornstal, D.M., Smith, A.M., & LaMott, E.E. (1995). A model of psychologic response to athletic injury rehabilitation. *Athletic Training: Sports Health Care Perspectives, 1,* 17-30.

This article offers a comprehensive framework for understanding the psychological responses of athletes to injury. Personal and situational factors influencing injured athletes' cognitive, emotional, and behavioral responses are discussed in depth.

Wise, A., Jackson, D.W., & Rocchio, P. (1979). Preoperative psychologic testing as a predictor of success in knee surgery: A preliminary report. *American Journal of Sports Medicine, 7,* 287-292.

Chapter 9: Documentation in Counseling

American Physical Therapy Association. (1995). *Criteria for standards of practice for physical therapy.* Alexandria, VA: Author.

Berni, R., & Readey, H. (1978). *Problem-oriented medical record implementation.* St. Louis: Mosby.

This text describes the POMR approach to medical documentation. It includes sections on how to implement the system, how various medical and allied health practitioners can use it, and how to evaluate it.

Bond, T. (1993). *Standards and ethics for counselling in action.* London: Sage.

Sports medicine professionals should read chapter 12, "Record Keeping," to gain an appreciation for the differences between medical and mental health documentation. This book is written from a British perspective but is still useful for U.S. readers.

Brown, E. (1982). Record content. In H. Schuchman, L. Foster, & S. Nye (Eds.), *Confidentiality of health records* (pp. 45-64). New York: Gardner Press.

This very useful chapter highlights the essential content of the medical record. Of special interest is the section on dual mental health records.

Dayringer, R. (1978). The problem-oriented record in pastoral counseling. *Journal of Religion and Health, 17,* 39-47.

This article describes the content of the problem-oriented medical record and provides examples for its implementation in a counseling setting.

Fulero, S.M., & Wilbert, J.R. (1988). Record-keeping practices of clinical and counseling psychologists. *Professional Psychology: Research and Practice, 19,* 658-660.

Grant, R.L. (1977). Can the problem-oriented system improve the delivery of psychosocial health care? Promises and caveats. *International journal of mental health.* Vol. 6, no. 2 pp 8-16.

Hartman, B.L., & Wickey, J.M. (1978). The person-oriented record in treatment. *Social Work, 23,* 296-299.

Heil, J. (1993). Referral and coordination of care. In J. Heil (Ed.), *Psychology of sport injury* (pp. 251-266). Champaign, IL: Human Kinetics.

This chapter outlines not only the steps to follow in helping sports medicine specialists make mental health referrals, but also the importance of the team approach to holistic care for the athlete.

Henry, P.F. (1994). Legal principles in providing telephone advice. *Nurse Practitioner Forum, 5,* 124-125.

This article contains useful legal guidance for those who provide medical advice over the telephone. The admonition to carefully document all such advice is highlighted in several places in the article.

Holmes, G.E., & Karst, R.H. (1989). Case record management: A professional skill. *Journal of Applied Rehabilitation Counseling, 20,* 36-40.

Iyer, P.W., & Camp, N.H. (1991). *Nursing documentation: A nursing process approach.* St. Louis: Mosby-Year Book.

This is an excellent text for any medical professional, although it specifically targets nurses. It contains a wealth of practical advice on medical record keeping and provides examples of forms that can be used for a variety of purposes.

Jacob, S., & Hartshorne, T.S. (1991). *Ethics and law for school psychologists.* Brandon, VT: Clinical Psychology.

This book is most appropriate for those sports medicine professionals who work in K-12 education. Chapter 4—"Privacy, Informed Consent, Confidentiality, and Record Keeping"—is particularly appropriate and applicable.

Keith-Spiegel, P., & Koocher, G.P. (1985). *Ethics in psychology: Professional standards and cases.* New York: Random House.

This is a comprehensive volume on ethical issues confronted by those who provide psychological services. Chapter 3—"Privacy, Confidentiality, and Record Keeping"—is helpful to sports medicine professionals who want to improve the documentation of their counseling contacts with athletes.

National Athletic Trainers Association. (1985). *Standards of professional practice.* Dallas: Author.

Perlman, B.B., Schwartz, A.H., Paris, M., Thornton, J.C., Smith, H., & Webber, R. (1982). Psychiatric records: Variations based on discipline and patient characteristics, with implications for quality of care. *American Journal of Psychiatry, 139,* 1154-1157.

Piazza, N.J., & Baruth, N.E. (1990). Client record guidelines. *Journal of Counseling and Development, 68,* 313-316.

This article delineates the essential components of the mental health record. It is written primarily for mental health professionals, but sports medicine specialists can improve their practice in this area by following the authors' advice.

Ray, R. (1994). *Management strategies in athletic training.* Champaign, IL: Human Kinetics.

This book describes the basic management functions that athletic trainers are expected to carry out in their daily practice. The chapter on information management provides sports medicine professionals with practical strategies for documenting the services they provide to athletes.

Reynolds, J.F., Mair, D.C., & Fischer, P.C. (1992). *Writing and reading mental health records: Issues and analysis.* Newbury Park, CA: Sage.

This book is a comprehensive treatment of the metal health record. Sports medicine practitioners will glean the most useful information from chapters 1, 5, and 6.

Soisson, E.L., VandeCreek, L., & Knapp, S. (1987). Thorough record keeping: A good defense in a litigious era. *Professional Psychology: Research and Practice, 18,* 498-502.

Thompson, R.A., & Sherman, R.T. (1993). *Helping athletes with eating disorders.* Champaign, IL: Human Kinetics.

Thompson and Sherman present a comprehensive approach to working with athletes who suffer from eating disorders. They speak about issues of confidentiality in chapter 5, "Treatment-Related Issues."

Walzer, R.S. (1989). Legal aspects of employing "counselors" in a clinical practice. *Connecticut Medicine, 53,* 147-151.

This article is especially important for athletic trainers and physical therapists who are employed by physicians and for physicians who employ other sports medicine specialists. It outlines the legal pitfalls of providing counseling in such a setting and highlights the importance of good documentation and communication with the supervising physician.

Chapter 10: Ethical Perspectives in Counseling

American Counseling Association. (1995). *Code of ethics.* Alexandria, VA: Author.

American Medical Association. (1980). *Principles of medical ethics.* Chicago: Author.

American Physical Therapy Association. (1991). *Code of ethics.* Alexandria, VA: Author.

American Psychological Association (1992). *Ethical principles of psychologists and code of conduct.* Washington, DC: Author.

Appelbaum, D., & Lawton, S.V. (1990). *Ethics and the professions.* Englewood Cliffs, NJ: Prentice Hall.

This book covers a broad range of ethical issues faced by professionals in many different disciplines. It is a particularly good reference for obtaining a concise presentation of ethical theory and important concepts that serve as a foundation for ethics.

Demos, G.D., & Grant, B. (1973). *An introduction to counseling: A handbook.* Los Angeles: Western Psychological Services.

Chapter 4 of this book is on the ethics of counseling. It includes an outdated version of the American Counseling Association Code of Ethics but is followed by an excellent summary of some important ethical principles for counselors.

Gorlin, R.A. (Ed.). (1990). *Codes of professional responsibility* (2nd ed.). Washington, DC: Bureau of National Affairs.

This reference includes the codes of ethics from a broad range of professions, as well as descriptions of the organizations and the context from which their codes are derived. It is a very good source from which to gain an appreciation of the ethics from diverse disciplinary perspectives.

Makarowski, L.M., & Rickell, J.B. (1993). Ethical and legal issues for sport professionals counseling injured athletes. In D. Pargman (Ed.), *Psychological bases of sport injuries* (pp. 45-65). Morgantown, WV: Fitness Information Technology.

This chapter is a good reference on the types of ethical issues with which the sports medicine practitioner should be familiar. It does a particularly good job of addressing issues that have both legal and ethical implications, and it addresses "Potential Traps" for which the practitioner serving in a counseling role should watch out.

National Athletic Trainers Association. (1995). *NATA code of ethics.* Dallas: Author.

Chapter 11: Counseling for Substance Abuse Problems

Alcoholics Anonymous World Services, Inc. (1976). *Alcoholics Anonymous* (3rd ed.). New York: Author.

American Psychiatric Association. (1994). *Diagnostic and statistical manual of mental disorders* (4th ed.; DSM-IV). Washington, DC: Author.

Beresford, T., Low, D., Adduci, R., & Goggans, F. (1982). Alcoholism assessment on an orthopedic surgery service. *Journal of Bone and Joint Surgery, 64A,* 730-733.

Brower, K.J. (1992). Anabolic steroids: Addictive, psychiatric, and medical consequences. *American Journal on Addictions, 1,* 100-114.

Brower, K.J., & Severin, J.D. (1997). Alcohol and other drug-related problems. In D.J. Knesper, M.B. Riba, & T.L. Schwenk (Eds.), *Primary care psychiatry* (pp. 309-342). Philadelphia: Saunders.

Brown, T.C., & Benner, C. (1984). The nonmedical use of drugs in sports. In W.N. Scott, B. Nisonson, J.A. Nicholas (Eds.), *Principles of sports medicine* (pp. 32-39). Baltimore: Williams & Wilkins.

Ewing, J.A. (1984). Detecting alcoholism: the CAGE questionnaire, *JAMA, 252,* 1905-1907.

Fleming, M.F., & Barry, K.L. (1992). *Addictive disorders.* St. Louis: Mosby.

A practical guide written to answer, "What should every health care professional know about the care of persons adversely affected by nicotine, alcohol, and other mood-altering drugs?" It includes specific chapters on drugs in sports, adolescent substance abuse, prescription drug abuse, and smoking cessation.

Hawks, R.L., & Chiang, C.N. (1986). Examples of specific drug assays. *National Institute on Drug Abuse Research Monograph Series, 73,* 84-112.

Kishline, A. (1994). *Moderate drinking: The new option for problem drinkers.* Tucson: See Sharp Press.

A self-help guide designed for at-risk drinkers and early problem drinkers. Includes tables for calculating blood alcohol levels from the number of drinks consumed for a given body weight and sex.

Miller, W.R., & Rollnick, S. (1991). *Motivational interviewing: Preparing people to change addictive behavior.* New York: Guilford Press.

An essential guide to motivating resistant patients. Filled with examples of what to say to patients who do not think they have a problem.

Moore, R.D., Bone, L.R., Geller, G., Mamon, J.A., Stokes, E.J., & Levine, D.M. (1989). Prevalence, detection, and treatment of alcoholism in hospitalized patients. *Journal of the American Medical Association, 261,* 403-407.

National Institute on Alcohol Abuse and Alcoholism. (1995). *The physicians' guide to helping patients with alcohol problems* (NIH Publication No. 95-3769). Washington, DC: U.S. Department of Health and Human Services.

Contains guidelines for alcohol screening and brief intervention by physicians. Single copies are available free from NIAAA, Scientific Communications Branch, Office of Scientific Affairs, Willco Building, Suite 409, 6000 Executive Blvd., Bethesda, MD 20892-7003. Telephone: (301) 443-3860.

Nuzzo, N.A., & Waller, D.P. (1988). Drug abuse in athletes. In J.A. Thomas (Ed.), *Drugs, athletes, and physical performance* (pp. 141-167). New York: Plenum.

Saunders, J.B., Aasland, O.G., Babor, T.F., de la Fuente, J.R., & Grant, M. (1993). Development of the Alcohol Use Disorders Identification Test (AUDIT): WHO collaborative project on early detection of persons with harmful alcohol consumption—II. *Addiction, 88,* 791-804.

Schuckit, M.A. (1995). *Drug and alcohol abuse: A clinical guide to diagnosis and treatment* (4th ed.). New York: Plenum.

This is a treatment-oriented book in which the chapters are divided by drug class. For each class of drug, it covers epidemiology, pharmacology, and emergency treatment of intoxication and withdrawal syndromes.

Skinner, H.A. (1982). The Drug Abuse Screening Test. *Addictive Behaviors, 7,* 363-371.

Vereby, K. (1991). Laboratory methodology for drug and alcohol addiction. In N.S. Miller (Ed.), *Comprehensive handbook of drug and alcohol addiction* (pp. 809-824). New York: Marcel Dekker.

Wadler, G.I., & Hainline, B. (1989). *Drugs and the athlete.* Philadelphia: Davis.

A well-written, comprehensive clinical book on drug abuse in sports. Topics covered include risk factors, specific ergogenic drugs, recognition, drug testing, clinical management, and legal considerations.

Yesalis, C.E. (Ed.). (1993). *Anabolic steroids in sport and exercise.* Champaign, IL: Human Kinetics.

This book provides essential, accurate information about the history, incidence, and physiological effects of anabolic steroids as well as the implications for treatment, prevention, and social policy that are useful when counseling potential or current users.

Chapter 12: Recognizing and Assisting Athletes With Eating Disorders

American College of Sports Medicine. (1987). Position statement on the use of anabolic-androgenic steroids in sports. *Medicine and Science in Sports and Exercise, 9,* 534-539.

American Psychiatric Association. (1994). *Diagnostic and statistical manual of mental disorders* (4th ed.). Washington, DC: Author.

Black, D.R., & Burckes-Miller, M.E. (1988). Male and female college athletes: Use of anorexia nervosa and bulimia nervosa weight loss methods. *Research Quarterly for Exercise and Sport, 59,* 252-256.

Davis, C., & Cowles, M. (1989). A comparison of weight and diet concerns and personality factors among athletes and nonathletes. *Journal of Psychosomatic Research, 33,* 527-536.

Davis, C., Kennedy, S.H., Ravelski, E., & Dionne, M. (1994). The role of physical activity in the development and maintenance of eating disorders. *Psychological Medicine, 24,* 957-967.

Dick, R.W. (1991). Eating disorders in NCAA athletic programs. *Athletic Training, 26,* 136-140.

In 1990, 803 NCAA institutions were surveyed concerning the number of student athletes who had experienced an eating disorder in the last two years; 61 percent responded. Results indicated that many more women than men had eating disorders and that eating disorders were more prevalent in lean (e.g., wrestling, gymnastics) as opposed to nonlean (e.g., volleyball, tennis) sports.

Enns, M.P., Drewnowski, A., & Grinker, J.A. (1987). Body composition, body size estimation, and attitudes toward eating in male college athletes. *Psychosomatic Medicine, 49,* 56-64.

Garfinkel, P.E., & Garner, D.M. (Eds.). (1987). *The role of drug treatment for eating disorders.* New York: Brunner/Mazel.

Mintz, L.B., & Betz, N.E. (1988). Prevalence and correlates of eating disordered behaviors among undergraduate women. *Journal of Counseling Psychology, 35,* 463-471.

This study examined the prevalence of eating disorders in female undergraduates by conceptualizing them on a continuum and found that over 60 percent of the sample reported an intermediate (subclinical) form of disordered eating. In addition, the study found a direct relationship between the level of disordered eating and psychological health, with greater eating disturbances being related to more body dissatisfaction, lower self-esteem, and greater acceptance of societal beliefs about attractiveness.

Mitchell, J.E. (1986a). Anorexia nervosa: Medical and physiological aspects. In K.D. Brownell & J.P. Foreyt (Eds.), *Handbook on eating disorders* (pp. 247-265). New York: Basic Books.

Mitchell, J.E. (1986b). Bulimia: Medical and physiological aspects. In K.D. Brownell & J.P. Foreyt (Eds.), *Handbook on eating disorders* (pp. 379-388). New York: Basic Books.

National Collegiate Athletic Association (1989). *Nutrition and eating disorders in collegiate athletics* [Video]. Kansas City, MO: Author.

Petrie, T.A. (1993). Disordered eating in female collegiate gymnasts: Prevalence and personality/attitudinal correlates. *Journal of Sport and Exercise Psychology, 15,* 424-436.

Petrie, T.A. (1996). Differences between male and female college lean sport athletes, nonlean sport athletes, and nonathletes on behavioral and psychological indices of eating disorders. *Journal of Applied Sport Psychology, 8,* 218-230.

The author examined male and female athletes and nonathletes to determine the potential influences of the athletic environment on behavioral and psychological indices of eating disorders and found that lean-sport environments are associated with athletes' preoccupation with weight and diet. In general, however, athletes are more satisfied with the size and shape of their bodies and feel more in control of and effective in their lives.

Petrie, T.A., Austin, L.J., Crowley, B.J., Helmcamp, A., Johnson, C.E., Lester, R., Rogers, R., Turner, J., & Walbrick, K. (1996). Sociocultural expectations of attractiveness for males. *Sex Roles, 35,* 581-602.

Petrie, T.A., & Stoever, S. (1993). The incidence of bulimia nervosa and pathogenic weight control behaviors in female collegiate gymnasts. *Research Quarterly for Exercise and Sport, 64,* 238-241.

Rosen, L., & Hough, D. (1988). Pathogenic weight control behaviors of female college gymnasts. *Physician and Sportsmedicine, 16,* 141-144.

Rosen, L., McKeag, D.B., Hough, D., & Curley, V. (1986). Pathogenic weight control behaviors in female athletes. *Physician and Sportsmedicine, 14,* 79-86.

Sherman, R.T., Thompson, R.A., & Rose, J. (1996). Body mass index and athletic performance in elite female gymnasts. *Journal of Sport Behavior, 19,* 338-346.

Stanton, R. (1994). Dietary extremism and eating disorders in athletes. In L. Burke & V. Deakin (Eds.), *Clinical sports nutrition* (pp. 285-306). Sydney: McGraw-Hill.

Sundgot-Borgen, J. (1993). Prevalence of eating disorders in elite female athletes. *International Journal of Sport Nutrition, 3,* 29-40.

Sundgot-Borgen, J. (1994). Risk and trigger factors for the development of eating disorders in female elite athletes. *Medicine and Science in Sports and Exercise, 26,* 414-419.

Swoap, R.A., & Murphy, S.M. (1995). Eating disorders and weight management in athletes. In S.M. Murphy (Ed.), *Sport psychology interventions* (pp. 307-329). Champaign, IL: Human Kinetics.

This chapter reviews the prevalence of eating disorders across athletic environments, identifies factors that might predispose athletes to eating disorders, and offers suggestions on recognition and treatment.

Thompson, R.A. (1987). Management of the athlete with an eating disorder: Implications for the sport management team. *The Sport Psychologist, 1,* 114-126.

Thompson, R.A., & Sherman, R.T. (1993). *Helping athletes with eating disorders.* Champaign, IL: Human Kinetics.

This book provides a comprehensive overview of eating disorders in sport, from a basic overview of what eating disorders are to issues regarding education and prevention to treatment.

Wilmore, J.H. (1991). Eating and weight disorders in the female athlete. *International Journal of Sport Nutrition, 1,* 104-117.

Wilmore, J.H., & Costill, D.L. (1987). *Training for sport and activity: The physiological basis of the conditioning process* (3rd ed.). Boston: Allyn & Bacon.

Wilmore, J.H., & Costill, D.L. (1992). Nutrition and human performance. In K. Brownell, J. Rodin, & J. Wilmore (Eds.), *Eating, body weight and performance in athletes* (pp. 61-76). Philadelphia: Lea & Febiger.

Wilson, G.T., & Eldredge, K.L. (1992). Pathology and development of eating disorders: Implications for athletes. In K. Brownell, J. Rodin, & J. Wilmore (Eds.), *Eating, body weight and performance in athletes* (pp. 115-127). Philadelphia: Lea & Febiger.

This chapter presents an integrated model to explain the development of eating disorders in athletes. This model focuses on the influences of the athletic environment, dietary restraint, and other factors, such as personality, family, or individual psychopathology.]

Chapter 13: Counseling Athletes With Nutritional Concerns

Gibson, R.S. (1990). *Principles of nutrition assessment.* New York: Oxford University Press.

This book is designed and written as a reference text on all aspects of nutrition assessment. It provides a comprehensive and detailed account of the major assessment methods—dietary, anthropometric, laboratory, and clinical—currently used.

Hedquist, A.M. (1993). Metabolic needs of exercise. In D. Benardot (Ed.), *Sports nutrition: A guide for the professional working with active people* (2nd ed.). Chicago: Sports and Cardiovascular Nutrition Practice Group, American Dietetic Association.

This section of the guide contains both the scientific explanations and practical recommendations regarding the physiology of anaerobic and aerobic exercise; fuel supplies for exercise; predicting energy expenditure; vitamins, minerals, and athletic performance; and fluid and electrolyte requirements of exercise.

Kleiner, S.M. (1993). Nutrition screening and assessment. In R.N. Matzen & R.S. Lang (Eds.), *Clinical preventive medicine.* St. Louis: Mosby-Year Book.

Written for medical practitioners in general, this chapter addresses the practical application of nutrition screening and assessment procedures for each stage of the life cycle.

Kleiner, S.M., Bazzarre, T.L., & Ainsworth, B.E. (1994). Nutritional status of nationally ranked elite bodybuilders. *International Journal of Sport Nutrition, 4,* 54-69.

Kleiner, S.M., Bazzarre, T.L., & Litchford, M.D. (1990). Metabolic profiles, diet, and health practices of championship male and female bodybuilders. *Journal of the American Dietetic Association, 90*(7), 962-967.

Laquatra, I., & Danish, S.J. (1988). A primer for nutritional counseling. In R.T. Frankle & M.-U. Yang (Eds.), *Obesity and weight control.* Rockville, MD: Aspen.

This chapter walks the practitioner through the counseling steps necessary to help a patient or client achieve behavioral and lifestyle changes.

Manore, M. (1993). Assessment of nutritional status. In D. Benardot (Ed.), *Sports nutrition: A guide for the professional working with active people* (2nd ed.). Chicago: Sports and Cardiovascular Nutrition Practice Group, American Dietetic Association.

This section serves as a primer on the fundamentals of assessing the nutritional status of active people. It contains chapters on medical and nutrition assessment, nutrient intake assessment, physical fitness assessment, body measurements, and computer programs for nutrition, diet, fitness, and body composition assessment.

McArdle, W.D., Katch, F.I., & Katch, V.L.(1994). *Essentials of exercise physiology.* Philadelphia: Lea & Febiger.

Michener, J.L. (1989). *Nutrition counseling: Translating research into practice.* Presented at the Opinion Leaders' Symposium for Rx Nutrition: Good Health in Practice, sponsored by University of Washington School of Medicine. Little Falls, NJ: Health Learning Systems.

Storlie, J. (1991). Nutrition assessment of athletes: A model for integrating nutrition and physical performance indicators. *International Journal of Sport Nutrition, 1,* 192-204.

This article serves as a seminal paper for the development of a nutrition assessment strategy tailored for athletes.

Tipton, C.M. (1990). Making and maintaining weight for interscholastic wrestling. *Sports Science Exchange, 2*(22).

An applied publication that specifically addresses the scientific basis and practical strategies for assisting and counseling wrestlers with their body weight goals.

U.S. Department of Agriculture & U.S. Department of Health and Human Services. (1995). *Nutrition and your health: Dietary guidelines for Americans* (4th ed.). Washington, DC.

A practical guide developed by the U.S. government to help the public plan a healthy diet.

U.S. Department of Health and Human Services, Public Health Service. (1988). *The Surgeon General's report on nutrition and health* (DHHS [PHS] Publication No. 88-50210). Washington, DC.

Chapter 14: Counseling for the Management of Stress and Anxiety

Alexander, V., & Krane, V. (1996). Relationships among performance expectations, anxiety, and performance in collegiate volleyball players. *Journal of Sport Behavior, 19,* 246-269.

Andersen, M.B., & Williams, J.M. (1988). A model of stress and athletic injury: Prediction and prevention. *Journal of Sport and Exercise Psychology, 10,* 294-306.

This review examined the literature about stress and proposed a theoretical model of stress and athletic injury. As the model describes, two mechanisms in the stress response affect athletic injury: increased general muscle tension and deficits in attention during stress. Personality, stress history, and coping resources affect the stress response. Psychological interventions also may affect the stress–injury relationship.

Bandura, A. (1995). Exercise of personal and collective efficacy in changing societies. In A. Bandura (Ed.), *Self-efficacy in changing societies* (pp. 1-45). New York: Cambridge University Press.

Bird, A.M., & Horn, M.A. (1990). Cognitive anxiety and mental errors in sport. *Journal of Sport and Exercise Psychology, 17,* 364-374.

Burton, D. (1988). Do anxious swimmers swim slower? Re-examining the elusive anxiety–performance relationship. *Journal of Sport and Exercise Psychology, 10,* 45-61.

Caruso, C.M., Dzewaltowski, D.A., Gill, D.L., & McElroy, M.A. (1990). Psychological and physiological changes in competitive state anxiety during noncompetition and competitive success and failure. *Journal of Sport and Exercise Psychology, 12,* 6-20.

Coddington, R.D., & Troxel, J.R. (1980). The effect of emotional factors on football injury rates: A pilot study. *Journal of Human Stress, 6,* 3-5.

Crocker, P.R.E., Alderman, R.B., & Smith, F.M.R. (1988). Cognitive-affective stress management training with high performance youth volleyball players: Effects on affect, cognition, and performance. *Journal of Sport and Exercise Psychology, 10,* 448-460.

Davidson, R.J., & Schwartz, G.E. (1976). The psychobiology of relaxation and related states: A multiprocess theory. In D.I. Mostofsky (Ed.), *Behavioral control and modification of physiological activity* (pp. 399-442). Englewood Cliffs, NJ: Prentice Hall.

Davis, J.O. (1991). Sports injuries and stress management: An opportunity for research. *Sport Psychologist, 5,* 175-182.

DeWitt, D.J. (1980). Cognitive and biofeedback training for stress reduction in university athletes. *Journal of Sport Psychology, 2,* 288-294.

Elko, P.K., & Ostrow, A.O. (1991). Effects of a rational-emotive education program on heightened anxiety levels of female collegiate gymnasts. *The Sport Psychologist, 5,* 235-255.

Faris, G.J. (1985). Psychological aspects of athletic rehabilitation. *Clinics in Sports Medicine, 4,* 545-551.

Targeted towards sports medicine professionals, this article provides information and guidelines for dealing with the emotional states of injured athletes. Guidelines for developing rapport, explaining the injury and recovery / rehabilitation process to athletes, addressing athletes' emotional reactions to injury, and teaching athletes to properly perform rehabilitation exercises are presented.

Flint, F.A. (1993). Seeing helps believing: Modeling in injury rehabilitation. In D. Pargman (Ed.), *Psychological bases of sport injuries* (pp. 183-198). Morgantown, WV: Fitness Information Technology.

This review describes how modeling can be used to enhance rehabilitation from a major injury. Modeling is described, then specific suggestions for implementing modeling in the rehabilitation environment are provided.

Girdano, D., Everly, G.S., & Dusek, D. (1993). *Controlling stress & tension: A holistic approach* (4th ed.). Englewood Cliffs, NJ: Prentice Hall.

This book describes the stress process and stress management techniques. A variety of techniques and exercises for learning and practicing them are provided.

Gould, D., Horn, T., & Spreeman, J. (1983). Sources of stress in junior elite wrestlers. *Journal of Sport Psychology, 5*(2), 159-171.

Gould, D., Jackson, S.A., & Finch, L.M. (1993). Sources of stress in national champion figure skaters. *Journal of Sport and Exercise Psychology, 15,* 134-159.

Gould, D., & Krane, V. (1992). The arousal–athletic performance relationship: Current status and future direction. In T. Horn (Ed.), *Advances in sport psychology* (pp. 119-142). Champaign, IL: Human Kinetics.

Greenspan, M.J., & Feltz, D.L. (1989). Psychological interventions with athletes in competitive situations: A review. *The Sport Psychologist, 3,* 219-236.

Hanson, S.J., McCullagh, P., & Tonyman, P. (1992). The relationship of personality characteristics, life stress, and coping resources to athletic injury. *Journal of Sport and Exercise Psychology, 14,* 262-272.

Hardy, C.J., & Riehl, R.E. (1988). An examination of the life stress–injury relationship among noncontact sport participants. *Behavioral Medicine, 14,* 113-118.

Ievleva, L., & Orlick, T. (1991). Mental links to enhanced healing: An exploratory study. *The Sport Psychologist, 5,* 25-40.

> *Psychosocial factors related to healing were examined in sports medicine clinic patients with knee or ankle injuries. The fast healers reported a greater commitment to healing, more feelings of personal control in healing, a more positive attitude, and more social support than the slow healers. The fast healers also used positive self-talk and implemented stress control, goal setting, and mental imagery.*

Jacobson, E. (1938). *Progressive relaxation: A physiological and clinical investigation of muscular states and their significance in psychology and medical practice.* Chicago: University of Chicago Press.

Jones, G., Hanton, S., & Swain, A. (1994). Intensity of anxiety symptoms in elite and non-elite sports performers. *Personality and Individual Differences, 17,* 657-663.

Jones, G., Swain, A., & Cale, A. (1990). Antecedents of multidimensional competitive state anxiety and self-confidence in elite intercollegiate middle distance runners. *The Sport Psychologist, 4,* 107-118.

Jones, G., Swain, A., & Hardy, L. (1993). Intensity and direction dimensions of competitive state anxiety and relationships with performance. *Journal of Sports Sciences, 11,* 525-532.

Kerr, G., & Leith, L. (1993). Stress management and athletic performance. *The Sport Psychologist, 7,* 221-231.

Kerr, G., & Minden, H. (1988). Psychological factors related to the occurrence of athletic injuries. *Journal of Sport and Exercise Psychology, 10,* 167-173.

Kolt, G.S., & Kirby, R.J. (1994). Injury, anxiety, and mood in competitive gymnasts. *Perceptual and Motor Skills, 78,* 955-962.

Krane, V. (1990). *Anxiety and athletic performance: A test of the multidimensional anxiety and catastrophe theories.* Unpublished doctoral dissertation, University of North Carolina at Greensboro.

Krane, V., Joyce, D., & Rafeld, J. (1994). Competitive anxiety, situation criticality, and softball performance. *The Sport Psychologist, 8,* 58-72.

Krane, V., Williams, J.M., & Feltz, D.L. (1992). Path analysis examining relationships among cognitive anxiety, somatic anxiety, state confidence, performance expectations, and golf performance. *Journal of Sport Behavior, 15,* 1-17.

Leddy, M.H., Lambert, M.J., & Ogles, B.M. (1994). Psychological consequences of athletic injury among high-level competitors. *Research Quarterly for Exercise and Sport, 65,* 347-354.

Lynch, G.P. (1988). Athletic injuries and the practicing sport psychologist: Practical guidelines to assisting athletes. *The Sport Psychologist, 2,* 161-167.

Lysens, R., Auweele, Y., & Ostyn, M. (1986). The relationship between psychosocial factors and sports injuries. *Sports Medicine, 26,* 77-84.

Lysens, R., Steverlynck, A., Auweele, Y., Lefevre, J., Renson, L., Claessens, A., & Ostyn, M. (1984). The predictability of sports injuries. *Sports Medicine, 1,* 6-10.

Mace, R.D., & Carroll, D. (1985). The control of anxiety in sport: Stress inoculation training prior to abseiling. *International Journal of Sport Psychology, 16,* 165-175.

Martens, R., Burton, D., Vealey, R.S., Bump, L.A., & Smith, D.E. (1990). Development and validation of the Competitive State Anxiety Inventory-2 (CSAI-2). In R. Martens, R.S. Vealey, & D. Burton (Eds.), *Competitive anxiety in sport* (pp. 117-190). Champaign, IL: Human Kinetics.

May, J.R., Veach, T.L., Reed, M.W., & Griffey, M.S. (1985). A psychological study of health, injury, and performance in athletes on the US alpine ski team. *Physician and Sportsmedicine, 13*(10), 111-115.

Maynard, I.W., & Cotton, P.C. (1993). An investigation of two stress-management techniques in a field setting. *The Sport Psychologist, 7,* 375-387.

Maynard, I.W., Hemmings, B., & Warwick-Evans, L. (1995). The effects of a somatic intervention strategy on competitive state anxiety and performance in semiprofessional soccer players. *The Sport Psychologist, 9,* 51-64.

Maynard, I.W., Smith, M.J., & Warwick-Evans, L. (1995). The effects of a cognitive intervention strategy on competitive state anxiety and performance in semiprofessional soccer players. *Journal of Sport and Exercise Psychology, 17,* 428-446.

McDonald, S.A., & Hardy, C.J. (1990). Affective response patterns of the injured athlete: An exploratory analysis. *The Sport Psychologist, 4,* 261-274.

McGrath, J.E. (1970). Major methodological issues. In J.E. McGrath (Ed.), *Social and psychological factors in stress* (pp. 19-49). New York: Holt, Rinehart, & Winston.

Palmer, S., & Dryden, W. (1995). *Counseling for stress problems.* Thousand Oaks, CA: Sage.

This book describes the multimodal-transactional model of stress. It also provides a variety of stress management techniques.

Passer, M.W., & Seese, M.D. (1983). Life stress and athletic injury: Examination of positive vs. negative events and three moderator variables. *Journal of Human Stress, 9,* 11-16.

Pen, L.J., & Fisher, C.A. (1994). Athletes and pain tolerance. *Sports Medicine, 18,* 319-329.

Petrie, T.A. (1992). Psychosocial antecedents of athletic injury: The effects of life stress and social support on female collegiate gymnasts. *Behavioral Medicine, 18,* 127-138.

Petrie, T.A. (1993a). Coping skills, competitive trait anxiety, and playing status: Moderating effects on the life stress–injury relationship. *Journal of Sport and Exercise Psychology, 15,* 261-274.

Petrie, T.A. (1993b). The moderating effects of social support and playing status on the life stress–injury relationship. *Journal of Applied Sport Psychology, 5,* 1-16.

Quackenbush, N., & Crossman, J. (1994). Injured athletes: A study of emotional responses. *Journal of Sport Behavior, 17,* 178-187.

Scanlan, T.K., & Passer, M.W. (1978). Factors related to competitive stress among male youth sport participants. *Medicine and Science in Sports, 10,* 103-108.

Scanlan, T.K., Stein, G.L., & Ravizza, K. (1991). An in-depth study of former elite figure skaters: III. Sources of stress. *Journal of Sport and Exercise Psychology, 13,* 103-120.

Smith, A.M., Scott, S.G., & Wiese, D.M. (1990). The psychological effects of sports injuries. *Sports Medicine, 9,* 352-369.

Smith, R.E., Smoll, F.L., & Ptacek, J.T. (1990). Conjunctive moderator variables in vulnerability and resiliency research: Life stress, social support and coping skills, and adolescent sport injuries. *Journal of Personality and Social Psychology, 58,* 360-370.

Thompson, N.J., & Morris, R.D. (1994). Predicting injury risk in adolescent football players: The importance of psychological variables. *Journal of Pediatric Psychology, 19,* 415-429.

Weiss, M.R., & Troxel, R.K. (1986). Psychology of the injured athlete. *Athletic Training, 21,* 104-154.

Williams, J.M., Haggert, J., Tonyman, P., & Wadsworth, W.A. (1986). Life stress and the prediction of athletic injuries in volleyball, basketball, and cross-country running. In L.E. Unestahl (Ed.), *Sport psychology in theory and practice*. Orebro, Sweden: Veje.

Williams, J.M., & Harris, D.V. (1998). Relaxation and energizing techniques for regulation of arousal. In J.M. Williams (Ed.), *Applied sport psychology* (pp. 219-236). Mountain View, CA: Mayfield.

Williams, J.M., & Roepke, N. (1993). Psychology of injury and injury rehabilitation. In R.N. Singer, M. Murphey, L.K. Tennant (Eds.), *Handbook of research on sport psychology* (pp. 815-839). New York: Macmillan.

Williams, J.M., Rotella, R., & Heyman, S. (1998). Stress, injury, and the psychological rehabilitation of athletes. In J.M. Williams (Ed.), *Applied sport psychology* (pp. 409-428). Mountain View, CA: Mayfield.

Psychological factors related to injury incidence and rehabilitation from injury are discussed. The authors emphasize a whole-person philosophy for working with injured athletes and describe psychological skills that can be taught to injured athletes.

Williams, J.M., Tonyman, P., & Wadsworth, W.A. (1986). Relationship of life stress to injury in intercollegiate volleyball. *Journal of Human Stress, 12,* 38-43.

Zinsser, N., Bunker, L., & Williams, J.M. (1998). Cognitive techniques for improving performance and building confidence. In J.M. Williams (Ed.), *Applied sport psychology* (pp. 271-342). Mountain View, CA: Mayfield.

Chapter 15: Counseling for Improved Rehabilitation Adherence

Bandura, A. (1977). Self-efficacy: Toward a unifying theory of behavioral change. *Psychological Review, 84,* 191-215.

Becker, M.H. (1979). Understanding patient compliance: The contributions of attitudes and other psychosocial factors. In S.J. Cohen (Ed.), *New directions in patient compliance* (pp. 1-31). Lexington, MA: Heath.

Beers, T.M., Jr., & Karoly, P. (1979). Cognitive strategies, expectancy, and coping style in the control of pain. *Journal of Consulting and Clinical Psychology, 47,* 179-180.

Caplan, R.D. (1979). Patient, provider, and organization: Hypothesized determinants of adherence. In S.J. Cohen (Ed.), *New directions in patient compliance* (pp. 75-110). Lexington, MA: Heath.

Caplan, R.D., Robinson, E.A.R., French, J.R.P., Caldwell, J.R., & Shinn, M. (1976). *Adhering to medical regimens: Pilot experiments in patient education and social support.* Ann Arbor, MI: Institute for Social Research.

DePalma, M.T., & DePalma, B. (1989). The use of instruction and the behavioral approach to facilitate injury rehabilitation. *Athletic Training, 24,* 217-219.

The authors assert that goal setting is a viable and practical means by which athletic trainers can enhance their effectiveness in rehabilitating sport injuries. Specific suggestions and means of assisting injured athletes to set goals are offered.

Duda, J.L., Smart, A.E., & Tappe, M.K. (1989). Predictors of adherence in the rehabilitation of athletic injuries: An application of personal investment theory. *Journal of Sport and Exercise Psychology, 11,* 367-381.

Evans, L., & Hardy, L. (1995). Sport injury and grief responses: A review. *Journal of Sport and Exercise Psychology, 17,* 227-245.

This article reviews the most relevant literature on the psychological responses of injured athletes in light of what is known generally about the grief response. Future research into grief models of imagery may offer the clinician useful information.

Fisher, A.C. (1990). Adherence to sports injury rehabilitation programmes. *Sports Medicine, 9,* 151-158.

The author offers a means of categorizing the myriad factors that enhance treatment adherence to simplify an understanding of this complex issue. A model of self-confidence is proposed as an umbrella concept from which strategies to promote adherence can be selected.

Fisher, A.C., Domm, M.A., & Wuest, D.A. (1988). Adherence to sports-injury rehabilitation programs. *Physician and Sportsmedicine, 16,* 47-50, 52.

Fisher, A.C., & Hoisington, L.L. (1993). Injured athletes' attitudes and judgments toward rehabilitation adherence. *Journal of Athletic Training, 28,* 48-54.

Responses from previously injured and rehabilitated athletes about their rehabilitation specifically and injury rehabilitation generally were compared with responses from certified athletic trainers. Both groups concur that rapport between athletic trainer and injured athlete, athletic trainer's support, athlete's self-motivation, and realistic pain appraisal by the athlete are important to enhanced rehabilitation adherence.

Fisher, A.C., Mullins, S.A., & Frye, P.A. (1993). Athletic trainers' attitudes and judgments of injured athletes' rehabilitation adherence. *Journal of Athletic Training, 28,* 43-47.

A survey investigation of certified athletic trainers led to the identification of important factors and strategies that promote injured athletes' rehabilitation adherence.

Fisher, A.C., Scriber, K.C., Matheny, M.L., Alderman, M.H., & Bitting, L.A. (1993). Enhancing athletic injury rehabilitation adherence. *Journal of Athletic Training, 28,* 312-318.

This article explains in detail several educational and motivational strategies to enhance rehabilitation adherence. The strategies are based on previous research findings from certified athletic trainers and injured athletes and on years of athletic injury rehabilitation experience.

Gould, D. (1998). Goal setting for peak performance. In J.M. Williams (Ed.), *Applied sport psychology: Personal growth to peak performance* (3rd ed., pp. 182-196). Mountain View, CA: Mayfield.

Green, L.B. (1992). The use of imagery in the rehabilitation of injured athletes. *Sport Psychologist, 6,* 416-428.

The author argues for a mind–body model for rehabilitation and demonstrates the application of imagery techniques to healing injuries.

Green, L.W. (1979). Educational strategies to improve compliance with therapeutic and preventive regimens: The recent evidence. In R.B. Haynes, D.W. Taylor, & D.L. Sackett (Eds.), *Compliance in health care* (pp. 157-173). Baltimore: Johns Hopkins University Press.

Recommendations are offered for the improvement and extension of knowledge and for the practice of health education. Of particular interest are the communication guidelines that sports medicine professionals are well advised to apply in disseminating information to their injured athletes.

Ice, R. (1985). Long term compliance. *Physical Therapy, 65,* 1832-1839.

Ievleva, L., & Orlick, T. (1993). Mental paths to enhanced recovery from a sports injury. In D. Pargman (Ed.), *Psychological bases of sport injuries* (pp. 219-245). Morgantown, WV: Fitness Information Technology.

This chapter discusses mental strategies for enhancing recovery from athletic injuries. Special emphasis is directed toward goal setting, healing mental imagery, and positive self-talk.

Lewthwaite, R. (1990). Motivational considerations in physical activity involvement. *Physical Therapy, 70,* 808-819.

Numerous factors relevant to injured athletes' motivation to adhere to their rehabilitation regimens are discussed. Goal orientations, perceived competence, and perceptual–affective experiences are arguably some of the most important psychological factors affecting rehabilitation adherence.

Ley, P. (1986). Cognitive variables and noncompliance. *Journal of Compliance in Health Care, 1,* 171-188.

Meichenbaum, D., & Turk, D.C. (1987). *Facilitating treatment adherence.* New York: Plenum.

This is the single best reference in the adherence literature. Factors predisposing athletes to treatment dropout are discussed, and preventive solutions are offered. Treatment adherence is addressed from a variety of treatment protocols.

Melzack, R. (1980). Psychologic aspects of pain. In J.J. Bonica (Ed.), *Pain* (pp. 143-154). New York: Raven Press.

The author, a well-known expert on pain, explains that the physiological explanation of pain contains implicit psychological concepts. Psychological strategies to alter pain perception and provide relief are discussed.

Pedersen, P. (1986). The grief response and injury: A special challenge for athletes and athletic trainers. *Athletic Training, 21,* 312-314.

The author identifies some of the cognitive, affective, and behavioral challenges facing injured athletes. The larger focus of the article is on the athletic trainer's role as facilitator of the grief response.

Pen, L.J., & Fisher, A.C. (1994). Athletes and pain tolerance. *Sports Medicine, 18,* 319-329.

The authors discuss acute and chronic pain, the impact of pain on performance, cognitive strategies to deal with pain, and implications for sport injury rehabilitation.

Pen, L.J., Fisher, A.C., Sforzo, G.A., & McManis, B.G. (1995). Cognitive strategies and pain tolerance in subjects with muscle soreness. *Journal of Sport Rehabilitation, 4,* 181-194.

Seligman, M.E.P. (1990). *Learned optimism: How to change your mind and your life.* New York: Pocket Books.

The ways in which people explain what happens to them creates and is created by their personal sense of optimism or pessimism. This book is required reading for anyone seriously interested in the role of self-confidence in all aspects of life.

Sluijs, E.M., Kok, G.J., & van der Zee, J. (1993). Correlates of exercise compliance in physical therapy. *Physical Therapy, 73,* 771-782. Commentaries by D.C. Turk (pp. 783-784) and L. Riolo (pp. 784-786).

A survey of physical therapists and their patients revealed that three main factors contribute to nonadherence in short-term, supervised treatment: barriers that patients perceive, the lack of positive feedback, and perceived helplessness.

Tuffey, S. (1991). The role of athletic trainers in facilitating psychological recovery from athletic injury. *Athletic Training, 26,* 346-351.

An understanding of athletes' responses to injury, as well as various psychological skills and strategies, is necessary to maximize the athletic trainer's rehabilitation efforts.

Weiss, M.R., & Troxel, R.K. (1986). Psychology of the injured athlete. *Athletic Training, 21,* 105-109.

In one of the early papers on the psychological aspects of injury rehabilitation, the authors address some factors related to coping with injury and offer some strategies to enhance rehabilitation adherence.

Wiese, D.M., Weiss, M.R., & Yukelson, D.P. (1991). Sport psychology in the training room: A survey of athletic trainers. *The Sport Psychologist, 5,* 15-24.

This study examined the attitudes and beliefs of athletic trainers toward the application of psychological strategies to injury rehabilitation, particularly communication, motivation, and social support.

Wiese-Bjornstal, D.M., & Smith, A.M. (1993). Counseling strategies for enhanced recovery of injured athletes within a team approach. In D. Pargman (Ed.), *Psychological bases of sport injuries* (pp. 149-182). Morgantown, WV: Fitness Information Technology.

This excellent chapter identifies counseling and psychosocial strategies that clinicians can use to enhance treatment effectiveness. Roles and responsibilities of various members of the sports medicine team are delineated.

Wilder, K.C. (1994). Clinicians' expectations and their impact on an athlete's compliance in rehabilitation. *Journal of Sport Rehabilitation, 3,* 168-175.

This article draws the parallel between student–teacher relationships and athlete–clinician relationships. Expectations that athletic trainers convey to their injured athletes tend to operate as self-fulfilling prophecies for adherence and rehabilitation outcomes.

Williams, S.L., & Kinney, P.J. (1991). Performance and nonperformance strategies for coping with acute pain: The role of perceived self-efficacy, expected outcomes, and attention. *Cognitive Therapy and Research, 15,* 1-19.

Chapter 16: Counseling Athletes With Catastrophic Injury and Illness

Asken, M. (1989). Sport psychology and the physically disabled athlete: Interview with Michael D. Goodling, OTR/L. *The Sport Psychologist, 3,* 166-176.

Asken, M. (1991). The challenge of the physically challenged: Delivering sport psychology services to physically disabled athletes. *The Sport Psychologist, 5,* 370-381.

The author presents an overview of the status of sport psychology issues and interventions with athletes with physical disabilities, including social and attitudinal aspects.

Berkman, L. (1995). The role of social relations in health promotion. *Psychosomatic Medicine, 57,* 245-254.

This article discusses the role of social support in health and disease status and outcome.

Bernstein, L., Bernstein, R., & Dana, R. (1974). *Interviewing: A guide for health professionals.* New York: Appleton-Century-Crofts.

Blinchik-Rybstein, E. (1979). Effects of different cognitive strategies on chronic pain. *Journal of Behavioral Medicine,* 2, (1), 93-101.

Brewer, B. (1991). *Athletic identity as a risk factor for depressive reactions to athletic injury.* Unpublished doctoral dissertation, Arizona State University, Tempe.

Brewer, B. (1994). Review and critique of models of psychological adjustment to athletic injury. *Journal of Applied Sport Psychology, 6,* 87-100.

Carney, R., Freeland, K., Rich, M., & Jaffe, A. (1995). Depression as a risk factor for cardiac events in established coronary heart disease: A review of possible mechanisms. *Annals of Behavioral Medicine, 17*(2), 142-149.

Case, R., Moss, A., Case, N., McDermott, M., & Eberly, S. (1992). Living alone after myocardial infarction: Impact on prognosis. *Journal of the American Medical Association, 267*(4), 515-519.

Cavaliere, F. (1995). EMDR remains controversial. *American Psychological Association Monitor, 26,* 8.

Charney, D., Miller, H., Licinio, J., & Salomon, R. (1995). Treatment of depression. In A. Schatzberg & C. Nmeroff (Eds.). *The American Psychiatric Press Textbook of Psychopharmacology.* Washington, DC: American Psychiatric Press

Chawla, J. (1994). Sport for people with disability. *British Medical Journal, 308*(June), 1500-1504.

Connell, C., Davis, W., Gallant, M., & Sharpe, P. (1994). Impact of social support, social cognitive variables, and perceived threat on depression among adults with diabetes. *Health Psychology, 1413*(3), 263-273.

Cooper-Patrick, L., Crum, R., & Ford, D. (1994). Identifying suicidal ideation in general medical patients. *Journal of the American Medical Association, 272*(22), 1757-1762.

Donellon, S., & Hagen, P. (1994, March 10). Outlook "positive" for Kruk. *Evening News*, p. D1.

Feibel, J., & Springer, C. (1982). Depression and failure to resume social activities after stroke. *Archives of Physical Medicine and Rehabilitation, 63,* 276-278.

Gil, K., Williams, D., Keefe, F., & Beecham, J. (1990). The relationship of negative thoughts to pain and psychological distress. *Behavior Therapy, 21,* 349-362.

Goodling, M., & Asken, M. (1987). Sport psychology and the physically disabled athlete. In J. May & M. Asken (Eds.), *Sport psychology: The psychological health of the athlete* (pp. 117-133). New York: PMA.

Heil, J. (1993). Specialized treatment approaches: Severe injury. In J. Heil (Ed.), *Psychology of sport injury* (pp. 175-193). Champaign, IL: Human Kinetics.

This chapter discusses psychological issues and approaches to severely injured athletes from hospitalization to accepting career termination.

Heyman, S. (1987). Counseling and psychotherapy with athletes: Special considerations. In J. May & M. Asken, M. (Eds.), *Sport psychology: The psychological health of the athlete* (pp. 135-156). New York: PMA.

This chapter discusses counseling approaches with athletes with an emphasis on how these may differ from general populations.

Hoffer, R. (1995). Ready, willing, and able. *Sports Illustrated, 83*(7), 64-73.

Horvat, M., French, R., & Henschen, K. (1986). A comparison of the psychological characteristics of male and female able-bodied and wheel-chair athletes. *Paraplegia, 24,* 115-122.

Kennedy, K. (1994). A second chance. *Sports Illustrated, 81*(16), 11-12.

King, K., Reis, H., Porter, L., & Norsen, L. (1993). Social support and long-term recovery from coronary artery surgery: Effects on patients and spouses. *Health Psychology, 12*(1), 56-63.

King, S. & Strain, J. (1994). Pain disorders. In R. Hales, S. Yudofsky, & J. Talbot (Eds.). *The American Psychiatric Press Textbook of Psychiatry.* Washington DC: American Psychiatric Press.

Kleinke, C. (1991). How chronic pain patients cope with depression. *Rehabilitation Psychology, 36*(4), 207-218.

Kubler-Ross, E. (1969). *On death and dying.* New York: Macmillan.

May, J., & Sieb, G. (1987). Athletic injuries: Psychological factors in the onset, sequelae, rehabilitation, and prevention. In J. May & M. Asken (Eds.), *Sport psychology: The psychological health of the athlete* (pp. 157-185). New York: PMA.

Mitchell, J., & Bray, G. (1990). *Emergency services stress.* Englewood Cliffs, NJ: Prentice Hall.

Mitchell, J., & Everly, G. (1993). *Critical incident stress debriefing (CISD).* Ellicott City, MD: Chevron Press.

Morgan, W., & Pollock, M. (1977). Psychological characteristics of elite distance runners. *Annals of the New York Academy of Sciences, 301,* 382-403.

Norris, F. (1992). Epidemiology of trauma: Frequency and impact of different potentially traumatic events on different demographic groups. *Journal of Consulting and Clinical Psychology, 60*(3), 409-418.

Ogilvie, B. (1987). Counseling for sports career termination. In J. May & M. Asken (Eds.), *Sport psychology: The psychological health of the athlete* (pp. 213-230). New York: PMA.

This chapter discusses issues and approaches to helping athletes accept the end of a career, whether due to injury or other factors.

Pantalon, M., Lubetkin, B., & Fishman, S. (1995). Use and effectiveness of self-help books in the practice of cognitive and behavioral therapy. *Cognitive and Behavioral Practice, 2,* 213-228.

Pedersen, P. (1986). The grief response and injury: A special challenge for athletes and athletic trainers. *Athletic Training, 21,* 312-314.

Price, S. (1995). The return. *Sports Illustrated, 83*(3), 21-26.

Reifman, A. (1995). Social relationships, recovery from illness and survival: A literature review. *Annals of Behavioral Medicine, 17*(2), 124-131.

Resnick, H., Kilpatrick, D., Dansky, B., Saunders, B., & Best, C. (1993). Prevalence of civilian post-traumatic stress disorder in a representative national sample of women. *Journal of Consulting and Clinical Psychology, 61*(6), 984-991.

Rosenfeld, L., Richman, J., & Hardy, C. (1989). Examining social support networks among athletes: Description and relativity to stress. *The Sport Psychologist, 3,* 23-33.

Santrock, J., Minnett, A., & Campbell, B. (1994). *The authoritative guide to self-help books.* New York: Guilford Press.

Smith, A., Scott, S., & Wiese, D. (1990). The psychological effects of sports injuries coping. *Sports Medicine, 9*(6), 352-369.

This paper discusses the psychological impact of injury on the athlete.

Smith, C., Fernengel, K., Holcroft, C., Gerald, K., & Marien, L. (1994). Meta-analysis of the association between social support and health outcomes. *Annals of Behavioral Medicine, 16*(4), 352-362.

Stone, A., & Porter, L. (1995). Psychological coping: Its importance for treating medical problems. *Mind/Body Medicine, 1*(1), 46-54.

Suinn, R. (1967). Psychological reactions to physical disability. *Journal of the Association for Physical and Mental Rehabilitation, 21,* 13-15.

Vernacchia, R., Reardon, J., & Templeton, D. (1997). Sudden death in sport: Managing the aftermath. *The Sport Psychologist, 11,* 223-235.

This paper describes the need for and nature of the critical-incident stress debriefing technique as applied to a sports team after the sudden death of a team member.

Weiss, M., & Troxel, R. (1986). Psychology of the injured athlete. *Athletic Training, 2,* 104-109, 154.

Wiese, D., Weiss, M., & Yukelson, D. (1991). Sport psychology in the training room: A survey of athletic trainers. *The Sport Psychologist, 5,* 15-24.

Athletic trainers were surveyed regarding their views of integration of sport psychology principles and techniques.

Wortman, C., & Silver, R. (1987). Coping with irrevocable loss. In G. Vandenboss & B. Bryant (Eds.), *Cataclysms, crises and catastrophes: Psychology in action* (pp. 185-235). Washington, DC: American Psychological Association.

Index

A

abdomen, 191
academic athletic counselors, 136-137
acceptance and adaptation, 296
acknowledging, 121
action skills, 71-73
action stage of change, 197
active listening, 69
adherence, 34, 276
    as a motivational issue, 277
    and athlete's characteristics, 277
    athlete–sports medicine professional interactions, 278
    ceiling effects encountered, 282-283
    commitment strategies, 278, 287-290
    competence strategies, 278, 279-283
    continuing contact with sport aiding, 288
    control strategies, 278, 283-287
    counseling strategies to promote, 278-290
    counselor's answers to questions, 281
    education about injury important to, 279-281
    factors influencing, 11, 38
    maintaining a positive approach, 282-283
    modeling helping, 287
    nature of program adherence, 277-278
    rehabilitation setting affecting, 277
    self-motivation improving, 34
    social support enhancing, 11, 46, 287-288
    variables affecting, 277
adverse consequences, from substance use, 181, 187-188
advice, in substance abuse counseling, 200
affective challenges faced by injured athletes, 276
affectively focused coping, 305-306
alcohol
    deaths related to, 228
    general equivalencies of alcoholic beverages, 185
    hazardous use of, 182
    testing blood alcohol levels, 193
alcohol screening, 184-187
American Counseling Association (ACA), 163, 164
American Medical Association (AMA), 163, 164
American Physical Therapy Association (APTA), 163, 164
American Psychological Association (APA), 163, 164
anabolic steroids, 183
Andersen, M.B., 27, 28, 29, 31, 33, 34, 42, 43, 84, 133, 138, 261, 262, 265
anorexia athletica, 210
anorexia nervosa, 101, 208
anthropometric weight analysis, 231-233. *See also*
    weight calculation of optimal body composition, 232
    health goals v. competitive goals, 233
    weight assessment tools, 231-232
anxiety, 258. *See also* depression
    cognitive anxiety, 262-263
    depression expressed as, 297
    direction of anxiety, 263
    distinguished from stress, 258
    following catastrophic injury or illness, 297
    interrelationship with stress and injury, 263-264
    multidimensional anxiety theory, 262-263
    need to address, 263
    reducing, 264-265
    somatic anxiety, 262-263
anxiety management, 264
    benefits of, 265
    cognitive anxiety management interventions, 269-271

effectiveness of, 264-265
    somatic anxiety management interventions, 271-273
Appelbaum, D., 162, 172
argument, avoiding, 198
Asken, M., 308
assertiveness training, 268-269
assessment, 132
assessment interview, 6
    athlete's circumstances affecting, 82-83
    counseling atmosphere for, 81
    counseling environment for, 76-77
    counseling styles used in, 77, 79
    demonstrating respect in, 81-82
    environmental considerations, 83
    ERAIQ used in, 77, 83-90
    establishing counseling relationship prior to, 80-81
    factors impeding effectiveness, 82-83
    factors promoting effectiveness, 80-82
    outcome evaluation following, 90
    overall impression of athlete's status, 88-89
    personal and professional characteristics of counselor affecting, 80, 83
    privacy essential to, 81
    Profile of Mood States used after, 82
    purpose of, 76
    time and place for, 77
    which athletes to interview, 76
    who should conduct, 77
association, to deal with pain, 286
athletes. *See also* injured athletes
    assigning value to sport, 84-85
    athlete-coach relationships, 99-100, 214-215, 220
    competitiveness a problem, 216
    counseling needed by, 11
    culture of risk affecting, 25
    fear of weight gain, 210, 218. *See also* weight
    female athletes feeling special pressures, 211-212
    female athletes' menstrual functioning, 217
    goal development for, 7
    goals of, 86
    health-related concerns of, 100-102
    inadequate diets of, 228
    at increased risk for eating disorders, 206-207, 211-212
    level of comfort in sport, 86
    nutritional advice needed by, 228
    pressures felt by, 101, 195
    professional athletes as models for, 97
    reasons for sports participation, 85
    relationships with management, 97
    reporting on stressors, 86
    self-identity in sport, 85
    sport ethic causing problems, 24-27, 51-52
    welfare conflicting with welfare of others, 172
    younger athletes at risk, 26-27
athletic equipment, 96-97
athletic identity, 34, 85, 112
athletic trainer
    communicating with sport management team, 219-220
    counseling role of, 15-16
    monitoring athletes with eating disorders, 220
    providing health education counseling, 104-105
    role in prevention of eating disorders, 213-214
    role in remediating eating disorders, 219-220
attending skills, 68-70
attentional disruption, 29

About the Editors

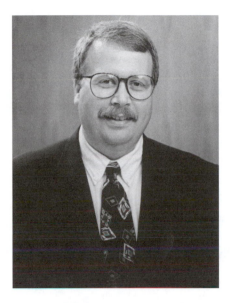

Richard Ray is coordinator of the athletic training program and associate professor of kinesiology at Hope College in Holland, Michigan. He has directed the school's sports medicine program since 1982 and is a recognized leader in the field of athletic training.

Counseling in Sports Medicine is the third Human Kinetics offering from Ray, who also penned the popular texts *Management Strategies in Athletic Training* and *Case Studies in Athletic Training Administration*.

Beginning in 1999, Dr. Ray will serve as editor of *Athletic Therapy Today*, and he has served as associate editor of the *Journal of Athletic Training*. He was chair of the National Athletic Trainers Association (NATA) Education Task Force and is a member and past president of both the Great Lakes Athletic Trainers Association and the Michigan Athletic Trainers Society (MATS). In 1993, Ray was named to the Educational Advisory Board of the Gatorade Sport Science Institute.

Ray received an MA in physical education from Western Michigan University in 1980 and an EdD in educational leadership from WMU in 1990. He graduated Summa Cum Laude in both graduate programs and was honored as a Graduate Research and Creative Scholar by the school in 1990. In 1995, Ray received the Distinguished Athletic Trainer Award from the MATS.

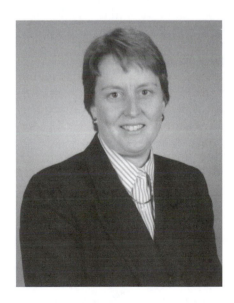

Diane M. Wiese-Bjornstal is an associate professor and director of graduate studies for the School of Kinesiology and Leisure Studies at the University of Minnesota.

Dr. Wiese-Bjornstal has taught and conducted research in sport psychology since 1989. Prior to that she was the head softball and volleyball coach at Northwestern College, Orange City, Iowa, and head softball coach at the University of Wisconsin-River Falls.

She is an editorial board member of the *Journal of Sport and Exercise Psychology*, *The Sport Psychologist*, *Journal of Applied Sport Psychology*, and *Research Quarterly for Exercise and Sport*. Her research on the psychological and sociological aspects of sport injury has been published in a variety of academic journals.

She is a member of the Association for the Advancement of Applied Sport Psychology (AAASP) and the American Alliance of Health, Physical Education, Recreation and Dance. In 1993, she received the Dorothy V. Harris Young Scholar/Practitioner Award from the AAASP. Wiese-Bjornstal earned an MS in physical education from Springfield College in 1983 and a PhD in physical education from the University of Oregon in 1989.

About the Contributors

Michael J. Asken, PhD, is with the Department of Physical Medicine and Rehabilitation at Pinnacle Health System's Polyclinic Medical Center in Harrisburg, Pennsylvania and is an adjunct Assistant Professor of Behavioral Science at the Pennsylvania State University College of Medicine, M.S. Hershey Medical Center. Dr. Asken is a Fellow of both the Division of Exercise and Sport Psychology and the Division of Health Psychology of the American Psychological Association. He is the author of *Dying to Win: Preventing Drug Abuse in Sport* and is co-author of *Sport Psychology: The Psychological Health of the Athlete.* Dr. Asken works with athletes at all levels and currently provides sport psychology consultation to the Harrisburg Heat and Hershey Wildcats professional soccer teams.

Britton W. Brewer, PhD, is an Associate Professor of Psychology at Springfield College in Springfield, Massachusetts, USA where he teaches undergraduate and graduate psychology courses, conducts research on psychological aspects of sport injury, and coaches the men's cross country team. He is listed in the United States Olympic Committee Sport Psychology Registry, 1996-2000 and is a Certified Consultant, Association for the Advancement of Applied Sport Psychology.

Kirk J. Brower, MD, FASAM is an Associate Professor of Psychiatry at the University of Michigan and is a Fellow of the American Society of Addiction Medicine (FASAM). He is the executive director of Chelsea Arbor Treatment Center, a joint venture of the University of Michigan Health System and Chelsea Community Hospital for treating patients with alcohol and drug problems. He is board-certified in the subspecialty of addiction psychiatry and the Director of the Addiction Psychiatry Fellowship Program at the University of Michigan. He has published and lectured extensively on the psychiatric and addictive effects of anabolic steroids, including meetings sponsored by the Big Ten Athletic Conference, the National Collegiate Athletic Association, and the U.S. Olympic Committee.

A. Craig Fisher, is the professor and chair of the Department of Exercise and Sport Sciences at Ithaca College. He has nearly 30 years of experience in his academic specialization, exercise and sport psychology. Dr. Fisher's most recent work has centered on various aspects of athletic injury rehabilitation adherence. The primary focus of his work relates to the construct of self-confidence as a mediator of adherence in athletic rehabilitation. He has published in a variety of medical, athletic training, and therapy journals. Outside of his teaching and research, Dr. Fisher is an avid golfer whose scores are a real testament to the power of maintaining a positive attitude.

Frances Flint has been a faculty member in the School of Physical Education at York University since 1977. She obtained her PhD from the University of Oregon in doctoral work that involved an integration of sport psychology and sports medicine focussing on the injured athlete. While at Oregon she earned certification as a Certified Athletic Trainer (NATA) and soon after as a Certified Athletic Therapist (CATA). She has developed the Sport Therapy Certificate Program at York for the education of future athletic therapists. Currently, Frances conducts research in the psychology of athletic injury and does consulting in sport psychology. Outside of the university setting, Frances has been a member of the Mission staff with the Canadian Olympic Association at the 1991 (Cuba) and 1995 (Argentina) Pan Am Games and the 1992 (Barcelona) Summer Olympics.

Diane M. Gardetto, MA, is a doctoral student in the School of Kinesiology and Leisure Studies at the University of Minnesota-Twin Cities, USA, specializing in sport psychology. Ms. Gardetto received her master's degree in sport psychology from Ripon College. Her research interests include the psychology of sport injury, eating disorders, women's issues in sport, and performance enhancement.

Christy Greenleaf is a doctoral student at the University of North Carolina at Greensboro, USA, studying sport and exercise psychology. Ms. Greenleaf received her master's degree in sport studies from Miami University of Ohio and her bachelor's degree in psychology from Bowling Green State University. Her research interest include peak performance, women's issues in sport, and body image. She is a former amateur and professional figure skater.

David Hough, MD was team physician and director of sports medicine at Michigan State University for 17 years prior to his death in 1996. He was a strong and capable advocate for the role of the primary care physician in sports medicine. He was a founding member of the American Medical Society for Sports Medicine and a fellow of the American College of Sports Medicine. He authored in excess of 125 scholarly articles and book chapters in addition to his many lectures.

Susan M. Kleiner, is the owner of High Performance Nutrition, a consulting firm specializing in media communications, project consulting, and sports and fitness counseling in Seattle, Washington. She is an Affiliate Assistant Professor of Nutrition at the University of Washington, and an Adjunct Member of the Sarah W. Stedman Center for Nutritional Studies at Duke University Medical Center. Dr. Kleiner is a national columnist and speaker on the subject of nutrition, sports, and fitness and has consulted with professional teams and elite athletes in all sports. In addition to her more than 200 published works, she is the coauthor of four books. She spends her leisure time living the good life with her family in the great outdoors of the Pacific Northwest.

Vikki Krane, PhD, is an Associate Professor with the School of Human Movement, Sport, and Leisure Studies at Bowling Green State University in Bowling Green, USA. She completed her doctorate in exercise and sport science at the University of North Carolina at Greensboro. Dr. Krane has served as a sport psychology consultant with elite youth sport, high school, and college athletes. She is a Certified Consultant, Association for the Advancement of Applied Sport Psychology, and has been honored with the Dorothy Harris Young Scholar/Practitioner Award (awarded by the Association for the Advancement of Applied Sport Psychology) and the Mabel Lee Young Scholar/Practitioner Award (awarded by the American Alliance of Health, Physical Education, Recreation and Dance). Her main research interests concern the relationship between competitive anxiety and athletic performance, and feminist issues in sport.

Peter V. Loubert, PhD, PT, ATC, is a member of the physical therapy faculty at Central Michigan University. He is a graduate of the University of Michigan where he received his PT degree, as well as a PhD in Anatomy and Cell Biology. He was awarded certification as an athletic trainer after completing the requirements at the University of Michigan. Dr. Loubert is a researcher in orthopaedic biomechanics and has been an active advocate for resolution of many of the professional issues of common interest and concern to physical therapists and athletic trainers.

Albert J. Petitpas, EdD, is a Professor of Psychology at Springfield College in Springfield Massachusetts, USA, where he directs the graduate training program in Athletic Counseling. He is a Fellow and Certified Consultant of the Association for the

Advancement of Applied Sport Psychology. He has provided consulting services to a wide range of sport organizations including the National Collegiate Athletic Association's Youth Education Through Sport Program, the United States Olympic Committee's Career Assistance Program for Athletes, the Ladies Professional Golf Association's Transitional Golf Program, and the United States Ski Jumping and Nordic Combined teams. His research and applied work focus on assisting athletes in coping with injury and other sport and career transitions.

Trent A. Petrie, PhD, received his doctorate in counseling psychology from The Ohio State University in 1991. He currently is an Associate Professor in the Department of Psychology and Director of the Center for Sport Psychology at the University of North Texas in Denton, Texas, USA. Dr. Petrie is a licensed psychologist, a Certified Consultant of the Association for the Advancement of Applied Sport Psychology, and a member of the 1996-2000 United States Olympic Committee Sport Psychology Registry. His areas of research include eating disorders, sport injury, and improving academic performance.

Jonathan H. Rootenberg, MD, FRCPC, is Staff Psychiatrist at Whitby Mental Health Centre in Whitby, Ontario, Canada, and a lecturer in the Department of Psychiatry at the University of Toronto. He also works for the courtesy staff at the Centre for Addiction and Mental Health, Clarke Division in Toronto.

Shelly M. Shaffer, PhD, completed her doctorate in 1996 at the University of Minnesota-Twin Cities, USA, with a major in kinesiology specializing in sport psychology. She received her master's degree in sport psychology from the University of Illinois, and her bachelor's degree in sports medicine and psychology from the University of Charleston. She has since worked as a grant writer in the Center for Research on Girls and Women in Sport in the School of Kinesiology and Leisure Studies at the University of Minnesota. Her research interests include the psychological and sociological dimensions of sport injury, and self-efficacy.

Roberta Trattner Sherman, PhD, received her doctorate in counseling psychology from Indiana University in 1982. She is co-director of the Eating Disorders Program at Bloomington Hospital in Bloomington, Indiana, a program she co-founded in 1988. Dr. Sherman also serves as clinician and consultant to the Indiana University Department of Intercollegiate Athletics. In addition to her clinical and consulting work, she conducts research, writes, and provides professional workshops on eating disorder. Included in her publications are two books she has co-authored entitled, *Helping Athletes With Eating Disorders* and *Bulimia: A Guide for Family and Friends.*

Aynsley M. Smith, RN, PhD, is a Sport Psychology Counselor and Research Coordinator in the Mayo Clinic Sports Medicine Center in Rochester, Minnesota, USA. As a counselor she works with the Mayo Sports Medicine team to assist injured athletes who have psychosocial issues that exacerbate injury and with injured athletes dealing with the effects of injury. Dr. Smith has both clinical and research interests in the psychology of injury and has published extensively in this area. She is also interested in performance enhancement and has worked with athletes and teams at all levels of participation from Pee-Wee to professional. Dr. Smith is listed in the United States Olympic Committee Sport Psychology Registry, 1996-2000 and is a Certified Consultant, Association for the Advancement of Applied Sport Psychology.

Tom Terrell, MD is an Assistant Professor of family medicine at the University of Maryland where his also serves as team physician. He is a graduate of Emory Medical School and has a graduate degree in biological anthropology from Cambridge University. Dr. Terrell served as a team physician for the 1996 Olympic Games. He has a strong interest in behavioral medicine and counseling issues. An author of both book chapters and articles in sports medicine publications, he is an active member of the American Medical Society for Sports Medicine, the American College of Sports Medicine, and the American Academy of Family Practice.

Judy L. Van Raalte, PhD, is an Associate Professor of Psychology at Springfield College in Springfield, Massachusetts, USA, where she teaches undergraduate and graduate psychology courses and conducts research on cognitive factors and sport performance. She is listed in the United States Olympic Committee Sport Psychology Registry, 1996-2000 and is a Certified Consultant, Association for the Advancement of Applied Sport Psychology.

Toni Schindler Zimmerman, PhD, is an Associate Professor in the Department of Human Development and Family Studies at Colorado State University in Fort Collins, Colorado, USA. She is the director of the master's program for marriage and family therapy at Colorado State University. Dr. Schindler Zimmerman has published numerous articles on sports and marriage and family therapy. Her primary interest is in examining how sports teams are like families and how interventions from family therapy can be applied to athletics. She also is actively involved in research and teaching in the area of gender equity.

Other Human Kinetics Books from Richard Ray

Management Strategies in Athletic Training
Richard Ray, EdD, ATC
1994 • Hardcover • 272 pp • Item BRAY0582
ISBN 0-87322-582-1 • $33.00 ($49.50 Canadian)

Case Studies in Athletic Training Administration
Richard Ray, EdD, ATC
1995 • Paper • 104 pp • Item BRAY0675
ISBN 0-87322-675-5 • $14.00 ($20.95 Canadian)

Other related books from Human Kinetics

Clinical Experiences in Athletic Training—A Modular Approach
Kenneth L. Knight, PhD, ATC
1998 • Spiral • 160 pp • Item BKNI0950
ISBN 0-87322-950-9 • $24.00 ($35.95 Canadian)

The Clinical Orthopedic Assessment Guide
Janice Loudon, Stephania Bell, and Jane Johnston
1998 • Paper • 239 pp • Item BLOU0507
ISBN 0-88011-507-6 • $29.00 ($43.50 Canadian)

Related Journal from Human Kinetics

Athletic Therapy Today
Frequency: Bimonthly (January, March, May, July, September, November)
Call for current subscription rates
ISSN: 1078-7895 • Item: JATT

To request more information or to order, U.S. customers call 1-800-747-4457, e-mail us at humank@hkusa.com or visit our Web site at www.humankinetics.com. Persons outside the U.S. can contact us via our Web site or use the appropriate telephone number, postal address, or e-mail address shown in the front of this book.

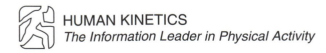

HUMAN KINETICS
The Information Leader in Physical Activity